MORTAL PERIL

MORTAL PERIL

❖ ❖ ❖

Our Inalienable Right
to Health Care?

RICHARD A. EPSTEIN

PERSEUS BOOKS
Cambridge, Massachusetts

Library of Congress Cataloging-in-Publication Data
Epstein, Richard Allen, 1943-
Mortal peril; our inalienable right to health care? / Richard A. Epstein.
p. cm.
Includes bibliographical references and index.
ISBN 0-201-13647-3
1. Right to health care—United States. I. Title.
RA395.A3E58   1997
362.1'0973—dc20   96-46024
CIP

Jacket design by Steven Brower
Text design by Karen Savary
Set in 11-point Minion by Vicki L. Hochstedler

1 2 3 4 5 6 7 8 9 10—03 02 01 00 99

❖   ❖   ❖

For Eileen,
Again

CONTENTS

❖ ❖ ❖

❖ ❖ ❖

Seen But Not Heard

On February 6, 1992, ABC's "Nightline" came in force to Mandel Hall, a large auditorium located at the heart of the University of Chicago campus. The telecast was scheduled as part of the university's centennial celebration. The topic for this ABC town meeting was the rising ground swell of public sentiment in favor of universal health care. "Nightline" staffers carefully orchestrated the happening to project the inevitable overthrow of the present unresponsive and patchwork system for providing medical care. Ted Koppel presided at center table with five carefully chosen experts on health care, all of whom supported some form of national health care coverage. Behind them on stage sat two rows of high powered experts and politicians, ready to jump in to air their views. Seated in front of the main table on the floor of the auditorium was a larger group of experts who were promised a good chance to speak their mind. I was placed in the fourth tier of participants assembled for the occasion, recruited only a few days before the session began. In light of my subordinated status, I was seated in the balcony near, but not at, a microphone handled by a tense "Nightline" staffer who was in constant two-way radio contact with the central production staff. The rules of the game allowed members of this fourth tier to speak if the staffer could persuade the central command unit that they had something to contribute. The fifth tier was located on the stage behind the second. It was there for show only, but barred from any speaking role. It was filled.

Nothing on the day was left to chance. Before the show went on the air, there was a short dress rehearsal that featured a forceful reminder by

Ted Koppel of the importance of civility in discourse. We then were treated to a short dry run of discussions, questions, and answers to get the feel of the hall, including one probing query by an earnest University of Chicago undergraduate who had the temerity to ask aloud why he should have to fund the health insurance costs of his grandparents' generation. A representative of the AARP fumbled with a reply that stated in essence that in the long run the student would benefit from the same system that imposed this short-term dislocation. Consistent with the norms of so much social accounting, no present-value calculations of benefits and cost were offered. It hardly mattered that the over-65 generation were large net recipients, and the under-25 generation large net payers.

Once the program went live, the mood changed. An unannounced video segment came first, and it featured the heartbreaking story of a young girl whose narrow escape from drowning left her in a permanent vegetative state. Her parents had exhausted their million-dollar health coverage policy and did not now know where to turn. The implicit message for the dialogue to follow was that this financial tragedy could be averted by a national health plan that supplied catastrophic coverage, without limitation. Sitting in my fourth tier I tried to persuade my reluctant staffer to let me gain access to the microphone that stood only five feet away to protest that outcome. No luck. My friends later told me that they saw me fidget while others spoke at the microphone. One or two wondered aloud why I suddenly became too shy to speak.

Shyness had nothing to do with it. My impatience stemmed from my inability to speak, as I am wont to do on public policy issues, against the grain. The received wisdom on the panel was that universal coverage was a moral given. The only question on the table was how to fund it. My hope was to inject a note of discord into this settled moral universe. The right reply to the parents, I wanted to say, was that *nothing at all* should be done to keep alive their child at public expense. The tragedy occurred with the initial near-drowning. All hope of recovery had past. The cost of care was enormous; its benefits, negligible, and the opportunities forgone, great. How many other children, I thought to myself, could receive food and education with the resources spent on prolonging one hopeless life by days or years? How many lifeguards or crossing guards could be hired to reduce the odds of similar tragedies? Why not commit resources to activities that promote human development and forestall human tragedy? Public support for children in a permanent vegetative state should not be on that priority list. We should suck in our gut and say no when asked to provide life support devices for those without hope of recovery. The short-term despair for some was justified by the long-term good that it produced for many.

That response would not have gone down well with the inner circle that dominated the discourse on "Nightline" that evening. Moral imperatives drove their discussion. The commitment was to transcend the constraint of scarcity that informs every other rational social debate. That panel started from the premise that medical care is so special that the lessons of economics drawn from the workplace and the household do not apply in health care settings. The panel believed that the application of standard business principles to health care disputes are the source, not the solution, to our most pressing problems. It displayed a strong preference toward government intervention, regarding market solutions, at best, as a last resort when all else failed.

I fall into a rival camp of beleaguered scholars who believe that the basic principles of human behavior and institutional organization do not magically cease to apply when health-related issues are on the table. Just recently, I was taken aback when at a faculty workshop a young doctor (with a Ph.D. in philosophy, no less) chided me as naive because my backward views on the physician/patient relationship presupposed scarcity. Scarcity is not an artificial assumption like complete information and perfect competition, designed to simplify the analysis at the cost of some accuracy in description. Quite the contrary, it is the inevitable constraint that any and all systems of social order must confront—before it confronts them. The brute truth of nature, which no editorial in the *New England Journal of Medicine* will be able to change, is that the best system of social control will be unable to satisfy all worthy ends, and it should not delude itself into trying.

Any analysis of health has to ask what system of organization works best to meet the needs of its citizenry. Markets are one powerful agency to match scarce resources to desired ends. Charitable activity is yet another. The former has well-nigh universal application, the latter is more restricted to the arts, education, and health—not necessarily in that order. The role of both markets and charitable institutions for handling health care was largely ignored, deprecated, or misunderstood in the "Nightline" presentation. The former was dismissed with such propositions that firms seek to maximize size and therefore cannot be trusted to provide medical care—a statement false as to markets, but truer as to government departments whose bureaucratic appetites can be easily replenished from the public purse. The system of charitable care that seemed so entrenched when my father practiced medicine in Brooklyn in the late 1940s and early 1950s has disappeared from view, a casualty of the system of government regulation ushered in by Medicare (for over-65 and disabled persons) and Medicaid (for poverty cases).

None of these thoughts, however, made it into public view on that "Nightline" show. In one sense, I wrote this book to set out in more systematic form the unfashionable points that I could not voice for even a second on TV. This book represents my sustained effort to demonstrate that the source of our collective anxiety begins with the elaborate and counterproductive schemes of entitlements that live off the illusion of abundance in the world of scarcity. It deals first with the grand questions of health care—chiefly the burning question of access to health care—that have not disappeared from the social stage since that "Nightline" town meeting some five years ago. It also explores a host of midlevel issues—organ transplantation, death and dying, and liability rules—that carry over some of the tensions evident in that "Nightline" show to problems of great intellectual interest and no little institutional importance.

Alas, this book is not rich in quick fixes for intractable problems. It is far easier to steer clear of trouble in the first place than to extricate a complex system from the pressures under which it labors. Yet the pillars of our present policy on health care have been etched in stone for over 30 years. It is no easy matter to design transitional schemes that allow us to escape from our past sins. It is already hard to find either the political or emotional willingness to bite the bullet on social security even though the only uncertainty in the debate is when the current system, with its archaic accounting principles, will fall into bankruptcy. And its offshoot Medicare faces the same unhappy prospect of gridlock on painful reform of a program that is scheduled to go bust within a matter of five or so years. I wish that I could offer solutions that could undo the past or rectify its errors. But even if that task is hopeless, I believe that there is some therapeutic value in pointing out where our previous policies have set the wrong headings. My hope is that others more adept in navigating the shoals of medicine and government can use it as a compass to make small-course corrections that could improve markedly the overall social situation.

Were this a purely legal book, I would make much of the maxim that "hard cases make bad law." In conventional adjudication, that maxim warns judges to beware of placing their sympathies for individual litigants above any concern for the long-term soundness of the legal order. The injured patient should not be allowed to recover just because he has been horribly hurt in routine surgery. The destitute tenant should not be allowed to remain in possession of her apartment just because she has no place to go. These all too human emotions do some good in helping the unfortunate, but they misunderstand the connection between charity and justice. Charity has to come from the physician or landlord. It cannot be compelled by any court conscious of the long-term dislocations its decisions might bring. The next would-be patient may find himself unable to get needed surgery because the doctor fears a large malpractice judgment. The next would-be tenant may never be able to rent suitable premises in the first place, because the landlord fears that she could not be evicted for nonpayment of rent. It is easy to feel compassion for visible, identified persons, but harder to understand the dangerous consequences of coercing, in the name of compassion, one person to help another. Compassion builds on empathy for the here and now. It is difficult to develop such empathy for statistical persons who cannot be identified in flesh and blood. But today's statistical lives become tomorrow's real people. The successful legal system never ignores the position of the parties before it, but it always asks itself whether the outcome it decrees in a single case is sustainable in the long run. Systems of coercion fail that test because they never explain how the coercion is to be limited once the compassion is brought into play. Systems of voluntary compassion are sustainable because the dimensions of the program are limited by the willingness of its supporters to give of their own resources, not those of others. No one should be against compassion. But everyone should be on guard against conscripting others into their compassionate causes.

Our inquiry is, in one sense, about the limitations on public expressions of compassion. As such, I examine more than the usual run of judicial decisions and venture opinions on the complex regulatory schemes now in place. Yet, as one moves from the more narrowly legal questions to the more broadly gauged social systems, the original insight holds good. Only the choice of maxim changes. "Hard cases make bad law" becomes a concern with "the unanticipated consequences of purposive action," to use Robert Merton's immortal phrase. Either way, the message is the same. Setting up practices that work for the here and now can plant the seeds for long-term disaster. Requiring hospitals to admit all patients to their emergency rooms reduces the long-term supply if these rooms are forced to close down for want of funds. Banning the sale of organs creates shortages that result in needless deaths. The inescapable message of the astute sociologist is no different from that of the cautious lawyer: beware of compassion unconstrained by awareness of long-term effects.

❖   ❖   ❖

The title chosen for this book is designed to reflect these many themes. "Mortal Peril" is not a phrase intended to boost reader confidence in the current array of legal reforms of the practice of medicine. Quite the opposite, it invites caution about the hidden consequences of reform which can backfire against its stated objective. The subtitle is a bit more nuanced in its application. Originally, I thought that "The Regulation and Reform of Health Care in America" helped capture the correct mood, by indicating, with barely concealed irony that the processes initiated for public protection could be the source of medical peril. The actual subtitle takes the same point from the opposite direction, and asks about the status of individual rights to health care.

The term "inalienable" has both positive and negative connotations. In its positive sense "inalienable" brings back shades of the opening sentence of the Declaration of Independence. "We hold these Truths to be self-evident, that all Men are created equal, that they are endowed by their creator with certain unalienable rights, that among these are Life, Liberty and the Pursuit of Happiness."

The word inalienable is a strong word, which suggests that these rights are so closely attached to the individual that they can never be removed by government, or at least by a well-functioning government. Health care was not on the original list, but it is easy to spin arguments that insist that so long as health care is fundamental to the pursuit of happiness, then, in an evolving legal universe, it has to be accorded the same fundamental status as life and liberty themselves. From there it is but a short leap to the proposition of universal access to health care, which is the position that I attack in the first half of this book.

The second meaning of inalienable is negative. In legal parlance an interest in property is inalienable if it cannot be sold or otherwise disposed by its owner. The inalienability of land is a fetter on commerce that can easily lead to idle and inefficient use of land, consequences which are bad both for its owner and for the larger society. The legal system therefore normally is reluctant to create interests that are by nature inalienable and is hostile to private efforts to impose clogs or restraints on alienation. Yet within the health care area, this presumption to is often reversed, so that restraints on alienation, including restrictions on freedom of contract, become the prized centerpieces of our policy on such matters as organ transplantation, euthanasia and assisted suicide, and tort liability. This book attacks these policies as well, and argues that the rights of self-control on matters of health care should be regarded as alienable, that is as subject to control and disposition by each individual. The subtitle is thus designed by indirection to question the regime of positive rights that is so much in vogue today, and by indirection to endorse a vision of the relationship between the individual and the state that is far closer to the sense of the original Declaration of Independence than the modern gloss that has been placed on it.

❖ ❖ ❖

A book of this length is not the product of a month or even a year. My initial involvement in medical issues began as a child when, long before the advent of managed care, I was lectured by my father, a practicing radiologist, on the ethical obligations of the physician. My own medical career was cut short for, as my mother noted, the young man who could not quite figure out how to hold a fork had little future as a surgeon. But my interest in medicine did not wane because of my inability to practice it. After coming to the University of Chicago in 1972, my interest in torts led me by degrees to write about the law of medical malpractice. From that early effort I was invited by Dr. Mark Siegler to speak at the Center for Clinical Medical Ethics in the university's Division of Biological Sciences. From there it was just a matter of time until I became attracted to other medical-ethical questions. Fate had it that in the summer of 1986 I served on the trustee-faculty committee that reorganized the University of Chicago Hospitals, which still benefit from the able leadership of their president, Ralph Muller. In the years that followed, I continued to speak and write about various topics in health care, including a presentation on "Why Is Health Care Special?" which I gave as Koch

Distinguished Professorship in Law at the University of Kansas in September 1991. That speech led to a generous grant from the Koch Foundation, which allowed me to begin work in earnest on this book in the fall of 1993. Thereafter, two grants from the John M. Olin Foundation, one in the spring of 1994 and the second in the fall of 1995, allowed me to bring this work to its conclusion. As usual, William Simon, Chairman of the Olin Foundation Board, and James Piereson, its executive director, gave me steadfast support and encouragement to pursue my own views on the subject. My personal debt to them on this and other occasions is enormous.

In the course of preparing this book, I have delivered parts of it at several workshops. At the University of Chicago, I presented various portions of the book in lectures organized by the Center for Clinical Medical Ethics, the Widener School of Law, Washington University School of Law, and the American Law and Economics Association. Various portions of the completed manuscript were reviewed by my colleagues. Arti Rai commented with great care and detail on the entire draft. I received helpful comments on portions of the manuscript from Mark Hall, Ralph Muller, and Lance Stell. David Cutler and David Hyman supplied me with valuable information on particular programs. My agent, Lynn Chu, supplied good advice and vigorous representation throughout the entire process. And Henning Gutmann, my editor at Perseus Books, has also lent his wisdom and encouragement in whipping the manuscript into final shape. My research assistants, Christopher Bowers, Jeffrey Greenblatt, Deborah Healy, and Annalisa Pizzarello, provided excellent research assistance on all phases of the writing of this book. My secretary Katheryn Kepchar helped assemble text and tables, more than one time. To all of them my thanks.

MORTAL PERIL

❖ ❖ ❖

Hard Truths and Fresh Starts

QUESTIONING ORTHODOXY

Health care, and the issues of life and death that surround it, have never been the ideal targets for disinterested reflection. The heated and protracted political struggles over the failed Clinton health plan in 1993 and 1994 virtually defined the first half of his Presidency. One year later, the tightly fought political struggles over the reform of Medicare led to a partial shutdown of the United States government. Yet within six months of that impasse, a Republican Congress celebrated the passage of legislation designed to encourage the portability of insurance coverage. At the same time, but on a different front, several courts initiated an enormous flap over the asserted constitutional right to physican-assisted suicide. These and other incidents all offer ample evidence that the debate over health care and policy continues to rank at the top of our overall social agenda. Implicit in the modern debates, both political and academic, is an agreement on ends and a disagreement on means. The protagonists of the debate all start from one grand working assumption, sometimes tacit and sometimes explicit, that health care is a "right" that should be made available to all Americans. The ensuing debate swirls only over the choice of means—what is the best set of policy instruments to satisfy the rights to which all citizens are entitled? This widely accepted claim about health care rights represents a broad acceptance of an enduring and legitimate government role in regulating and financing health care. Lost in the shuffle is any serious consideration of some alternative conception of individual rights and responsibilities that, as a matter of first principle, denies the government any large or distinctive role in the health care arena.

1

In this book, I seek to fill this unoccupied space and to expand the debate over health care to cover ends as well as means. I hope by argument and example to show that the conventional wisdom, accepted by most academic writers and by both political parties, is wrong insofar as it postulates large government solutions to the persistent problems in health care access and delivery. As so often happens, the case for government intervention is couched in both moral and economic terms. The moral argument is, quite simply, that all persons are entitled to some minimum level of health care by virtue of their participation in society.[1] No one believes that the right to health care is so absolute that it sweeps aside all claims to food, clothing, or shelter. Yet by the same token, the scope of a more circumscribed duty turns out, at a philosophical level, to be well-nigh indefinable, no matter how many times we intone the words "reasonable," "decent," "basic," "adequate," or "necessary."[2] Likewise, a question of correlative duties to the decent minimum is neatly suppressed.

On the economic front, the argument for the right to health care is made on grounds of exceptionalism. The health care market has special problems of monopoly, information deficits, volatility, uncertainty, surprise, insurability, and inequality of bargaining power that do not plague ordinary competitive markets.[3] The upshot is said to be pervasive market failure and gross maldistribution of health care resources. The response to the perceived market failure is regulation that responds to information deficits and structural problems. The response to the maldistribution problem is cross-subsidy from rich to poor or from healthy to sick brought on by a wide range of government programs.

This two-pronged attack on markets, however, never plays out as it is supposed to. The effort to neutralize market failure by regulation brings in its wake government failure that only exacerbates problems of information, uncertainty, and monopoly. Income disparities are hard to rectify through government action. All too often, health reforms transfer wealth from individuals in their 30s, burdened with heavy taxes and the expenses of raising families, to their more affluent elders with clogged arteries who could have and should have taken better care of their own health. The shift, moreover, is hardly a zero-sum game. Some fraction of the taxes disappears in administrative overhead. Still more wealth disappears in excessive consumption and distorted incentives. In large measure, state intervention in health care markets yields outcomes no different from those found elsewhere. Noble intentions quickly lead to an endless tangle of hidden subsidies, perverse incentives, and administrative nightmares which in the long run often backfire on its intended beneficiaries, if not in the first generation, then like social security, surely in the second. Government schemes are organized Ponzi operations that eventually go broke by using the capital of later contributors to satisfy the obligations to earlier plan participants.[4] This chronic travail over health policy in the United States is not a mysterious occurrence, wisely chalked off to unanticipated glitches in executing some well-conceived plan for government participation in health care delivery. Rather, the root cause of our social difficulty lies in the mistaken assumption that any well-functioning health care system requires, or must tolerate, a major infusion of government inputs and control.

The pattern that unfolds is a familiar one. Time and time again, the policy issues on health care draw us back to large questions of the proper methods of social organization. At one level, the choices seem to concern the proper "mix" of government control and private initiative. In responding to that question, no defenders of larger government activities would defend their position in the name of socialism, given its evident systemwide failure in Eastern Europe. Nonetheless, carefully purged of their historical antecedents, certain remnants of a discredited socialism creep back into their debate. The modern positions on health care emphasize the "right to" and never the "freedom from." List all the good things in the world, and everyone has a right to all of them: a right to housing, a right to education, a right to a job, and, in apparent defiance of the laws of nature, a right to life itself. This conception of individual welfare rights survives on the naive belief that government can continue to fund the right without dictating the plan of service. Yet the protection of these newly minted positive rights invests government at all levels with vast powers to tax, to regulate, and to hire and fire the very individuals whose rights it is duty-bound to protect.

And by what right? Before we look at the matter of technique, it is wise to confront the prior issue of principle. The expansion and ossification of government powers continues apace because its foundations are rarely questioned in polite company, let alone rejected after open and thorough debate. Programs are introduced with political fanfare trumpeting the rights they create and the benefits they provide. Coupled with the grander pronouncements is a serene assurance that we can square the circle by controlling their correlative costs; that we can achieve, in a word, universal access and cost-containment simultaneously. Programs born of such principles expand with time beyond our worst fears until they devour resources that by any sane reckoning are better spent on other human needs. Yet, even in failure, these expansive programs create expectations that our available resource base, both human and physical, cannot sustain. Today political forces have moved too far for it to be within anyone's power to devise a set of transition rules that can rationalize priorities and cut the fat out of the system without causing material uncertainty and hardship to a substantial portion of the population. The only questions on the table are how much pain is unavoidable and who will shoulder it and in what proportions.

We need a change in course. We must be careful not to decree legal rights to housing or health care. We must focus more on the flip side of rights: their correlative costs. We must face the possibility that someone may have to "do without" in a world of scarcity. We can no longer start our public debate with the false but comforting assumption that our social abundance can support social safety nets and minimum entitlements to everyone in society. We can no longer declare that certain rights are special and thus immune from critical challenge and review.

BACK TO OUR COMMON LAW BASICS

To attack the present complacency, we must strip away our current illusions and rethink fundamental questions at the very point where ordinary political discourse ends. This task is as necessary as it is unpleasant. Toward that end, I trace in this book the evolution of rights from the traditional (or common law) accounts of negative liberty to the more modern accounts grounded in the recognition of an affirmative right to health care. In conducting this examination, I think that it is important to take a firm stand where ordinary politicians of both parties fear to tread, and to argue that philosophical questions of health care do not begin and end with the passionate observation "that you can't just let anyone die." The short answer is that you can, and indeed in some cases, you should. The longer answer requires a reconstruction of the basic system of rights and duties—one that goes far beyond health care, but ultimately embraces it.

Putting the emphasis on first principles leads quickly to a fork in the road. Is it better to stress health first, and then turn to rights? Or to stress rights first, and then turn to health? In a perfect intellectual universe, these two paths of exploration should converge on the same set of prescriptions. But the frictions of practical reasoning make it likely that the outcome of our deliberation will turn on the choice of starting point. Those who treat health as the dominant locus have a partiality for the field and want to give it pride of place in competition with other goods and services. Armed with their institutional bias, they believe that the field of health should attract greater resources than other areas, for example, education and nutrition, and they are likely to invent or endorse schemes of regulation that require extensive subsidies of health care. Their claims of medical or bioethical expertise can then be used to deflect or defeat an outsider's criticisms of their policy choices. Physicians and health care policy analysts of various stripes fall into this class of preferred thinkers.

Analysts who begin with the generic question of rights and duties are far more likely to be relatively agnostic about the ultimate pattern in the distribution of goods and services that emerges from a sound system of legal rights and duties.[5] Although abstract theorists may lack detailed knowledge on the specifics of health and related fields, they can avoid the correlative risk of intellectual capture, a risk ominously similar to that of regulatory capture. As in so many other policy debates, the virtues of an outsider are easily underappreciated: a broad command of theory and its application in neighboring areas form a useful corrective against the enthusiasms of special pleading.

The best way to undertake this inquiry into rights is to recall the simple observation that rights do not exist in a vacuum. To create a right in A is to impose a correlative duty on some other person. That person may be specifically identified, as when A has the right to collect $10 from B. But all too often, the identity of the person who bears the correlative duty is concealed. The most common tactic used to achieve that false separation is to interpose some impersonal entity between the holder of the right and the bearer of the correlative duty. Thus the correlative duty to A's right could fall on some corporation or on the government. But no person has, functionally speaking, a claim against abstract legal entities, no matter how congenial that mode of thought. These legal entities are composed of individuals, and it is on all or some of their members that any correlative duties fall. Corporations and governments are legal vehicles to facilitate the organization of shareholders and citizens. When the state imposes duties on these entities, the burdens always fall to individual members, often without their consent. A full analysis of any proposed system of rights and duties can only take place after the abstract middlemen are removed from the picture, thereby linking the individuals on whom their duties devolve to the persons who hold the correlative rights. Once that linkage is made, it then becomes apparent that any claim of right carries with it correlative costs. The sensible approach to any claim of right necessarily asks about the *net* social advantage that accrues from its recognition relative to some rival form. In each case, it is necessary to see the size of the gain caused by creating the right and the size of the loss caused by imposing the correlative duty. As a minimum condition, the creation of a given right and its correlative duty only makes sense if the gain is greater than the loss by some agreed standard of measurement, be it utility or wealth.[6]

To undertake this investigation, it is useful to outline two rival conceptions of rights and their correlative duties. The first of these is the common law system of individual rights and duties, which for convenience I will sometimes refer to by the common, if somewhat misleading, name of negative rights. Within that system, the basic correlative duties stress forbearance and noninterference, or "freedom from" the actions of others. The rival "rights to" tradition travels under the name of welfare or positive rights.[7] These rights speak of the end states that individuals desire: health, education, and housing. Their correlative duties of support are targeted not to particular individuals but to the government or the state. The system builds in extensive amounts of taxation at the ground floor and expects that some individuals will take more from taxation than they give, whereas others will do the reverse. Systems of positive rights thus frequently contemplate the use of government force to redistribute wealth from those who need it least to those who need it most.

The distinction between the two views can be most easily grasped by unpacking what it means to talk about the right to life. Thus, within a system of positive rights, any individual can turn to other people in order to obtain the wherewithal to continue to survive and flourish. The precise limits of the right are difficult to set. As has been pointed out countless times, no society can afford to spend all of its wealth to prolong a single life for a single day; nor can it afford the more "modest" goal of spending all its wealth on health care, to the exclusion of all other ends. The failure to include costs in the equation leads to an extravagant overcommitment to issues of health care, which we try to moderate by casting the claim in terms of decent minimums, not absolute rights. Yet, a soft political landing is difficult at that intermediate point. The minimums required can move imperceptibly up to the medians, and the budgetary pressures can grow apace. Yet no observable limits on the process can take place so long as the basic commitment to redistribution of wealth through state force is in place.

In contrast, the tradition of negative rights, whatever its flaws, at least avoids the sin of extravagance. To be sure, the right to life has universal correlative duty in a system of negative rights: no other person is entitled to kill me, at least not without my consent, which is not likely to be forthcoming, given my interest in self-preservation.[8] Here the universal nature of the obligation is critical to its overall success. If even a small number of people were allowed to kill me with impunity, legal protection from all the rest would count for very little. I would take very little comfort from the fact that others have to respect my bodily integrity. A person can only be killed once. Yet, by the same token, the structure of any negative obligation does not become more complex when it is made universal and reciprocal. Forbearance is forbearance whether demanded by *or* of one, a thousand, or a billion. Nor does that content shift with a change in the wealth or preferences of any individual or of society as a whole. The stability of the forbearance norm in turn makes its communication to the public easy. Once the message is delivered, it need not be modified and redelivered to take into account changed circumstances. Whatever turmoil is observed in the domain of positive obligations, no legal system has ever thought it fit to repeal the prohibitions against murder or theft. The overall utility of a system of negative rights should be apparent, and so too its lexical priority over any system of positive rights.

The second component of a system of negative rights is that no stranger—parents and child are a different matter—has a correlative duty to support me with food, clothing, and shelter, let alone health care, even when my own resources are insufficient to guarantee survival. To obtain what I need, I can refashion my possesions for my own advantage, or, more commonly perhaps, make contracts with specific people to purchase what I cannot produce myself. Unlike property rights, these contractual rights do impose positive obligations for care and assistance.

They are directed not against society at large, but against persons who have singled themselves out for special treatment by having assumed special undertakings.

What is true of life is also true of labor. At common law, my right to my own labor only meant that other persons could not use force or defamation to keep me from selling that labor to a willing buyer.[9] But full protection of this right does not create in other people the correlative duty to give me a job, or to make sure that their job offers comply with some socially determined minimum standards on wages, benefits, and working conditions. I am the best judge of my own situation and the best guardian of my own self-interest, not because I possess infallible instincts, but because I have better motivation and more knowledge about my own welfare than anyone else. In turn, other people protect themselves by weighing the offers that they want to make or accept: so long as both parties voluntarily consent to an arrangement, who should be regarded as a loser? Behind the common law position lies the accurate economic assumption of mutual gains from trade, gains that can be dissipated when government throws obstacles in the path of those who do have knowledge of their own needs.

A PRIMER ON NEGATIVE RIGHTS

The basic legal framework for a world of negative rights contains four central components, which I have elaborated in my book *Simple Rules for a Complex World*:

- ❖ Rules for the self-ownership both of one's person and one's labor
- ❖ Rules for the acquisition for property in external things
- ❖ Rules of contract law to secure the advantages of exchange both for capital and services
- ❖ Rules for the protection of both liberty and property from aggression and deception by others[10]

The question that one asks is, why should this set of rules command allegiance in political and legal debate? There is no clean answer to this question, for simply articulating the system of negative rights is not to justify it. How then might that general system be justified? The answer is, by the beneficial consequences that are on average generated by its consistent long-term application. Let us review the bidding.

The first rule speaks of autonomy, or self-rule, for all individuals within a legal system.[11] This familiar philosophical principle claims universal application to all persons, regardless of origin or circumstance. The autonomy rule gives each person a right of self-determination over what should be done to or with his or her own body. Although often treated as a self-evident truth, the principle of autonomy can be denied without fear of self-contradiction. Logic is not the reason why this abstract principle exerts so great a hold on our moral imaginations. Rather, the explanation is found in the beneficial consequences that flow from its consistent application. Those consequences in turn are only revealed by examining and rejecting the alternative systems of consistent rights that might be substituted in its place. The alternative to consistency is, quite literally, a collision course between separate persons. Inconsistent rights give both north-south and east-west traffic a green light at the same time all the time. Any takers?

Within the domain of consistent regimes, the alternatives quickly reveal themselves to be unpalatable. One possible legal regime posits that no individuals can have any rights in their own persons no matter what. Here there is no difficulty with inconsistent or overlapping rights. Rather there are no rules of the road at all. Because there are no legal rights, it follows that there can be no wrongs. Or, if you prefer, everyone has the legal right to do exactly what he wants so long as he can get away with it. "Where there is no common power, there is no law; where no law, no injustice. Force, and fraud, are in war the two cardinal virtues."[12] Killing may take place as a matter of course, but murder is by definition now impossible. It is just from this world, however described, that all brands of social contract theory, from Hobbes to the present, have sought refuge and escape. Is there anyone who thinks that we are all made better off by mutually renouncing our respective rights to security of the person? One favorite heuristic device asks you to place yourself behind a veil of ignorance, so that you do not know whether you will kill or be killed.[13] Do you want a world in which you can kill with impunity when others can do the same with you? There is no need to answer.

Other possibilities are no better. Slavery is a system of rights in persons that give some individuals rule over both themselves and other individuals. Yet it denies to some individuals even the rudiments of self-rule. There is widespread moral revulsion to this system, and its undesirable consequences are also revealed by a thought experiment similar to the one just invoked to reject a normative universe that shuns any limits on human action. Put yourself in the position where you know that you have a 50 percent chance of being a slave and a 50 percent chance of owning one slave—or if it matters, a 20 percent chance of owning four slaves and an 80 percent chance of becoming one of those slaves. Do you prefer these odds to a world where all individuals enjoy rights of self-determination? For some people, owning slaves itself would be a huge negative, and for them the choice is so easy that they do not have to calculate the odds. But even for those prepared to own others—and there have been many throughout history—the prospects of being owned are surely far worse.

It is no accident that slavery is an institution imposed on outsiders, on persons of different races or nationalities, by conquest. Even when allowed as a matter of law, it was not practiced within clans or racial or religious groups. The antebellum South was not known for its white slaves or black slave owners. And most significantly, it never arose by voluntary contract. It is for good reason that it is so easy to ban the enforcement of a contract that we are never likely to see. But we should not be too hasty in conflating the contractual slavery with the involuntary slavery. The closest we get to contractual slavery is indentured servitude for limited periods of time, where the advantages to the servant in either training or transportation often proved decisive. We should take our cue from history. Faced with genuine uncertainty as to your future station in life, you will pick autonomy as your baseline every time. The question of whether these rights over one's person should be regarded as inalienable is a distinctly second-order problem that turns on such questions as whether allowing the contract to be created or enforced permits certain forms of coercive transactions that could not be easily detected or countered on a case-by-case basis.[14]

The most controversial alternative to individual self-rule attacks the principle on the grounds that it allows each person to control his or her own talents, whose natural distribution does not conform to any known moral criteria. But once again this alternative requires some complex scheme of ownership where each person has, as it were, a part claim in the output of all other persons within the same community. At some level, everyone recoils from this conception. Must we have the consent of others to choose whom to marry and what to buy? And which persons have claims over our bodies and our labor once these are treated as a matter of common resources? No doubt, most of us recognize some claim of sorts that the less fortunate have against the more fortunate— an issue that is addressed in full in Chapters 11 and 12. However, even before we deal with this proposed exception at length, everyone senses that a world in which no choice can be made without the consultation or approval of some undifferentiated group of strangers is intolerable. The process of decision making for everyone is vastly facilitated if each person is treated as the owner of both his or her body and labor. The extent to which this assumption carries over is critical to our discussion of organ transplantation and death and dying found in Parts One and Two.

But what can be done with the labor that we separately possess? One important function of the legal system lies in assigning owners to natural resources. These property rules sometime call for individual ownership of land and movable property, and sometimes, as with air and water, point in favor of systems of common ownership. The key tradeoff in all cases involves a comparison of two kinds of costs. A system of private property imposes costs on the individuals who are excluded from resources they need. A cost of the system of common ownership is that we must design a system of collective governance to decide who can do what with the common property. The relative costs of exclusion and coordination vary with the nature of the resource under consideration. A book devoted to health need not explain how these tradeoffs work out with common resources such as water, air, oil, and gas; for our purposes, the key resources are land and chattels. Here the rule of exclusive rights has the same benefit as the autonomy principle because it allows a single owner to decide what will be done with given resources without having to procure the consent of other persons. Decisions to sow today can be made in the confidence that you can reap tomorrow. So long as all persons possess that right, the gains from exclusion will also be widespread. For land and chattels, the costs of collective ownership become very high very rapidly, as is revealed in our discussion of the positive rights to health care found at the outset of Part One.

Having exclusive rights also facilitates trade between individuals for both labor and property. The third rule of voluntary contract allows every person to surrender labor or property (secured by our first two rules) in exchange for something to which he attaches greater value. The moral impulse for keeping promises is grounded in the proposition that gains from trade accrue to all contracting parties. An alternative world that denies trade destroys the possibility of division of labor and limits the return on capital to its value in the hands of its present owner. Yet who benefits systematically when exchange values are systematically lost? Once again, our political behavior reveals the tenacity of our social judgments. No one favors any universal restrictions on exchange. The proponents of restraint will isolate some particular transaction (rent control, minimum wages) for special treatment while conceding the forcefulness of the general rule. Those special pleas for limiting exchange are valid to the extent that they can point to some foul play or improper behavior in the contracting process. Fraud and duress are out of bounds in all contexts, and in some cases affirmative obligations to disclose, such as those found in the law of informed consent, may also play a part. But arguments about exploitation based on superior wisdom, position, or wealth should be firmly rejected as a roundabout way to undercut the basic principle of mutual gains from trade whenever the supply of potential trading partners is large. The ability to enter and exit a market provides far greater protection to individual choice than any government interference in contractual relationships.

Of special importance to a book on health care is the proposition that the institution of contract and exchange does not fully exhaust the class of voluntary transfers. In addition, the system allows for full charitable giving, without the receipt of any quid pro quo. It may well be that the correct legal rule does not allow any donee or charitable recipient to enforce a bare promise to make a gift, even if it is in writing.[15] The dangers of impetuous promises, false claims, or social pressures might make it desirable to legally enforce gift promises. But for these purposes, the key point is that no legal rule should prevent people from following through on their promises where they see fit, such that once money has been paid over, it cannot be recovered from the donee except for cause, as in cases of fraud or duress. The rule that protects completed gifts is sufficient to allow the emergence of the strong charitable sector, so critical to any health care system. Although the modern law usually protects both gifts and exchanges, it does not do so in a number of areas so critical to health care generally. Thus prohibitions on exchanges are important in three key areas: the legal rules that regulate organ transplantation, death and dying, and the imposition of liability for professional and hospital malpractice. These subjects are discussed in Part Two.

The first three rules of the system of negative rights set out what individuals can do. These rights of autonomy, property, and exchange have distinct correlative duties, which coalesce in the fourth rule that prohibits the use of force or deceit (as with defamation) to interfere with the rights as stated. The logic of this fourth rule lies in the universal preference for security relative to the right of unbounded freedom of action, including aggressive behavior. The exceptions to the rule against the use of force, dealing with the issues of self-defense, are designed to reinforce the basic prohibition, not to undermine it. People will be less willing to attack if they know that others enjoy the right to use force in self-defense. But this basic rule does have a flip side. The prohibition on the use of force is not the same as a duty to rescue other individuals, that is, to use your labor and property for their advantage. Here the common law did not flinch at the hard case when it recognized a right, but not a duty, to rescue other people in a position of imminent peril, even for rescues that could be accomplished at little cost or inconvenience to the rescuer.[16] The defense of this no-duty rule rests on the proposition that some good actions cannot be compelled. It tolerates the no-rescue rule largely because efforts to coerce benevolence may turn out to be more counter-productive than efforts to foster an environment where people who want to help can do so without fear of state entanglements. Within the health care area, no one can find any movement to relax the prohibition against the use of force. Nor is there any effort to limit or block charitable giving. But the failure to impose a legal duty to rescue has been intensely debated because it is easy to see the potential gains that could be created by having some duty to assist in conditions of imminent peril. That topic is taken up extensively in the discussion of emergency care in Chapter 4.

POSITIVE RIGHTS AT COMMON LAW

The first four rules in this system seek to create clear, certain rules of individual and property ownership, to enforce and protect exchange and gift relationships in accordance with the intention of the parties, and to prevent the forms of aggressive and asocial private behavior that might undermine these rights. Yet this thumbnail sketch of the common law system is incomplete because it has not yet addressed the two basic exceptions to the general rule, exceptions that bear heavily on assertions of a general right to health care. The first is a variation on the issue of necessity in rescue cases. The second concerns the obligations of common carriers, innkeepers, and, by statutory extension, natural monopolies to provide service to all comers. These two cases show how the legal system can organize a limited retreat from a thoroughgoing principle of individual autonomy while still maintaining a powerful bar against the redistribution of wealth or property. The linkage between positive rights generally and redistribution is hardly fortuitous—redistribution cannot happen in a regime of negative rights—but, by the same token, it is not logically necessary. That connection can be severed by invoking the principle of just compensation that at once supplies a sensible response to market failures in coordination without embracing principles of wholesale redistribution.

PRIVATE NECESSITY

One evident consequence of the four rules stated previously is that A's need is never the source of B's legal obligation to provide assistance or care. But at the same time, the common law took this categorical stance against the conscription of personal services. It did allow one person to use someone else's property to save himself from imminent peril, as when A moors his boat at B's dock without her permission in the midst of a storm.[17] The common law allowed A to seize B's property to obviate the risk that she would hold out for the small fortune that A might pay to save his life. Yet A's right to enter the property is conditioned on his willingness to compensate B for the (normally trivial) rental value for use, and, more importantly, for any property damage attributable to A's self-help.[18]

At first glance, these necessity cases seem to contain the germ of a welfare right to assistance in time of need, and thus a rationale for a positive right to health care for all. If B's dock can be impressed into service against her will when necessity calls, why cannot general tax revenues be used to fund care for persons in need of health care? In many ways, the taxation alternative is far less intrusive than forced entry onto specific property. Taxation can be planned for in advance, and its form and amount can be debated extensively by democratic institutions. The funding can be obtained, not from the hapless individual whose property is needed on the spur of the moment, but by broad-based taxes collected from virtually all productive members of society.

Yet redistributive taxation is not justified by the common law rules on necessity. The privilege created by necessity imposes on A the correlative duty to pay just compensation for harm caused and property used, no matter how noble the cause. Indeed, even if A's privilege to use B's property were not conditional on payment of compensation, it would still not provide an analogy to redistributive taxation. In a world in which necessity is a chance event, everyone's compensation comes from the *like ability* to use someone else's property if faced with a similar necessity of his own. This rule works tolerably well because few people are likely to take foolish risks just to avail themselves of the necessity privilege. Stated otherwise, the uncompensated right to use someone else's property in time of peril does not threaten the stability of the overall system, even if compensation were not required, as it now generally is.

On matters of health, however, the system of guaranteed access works in a very different fashion. No longer does the system of forced exchanges create the win/win relationship. Instead the open-ended system of entitlements shifts wealth from young to old, and, for just that reason, as often from poor to rich as from rich to poor. The system of coerced transfers fosters win/lose relationships where the winners get far less than the losers sacrifice. In principle it seems possible to craft a positive right to health care that is both universal in its reach and limited in the coverage it offers. But the tug and pull of political pressures never permit the orderly unfolding of this ethical program. Unfortunately, in practice, the patterns of wealth transfer spawned by these political pressures show virtually no resemblance to the idealized theories of redistribution spawned by elevating health to the status of a special good. Huge sums of money are poured into the last weeks and days of life, money that would do far more for the health of the nation if left in the pockets of young parents to spend on the nutrition and education of their children. The use of taxation and regulation therefore strays far afield from the common law necessity principle, which only allows forced exchanges to neutralize the difficulties when one person can forcibly exclude others from his land when there is quite literally no other place to go. The use of the necessity principle owes its existence to the absence of multiple trading partners in unanticipated crisis situations. The necessity principle does not extend to forced exactions from those with property to those in need. Redistribution on grounds of wealth or need forms no part of its rationale.

Furthermore, the modern entitlement to health care covers a far broader domain. Often health care is demanded, not for reasons of strict necessity, but because its benefits are said to be greater than its costs. Yet the necessity rule has been fashioned to avoid that slippery slope. The doctrine of necessity is designed to isolate those situations in which the gains from private coercion far exceed its costs, and is to that extent frankly utilitarian in its origins. But the rule itself, when couched in the language of necessity, does not incorporate the language of costs and benefits, lest it be watered down into a rule of relative convenience. If you are out of town, I cannot take your bicycle from your garage just because I am late to a business appointment, even if my short-term gain is greater than your short-term cost. The necessity doctrine does not make any explicit straight-up comparison between the loss inflicted on you and my anticipated gain. It resists those extensions because of the way in which they would obviously destabilize the entire system of property rights so necessary to secure productive investment and voluntary exchange. Accordingly, the privilege should not be expanded beyond its narrow common law context, for to do so would give me a strong and insidious incentive to neglect prudent steps of private planning in the hope that I could always bail myself out at your expense. Contracting *in advance* is far better than negotiating spot transactions under emergency conditions. The necessity doctrine does not justify any general health care entitlement.

COMMON CARRIERS, PUBLIC UTILITIES, AND THE DUTY TO TAKE ALL COMERS

The second principled breach in the common law wall of individual autonomy concerns the obligations of common carrier and innkeepers, which in turn were extended during the nineteenth century to public utilities, such as gas, power, and light. These establishments were said to be "affected by the public interest."[19] So limited, the owners of these facilities could not use the absolute right to exclude potential customers as a lever to charge them whatever price they pleased. The common carrier was obligated to charge not what the market could bear, but only a reasonable price.[20]

The explanation for this apparent reversal of the general rule of freedom of contract and association—including the freedom not to contract and not to associate—lies in the monopoly power these owners have over their customer base. Lord Ellenborough was emphatic on the point as early as 1810: "There is no doubt that the general principle is favored in both law and justice, that every man may fix what price he pleases upon his own property or the use of it; but if, for a particular purpose, the public have a right to resort to his premises and make use of them, and he have a monopoly in them for that purpose, if he will take the benefit of the monopoly, he must as an equivalent perform the duty attached to it on reasonable terms."[21] That power, when created and fortified by exclusive state franchise, could allow these owners to extract different prices for the same services from similarly situated persons.[22] The prohibition against "unfair" discrimination does not rest on any ad hoc conception of fairness and minimum access to needed services. It rests solely on the need to limit the monopoly power created in markets that are occupied by a single supplier.

It is best to begin by noting the efficiency justifications for the standard rule requiring services to be provided at nondiscriminatory prices. The price discrimination game always consumes real resources, and, as typically played, it often leads to undesirable social outcomes. An unregulated seller will demand that most consumers pay prices in excess of the competitive rate. Sometimes the seller guesses correctly, and the deal goes through: the more the consumer pays, the more the seller receives. But even this transaction has the added cost of computing separate price schedules for different classes of consumers. The social losses, moreover, are only compounded because the discriminating monopolist could incorrectly guess the reservation price of some potential consumers. Setting some prices too high means that some mutually beneficial transactions are lost forever. Competitive markets eliminate both these risks. There is no jockeying over price and no setting of artificially high prices that some consumers are nonetheless willing to pay.

The strategic games of the clever monopolist thus offer a prima facie justification for some state control; yet even here the costs of legislative or judicial intervention can rise to levels that nullify the gains from government action. One limited response, easily imposed by courts, is a nondiscrimination rule. This rule places no dollar limitations on the prices charged but insists that all persons in the same class be charged the same price. But the qualification of "the same class" shows that the antidiscrimination constraint has no redistributivist impulse. Individuals whose cost of service to the regulated firm are about comparable fall into the same class and can be charged the same prices, even if the services rendered are worth more to some consumers than to others. By the same token, if it costs different amounts to supply different consumers the same good, there should be some cost-justified discrimination between individuals in order to avoid the subsidy of one class by another. A good that costs $10 to supply to one group and $20 to another should not be supplied to both groups at $15.[23] This basic principle carries over to health care as well, where the cost of service can vary enormously. Of course, it may be impossible to identify groups whose members are all identical. But it should be possible to define groups so as to minimize the cross-subsidies, as when life insurance customers are grouped, usefully but imperfectly, by age.

An antidiscrimination rule does not, however, supply a perfect antidote to the potential dangers of monopoly pricing: each group of customers could be charged a monopoly price by, as it were, a nondiscriminating monopolist. Direct rate regulation is the stronger medicine used to counter that risk. But, like all strong medicine, it introduces a different set of heavy costs that compromise its efficacy.[24] Regulators have to incur substantial administrative costs to squeeze out the residual elements of monopoly profits. Yet their exuberance can stifle entry and innovation by new firms that could erode the monopoly from without. Monopoly regulation easily shades itself into monopoly protection. Yet the dangers of regulation do not lead down a single path. The same regulators that can protect one industry can wield their official power to confiscate the capital of a regulated firm by setting its rates below those needed to allow the firm a reasonable rate of return. The constitutional rules that are invoked to guard against this possibility offer only uncertain protection, for the initial tilt under rate of return is now heavily in favor of the state,[25] a point that bears heavily on Medicare's schemes of rate regulation, covered in Chapter 7.

For the moment, there is no reason to labor the difficulties of rate regulation. The simple point is that rate regulation makes sense, if at all, as a counterweight to monopoly power. The system is *not* justified by any effort at redistribution from those who could afford to pay for their services to those who could not. The inn had no free rooms for those who could not pay the standard price. To be sure, elements of redistribution can be easily introduced into modern systems of rate regulation. Some customers could be asked to pay for rooms at the inn that are occupied by others. Or, in a more modern vein, safe drivers could be required to subsidize risky drivers, or commercial telephone users could be asked to subsidize residential users. But these cross-subsidies cannot be justified in the name of curbing and limiting monopoly power. They must stand or fall on a candid assessment of their redistributive purpose.

Health markets may be subject to many imperfections of information and insolvency, but systematic private monopoly power is typically not one of them. The number of hospitals, health care groups, and individual physicians that engage in the practice of medicine and the related arts preclude the emergence of monopoly. Where pockets of private monopoly survive, the antitrust laws, which are outside the scope of this book, should be able to restrain their horizontal price-fixing activities.[26] In addition, the types of goods and services subject to regulation differ radically as we move across different sectors of the economy. The traditional obligation on innkeepers and common carriers was to provide a set of standardized services at standardized prices. Telephone companies provide access to lines; electric companies provide kilowatt-hours. Even in this variable context, hidden variations (phone calls on Sunday are not phone calls on workdays and so on) make sound regulation far trickier than the uninitiated might suppose. But the choice of a telephone company is never as personal as the choice of a physician. From every point of view, traditional rate regulation cases, complex as they are, present relatively few of the problems of controlling the quality and quantity of care—difficulties that do not disappear as the arena shifts from unregulated to regulated prices.

The state regulation of health care and services thus differs from the classical forms of common carrier regulation—themselves hardly unambiguous models of success—on both the benefit and the cost side. The monopoly problem is far weaker, and the costs of state intervention are far higher. In light of these dual factors, the best social strategy is for competition to flourish, so that higher levels of access flow from lower costs of entry. That outcome is best achieved by removing legal barriers to entry, whether in the form of licensing laws or certificates of need. If that proves insufficient, it may be appropriate to (cautiously) invoke the antitrust laws against horizontal arrangements in the health care business. Public expenditures of any sort need not be made. To implement this program, the traditional regulation of common carriers and public utilities affords no systematic justification for a regime of positive rights in health care. The case for positive rights to health care does not turn on either autonomy or efficiency, but on redistribution on the basis of need, pure and simple.

AUTONOMY, TWICE VIOLATED

The central thesis of this book is that the rules of the game as have just been laid out are more likely to lead to a sensible regime for the reform and regulation of health care than the dominant regime. To make out this claim, I shall examine various ways in which these principles have been offended across broad areas of medical regulation. The initial focus is on the question of whether positive rights of access to health care make sense as a matter of philosophical, economic, and legal principle. The issue here is not only theoretical because the American health system has, at least for the past 30 years, treated access to care as its starting point for analysis. That starting point is often defended on the grounds that adequate provision of health care resources is necessary to allow patients to make responsible and autonomous choices. Yet in so doing, it treats the ultimate good solely as the preservation of patient autonomy, to the derogation of the principles of freedom of contract and association that normally apply to all individuals in civil society. "A party has a right to select and determine with whom he will contract, and cannot have another person thrust upon him without his consent."[27] The proposition does not, and should not, apply only to ordinary individuals. It applies to all parties, business or charitable, so long as they do not occupy any monopoly position.[28] Autonomy is a generative concept that protects both individual and institutional choices equally.

The first half of this book investigates that assault on the autonomy principle, which comes in the form of a demand for forced association, which, in the absence of monopoly, operates as a vehicle for the forced redistribution of wealth. It begins by taking dead aim on the justifications offered for creating positive rights to health care. Chapter 1 begins by developing the strongest possible case for the creation of positive rights—a showing that the maximization of wealth brought about by markets is not equivalent to a maximization of utility that should be our general social objective. Chapter 2 seeks to undermine that conclusion by showing the practical difficulties that beset any effort to transform a strong moral intuition into a protected legal right.

The arguments offered are not advanced as deductive certainties, but as empirical propositions, capable of being tested in particular contexts. Chapter 3 takes up that empirical challenge by criticizing the use of positive rights as a response to the question of demanded care for futile treatment, and in turn proposes a number of methods to prevent exaggerated claims of patient autonomy from commandeering resources better spent on other causes. Chapter 4 continues the critique by looking at the mishaps that arise from requiring hospitals, when the principle of institutional autonomy is rejected, to supply emergency care to individuals in an unstable condition or active labor.

The analysis is further extended in Chapters 5 and 6, which tackle the question of cross-subsidy and redistribution through the mechanism of antidiscrimination laws. They show the unfortunate consequences of those forays in connection with such important questions as genetic discrimination, community rating, and required coverage for pre-existing conditions.

The claims for positive rights are not confined to individual transactions; they apply to larger institutional settings as well. Chapter 7 discusses the vast array of problems created under the Medicare system. Chapter 8 attempts to explain why the effort to create universal and comprehensive health care under the Clinton Health Security Act proves that even the idea of positive rights comes up against powerful political limitations, albeit too little and too late.

The second half of the book deals with the flip side of the autonomy principle captured in the terms self-determination and individual choice. It examines the right to enter into contracts or arrangements with other parties free of the interference by third parties, and the limitations that should be imposed on contractual freedom to deal with the risks of incompetence and undue influence. Once again the modern defense of the principle of patient autonomy reveals sharp inconsistencies about the matters left to individual choice and those which are subjected, mistakenly in my view, to collective control. Accordingly, Part Two concentrates on three topics: organ transplantation, euthanasia and physician-assisted suicide, and liability for medical injuries.

The first four chapters of Part Two deal with the many issues that surround the question of organ transplantation and seek to show why a simple combination of ordinary rights of autonomy and exchange, taken together, strongly favor removing the prohibition against the sale of organs. Yet the prohibition on private transactions remains in force today, with unfortunate consequences for the procurement and distribution of organs. In fleshing out this theme, Chapter 9 deals with the general principles of alienation, with special reference to the problems of baby-selling and surrogate motherhood, the closest analogies to organ transplantation. Chapter 10 introduces the discussion in connection with organ transplantation. Chapter 11 examines the supply side of the market for organs. Chapter 12 picks up the demand side.

The most controversial issue today is that of death and dying, where the autonomy principle plays a key role. Unfortunately, its legal invocation is mixed and wavering. At one level, the principle is correctly invoked to allow patients to refuse medical treatment for whatever reason they see fit, even if the consequences should prove fatal to them. But at the same time, the force of the autonomy principle has been regrettably denied when the controversy turns to active euthanasia and physician-assisted suicide. The common law courts and state legislatures, which should be most responsive to these claims, have, by and large, turned a deaf ear. But recent developments, dating only from the first half of 1996, have taken a very different turn by invalidating on constitutional grounds the legal prohibitions on assisted suicide, without upsetting the traditional ban on active euthanasia. Chapters 13 through 17 investigate the many facets to this high-profile issue. Chapter 13 uses the autonomy principle to defend the practice of active euthanasia. Chapter 14 extends the analysis to the prohibition on assisted suicide, which implicates not only individual autonomy, but also the contractual norm of voluntary cooperation. Chapter 15 addresses objections to both active euthanasia and assisted suicide on grounds of abuse, with special reference to the common Dutch practice, which I defend against its many critics. Chapter 16 switches ground and concludes that notwithstanding the substantive case for both active euthanasia and assisted suicide, the case to constitutionalize all or part of this program is subject to fatal intellectual objections. Chapter 17 rounds out the picture by defending, but not on constitutional grounds, the cautious use of active euthanasia for incompetent patients.

Medical services are normally provided by consensual arrangement. Yet everywhere, there are restrictions on the scope to which responsible parties can contract out of tort liability for medical and hospital malpractice. The last three chapters urge a reversal of those policies and the adoption of a regime of free contract for both purchased and charitable care. Chapter 18 explores the basic history of medical malpractice liability and concludes that it is better judged by contractual principles of voluntary exchange. Chapter 19 then argues that the inefficiency of the current legal regime on medical malpractice supports that prior judgment. Chapter 20 then rejects other proposed solutions to the malpractice question, such as medical no-fault insurance, which substitute one inappropriate response to medical injury for another.

Throughout these various discussions one theme stands out. The simple and compact set of common law rules does a far better job of providing health care than the endless set of legislative and judicial innovations of our day. Taken in isolation, the social system can survive this reform or that. But taken together, the full range of reforms poses a mortal peril to the very ends they are supposed to advance: the health and prosperity of society. My criticisms are directed less to the good will of their proponents and more to the actual and observed consequences from 30 years of ceaseless legal experimentation with greater measures of government control. I doubt that most people will agree in full with my diagnosis. I suspect that many will find policy recommendations too radical for their own liking. But the accumulation of evidence about the failures of various health reforms cannot be ignored. The field of health may be special, but not so special as to be immune from the proposition that unintended consequences can sink the most high-minded of plans.

PART ONE

❖   ❖   ❖

Access to Health Care

❖   ❖   ❖

CHAPTER I

A Positive Case for Positive Rights

This normative inquiry into the principles for allocating health care has received a definitive answer within the framework of the classical common law. But it is one thing to invoke the common law system as a description of the current situation, and quite another to defend it against all comers. When used to deny access to health care, the autonomy principle could be attacked as remote and egotistical. The efficiency principle can be attacked as harsh and cruel. The common law tradition can be viewed as a warmed-over view of some discredited natural law theory, easily dismissed as obscure, high-falutin', or politically naive. Today any set of rights to protect life, liberty, and property is no longer regarded as either self-evident or inalienable, much less as necessary truths demonstrable by pure reason. We live in an age that asks the insistent and instrumental questions: what set of legal rights does society want to institute to govern itself, and why?

Judged by this pragmatic test, the traditional common law framework counts as a social and political failure. At best, it lurks as a background principle that much-desired complex legislative and administrative schemes can easily and frequently displace. Government interventions may, when thought socially wise, force associations on unwilling parties and subject them to taxes designed to benefit others. This shift in emphasis is well marked by the changes in political discourse. When founded in 1954, the Department of Health, Education, and Welfare contained the term "welfare," as if to suggest that public assistance was a privilege conferred by the state and not a positive right. Twenty-six years later, in 1980, President Carter by executive order split HEW into two departments. The larger piece was not called "The Department of Health and Welfare." It was called Health and Human Services. A coincidence perhaps? But more likely, the change was deliberately chosen to foster and reflect the newer social understanding that human services were received as of right, not as of public grace.

Terminology matters in the hurly-burly of political debate. And it also matters in academic settings. The person who controls the name often controls the agenda: just think of the shift from "sex" to "gender" in the modern discourse over feminist issues, or from "Negro" to "black" to "African-American" in 30 years of race relations. But like the issues of sex and race, questions of health and welfare are too important to be resolved solely by the names and labels that public officials place on government programs. The political battles of the previous decade or century do not explain or justify their outcomes. What is needed first is a theoretical discussion of whether the elevation of health care as an affirmative right makes intellectual sense, regardless of its magnetic appeal in the political realm. The details of individual programs have been, and will continue to be, subject to constant tugs from warring political factions. Yet none of these short-term fixes, including our own desperate maneuvers, is likely to be correctly undertaken unless and until we answer collectively some fundamental questions of philosophy and economics. The wrong conceptual apparatus always leads to the wrong practical choices, no matter how much data is accumulated and analyzed. This chapter addresses the philosophical underpinnings of the principles of forced association and forced redistribution and finds them wanting. The following chapters translate this abstract doubt into concrete examples by showing how implementing a regime of positive rights has provoked crises and dislocations in the market for health insurance and in the direct provision of health care.

In dealing with the positive rights to health care, one possible approach treats the status of the right of health care as a deductive rather than an empirical question. The distinguished philosopher Bernard Williams made one succinct argument for the affirmative right to health care when he wrote: "Leaving aside preventive medicine, the proper ground of distribution of medical care is ill health: this is a necessary truth."[1] Why the proposition is true, let alone necessary, was left unexplained. Williams's formulation, for example, does not take into account how people come to need their medical care and thus is utterly unresponsive to the question of how the distribution of treatment might influence the utilization of medical resources, which for any point of view should rise at least to the level of a relevant consideration. Even so, the recognition of a right to health care is often thought to be a logical necessity, so much so that "an irrational state of affairs is held to obtain if those whose needs are the same are treated unequally, when needs are the ground of the treatment."[2] But once again, no explanation is offered of how "necessary" truths fund the massive entitlements that they create.

The more powerful defenses of the affirmative right avoid appeals to necessary truths and stress the enormous intuitive appeal to the ideal of positive rights. Alain Enthoven begins his influential defense of managed competition not with an economic analysis of the various alternatives, but with his moral declaration of why the good society must provide for the health care of its citizens. He writes:

> *Decent minimum.* A just and humane society can define a minimum standard of medical care that ought to be available to all its members; essentially all the 'cost-worthy' medical care that can effectively prevent or cure disease, relieve suffering and correct dysfunction. By 'cost-worthy' I mean a standard of care that equates marginal benefits and marginal costs for people of *average* incomes in that society. Denial of anything up to that standard is morally unacceptable. Care above that standard can be considered a discretionary luxury whose availability can be left to the reward system. . . . Defining such a standard is difficult or impossible to do in theory. There are endless dilemmas and paradoxes for those who want to explore them. Somehow societies cut through them and make decisions. They build a kind of 'case law' of norms of treatment. What is difficult in theory is feasible in practice. A test might be to ask economically self-sufficient people: 'Can you personally look at the sick person and the care he is receiving and say that you are morally comfortable with it? If your family were impoverished and in need of care, would you consider this standard to be fair treatment?' In other words I would base this on the golden rule: treat others as you would have them treat you. No person should be

denied the decent minimum standard of care because he or she cannot pay, and no person should be subjected to extreme financial hardship to pay for it, such as having to 'spend down' to poverty before receiving public assistance.

Moral obligation to help the poor. The economically self-sufficient have a moral obligation to help those who are unable to maintain decent living standards on their own. I believe this principle can be grounded in the enlightened self-interest of the economically self-sufficient who do not want to have poverty or disease in their midst. But, beyond that, it is part of being a decent, moral human being to want to help relieve the suffering of others. Access to a decent minimum level of medical care is a precondition to 'life, liberty and the pursuit of happiness.' Governments exist to secure these rights for all their citizens.[3]

Enthoven thus defends the right to health care by appealing to the same egalitarian principle used to support social minimums for food, clothing, shelter, and education. Difficulties of implementation are not ignored, but they are addressed only *after* establishing these social minimums in principle. The remaining task is to work out the subsidies and transfers necessary to put the system into operation. It is as though jobs, housing, and health care are sacred, or as is sometimes said, primary goods whose satisfaction comes first. Their priority exempts them from the usual calculations based on scarcity and competition, which continue to apply to some second tier of less privileged goods and services.

This widespread moral intuition that health care is a good prior to the market can, however, be subjected to rational challenge. The first step in the analysis is to isolate the strongest arguments *for* a positive right to health care. Two arguments merit serious attention. The first rests on our ability to make interpersonal comparisons of utility—the type of comparisons that are not captured by any market. The second is to treat the provision of health care to needy individuals as a classical collective or public good. Some weight has to be attached to both these arguments because clearly we possess, and act on, some powerful intuitions in dealing with health care questions. On matters of health care, side by side with the market an extensive network of voluntary charitable organizations that are, and should be, a part of any decent society. But the key to the argument lies in the futile efforts to transform that moral intuition into a legal right. These difficulties include defining and enforcing the appropriate set of entitlements; the massive deformations that the political process places on any such system; and the willingness of private individuals, with less than charitable motives, to game the system for their own advantage. These problems necessarily pose enduring obstacles to any system of state-provided health care. In the end, the sum of these practical considerations is strong enough to abandon the coercive pursuit of public benevolence—a conclusion to which most experts take strenuous exception. But even if that radical conclusion is rejected, the cumulative weight of these objections should counsel us to regard public provision and financing of health care as a last resort of limited utility—a small piece of any overall approach to health care. But first it is best to turn to the components of the positive case.

WEALTH OR UTILITY?

On balance, I think that the strongest theoretical argument *in favor of* a welfare right in health care, or anywhere else, is one that exploits the wedge between maximizing social wealth and maximizing utility. To be sure, these two systems have much in common. Both approaches seek to identify the proper *social* end of social institutions, and to devise a system of individual rights and duties that edges us closer to that desirable social state of affairs. It is all too easy to slip into the common error that both kinds of theories are narrowly economistic; that they glorify greed or profit; or that they ignore various noneconomic values such as human dignity.

These misconceptions misunderstand the central aspirations of both approaches. A wealth maximization theory implies that a society that is prosperous is superior to one in which people are poor: and although that simple characterization does not immunize the theory from criticism, it certainly states a social objective that, other things being equal, is laudable in itself: who would want to affirm the importance of poverty as a social objective? And who thinks that we can raise up the condition of the poorest in society without assuring some general economic prosperity? In contrast, a utilitarian theory seeks to maximize a more elusive goal of human happiness—one that is harder to measure for any individual and harder to sum across separate and distinct individuals. My $5 and your $10 may sum to $15, but my 5 utils and your 10 utils—assuming we can count them—don't seem to sum at all. Wealth is easily compared across individuals; utility is not.

We can hardly denounce, however, a theory that allows individuals to convert raw inputs (time, labor, capital) into outputs to which they attach subjective value. Over a broad range of cases, the two theories tend to converge on the shape of legal institutions: both systems prefer a competitive market to a monopolistic one, and both systems offer stronger justifications for that conclusion than can any rival theory that celebrates individual autonomy as an end in itself, or any commitment to egalitarianism. In ordinary conversations, most individuals try to justify human actions and social institutions by pointing to their desirable consequences either in the individual case or over a broad class of similar cases. As such they tend to stumble into one of these two camps, often without troubling to distinguish between them. So the discussion of the tensions between these two theories is not meant to glorify the cruel and the heartless, but to sharpen the inquiry into the status of health rights. Sometimes the system of common law rights is said to be flawed because of its bias toward wealth maximization. Under wealth maximization, individual preferences count only if they are backed by dollars, that is, backed by the willingness *and* the ability to pay. Preferences, however genuine, that are unmediated by wealth just do not count. It is not enough to say that *if* I had money, or more money, I would surely spend it first on medical care and afterwards on entertainment. Without wealth, my preferences or desires do not enter into the social calculus at all.

Matters are very different when utility is the ultimate test of the soundness of social institutions. Now wealth is relegated to a useful but subordinate status: it becomes simply one imperfect means to grope our way through the legal and institutional arrangements that maximize human happiness. That some persons lack wealth to buy goods and services interposes an obstacle to measuring their needs and satisfactions. But although faulty measurement may require compromises on matters of social policy, the problems it raises are only instrumental and not moral. The welfare of certain individuals does not just disappear from the social map because they cannot vindicate their preferences in dollars. They continue to have needs and desires, hopes and fears. Their utility moves up and down as they become happy or sad, hungry or well fed, and sick or healthy—even if they are broke.

With utility as the ultimate touchstone of human institutions, wealth frequently functions as its convenient proxy. Any doubters should ask how we could run a system of taxation tied to increments of utility and not increments of wealth—which is what the income (literally, that which "comes in") tax necessarily measures.[4] Generally persons with greater wealth are happier than those with lesser wealth, but of course the correspondence is far from perfect. Personal illness, a death in the family, or a betrayal in business often reverse the relationship in particular cases: the rich can become miserable. Imputed income from nontaxable sources—good family life, religious beliefs, optimism about the future—may be greater for persons with low income than for those with higher ones. The struggling author may take more pride in her work than her wealthy colleague who has sold out to market pressures. But so what? All these complications have to be ignored in operating a vast impersonal system of income tax collection.[5] The inevitable variations between the law's proxy and the social ideal are likely to wash out over time when thousands of individual transactions are aggregated into some social whole, for the people who have lost on one throw of the dice may well have won on the next. The massive intrusion into private affairs that is necessary to monitor, say, the utility of a good or a bad marriage would destroy the fabric of that relationship. Taxation for all persons is rightly confined to transactions with readily realizable market values, even at the cost of some inequity and distortion of incentives from inducing activities into tax-free areas of endeavor. The best antidote to inequity in the incidence of taxation is to lower the level of taxes in order to minimize the negative incentives on production and to temper tax evasion. A recalibrated tax keyed to individual utility as such is just not in the cards.

In other cases, moreover, the proxy problem is relatively unimportant because standards of wealth and utility tend to move hand in hand. The exhibit-in-chief is the voluntary contractual arrangement. The judgment about utility rests on the observation that each party consents to the transaction only because by his subjective lights he prefers what he receives to what he surrenders. No matter how often it is repeated, this sentence of Thomas Hobbes is worth quoting again: "The value of all things contracted for, is measured by the appetite of the contractors; and therefore the just value, is that which they be contented to give."[6] Even if we, the public, as external observers, cannot tell why people enter into particular exchanges, they know how to make these decisions for themselves. To advance their own self-interest, why would they consent to any transaction that leaves them worse off than before? Indeed this framework recognizes certain principled exceptions. The term "voluntary" is designed to rule out conditions—duress, fraud, undue influence, and incompetence—which, if present, substantially reduce the likelihood of mutual gains from trade.

Likewise transactions to create and exchange goods and services normally increase the productive wealth of the economy. The buyer can make greater use of the thing acquired than the seller. How has wealth been increased when one family moves into a house that another has just vacated? The ability to sell increases willingness to buy and thus increases the chances that the house will be built in the first place. This resale option, often stressed by skilled brokers, induces sellers to forecast the needs of both immediate and subsequent purchasers. Theories of wealth and utility both endorse freedom of contract as the basic organizing principle between consenting adults. There is a strong lesson here about current health law structures: to insist on a positive right to health often goes hand in hand with the parallel decision to bar many kinds of private contracts. That was the lesson with organ transplantation, euthanasia, and medical liability, where interference with contract came at a high social price.

The correspondence between wealth and utility is thus well-nigh complete when successful voluntary transactions *do* take place between the parties. The conceptual problem becomes more clouded when certain transactions do *not* get completed because the prospective buyer lacks the necessary funds. In his usual blunt fashion, Judge Richard A. Posner offers an illustration of the hard case for markets. A pituitary extract is of modest use to the child of a rich family, and of great use to the child of a poor family, who without it will become a dwarf. "In the sense of value used in this book, the pituitary extract is more valuable to the rich than to the poor family, because value is measured by willingness to pay; but the extract would confer greater happiness in the hands of the poor family than in the hands of the rich one."[7] His choice of examples reveals his surprising willingness to embrace the wrong measure of social well-being by treating wealth as dispositive and happiness as irrelevant— a far cry from regarding wealth as a proxy for the utility. Posner himself is aware of the limitations of his argument but stubbornly refuses to make any conceptual adjustments in order to deal with the matter.[8]

It is here that the denunciations of wealth maximization are likely to reach their crescendo. But before these are embraced, note one possible defense of Posner's position: the resort to a tenet of formal economic theory that declares all interpersonal comparisons of utility to be conceptually impossible. On this view, it is idle even to attempt to compare the position of the poor potential dwarf with that of the rich child. Throwing up one's hands on utility comparisons often has a sensible functional role. It says that it is preferable to use market exchanges instead of coercive arrangements to reach any chosen end. After all, what moral argument could be raised for banning transactions that leaves both sides better off than before? Offsetting negative consequences to third persons are one credible answer. That issue surely looms large with pollution and drunk driving, but not with the rendering of ordinary services to health care.[9] The people who *do* pay cash have made some honest revelation of the minimum value that they attach to the services received. Talk is cheap, especially when dissimulation produces private gain. Thus to opine as a matter of public faith that the utility of the present tenants in rent-controlled housing is greater than that of potential renters is an open invitation to social disaster. If the current occupants attach greater weight to where they live, they should eagerly pay in dollars the rent sufficient to keep outsiders away because as a group their wealth constraints are no greater than those of the rival group. To make utility the coin of the political realm is to invite piteous tales of woe, exaggerated for the partisan purpose for which they are made. Using dollars in open markets muffles the rhetorical din and forces persons to reveal honestly the strength of their preferences in a common medium understood by all. "Put your money where your mouth is" is a coarse reminder of a high philosophical truth. If the tax collector cannot measure utility straight up, neither can the regulator who is all too likely to succumb to the demands of local residents (and voters) and to overlook or undervalue the preferences of outsiders. Direct political measurements of utility tend to destroy utility itself. The wealth proxy has a lot to commend it in straight utilitarian terms.

Resorting to wealth measures does not commit us to the necessary truth that all interpersonal comparisons of utility are logically impossible. To be sure, it is easy to construct examples of persons with greater wealth who attach more value to their marginal dollars than do persons with lesser wealth. Posner for one is quite content to draw a somewhat distended graph that exhibits just this relationship.[10] But it is far easier to draw graphs depicting the diminishing marginal utility of wealth than it is to be confident that a fixed increment of money means less to the poor person than the rich one. However, the usual relationship between wealth and utility is not a dark secret known only to antimarket moral philosophers and enlightened political theorists. A huge portion of charitable giving is predicated on just this insight, namely that the poor need the help that the rich are able to give. It is therefore regrettable that so many academics regard charitable responses as occupying only a tiny corner of the social space. It is also mystifying when the historical record, in health care and elsewhere, reveals a rich profusion of charitable enterprises that flourished even—better, *especially*—at the height of laissez-faire. Around the turn of the century, charitable hospitals in active operation numbered perhaps as many as 2,500.[11] Religious organizations, friendly societies, and all sorts of associations organized them. Yet the role of charitable support does not receive so much as a mention from Enthoven, or indeed from philosophers of similar political orientation. The only human interactions they envision are market exchanges or coerced exactions.

This extensive practice of charitable giving, however, does not rest on some philosophical mistake easily unmasked by classical economic theory. Rather the continuous outpouring of charitable behavior flows from the evident ability of both wealthy and ordinary people to compare their own welfare with the welfare of unidentified strangers in need and to resolve their internal conflicts *against* some narrow conception of their own economic self-interest. On a daily basis, the theoretical barrier to comparing utility between persons quickly crumbles. Left in its place are a host of thorny empirical issues. Which people should receive what assistance? Should it be direct or through specialized organizations? How much should be given? These particular inquiries arise precisely because charitable endeavors are not doomed by the conceptual hurdle that the pure economic model erects. We routinely make interpersonal comparisons of utility in favor of families, friends, and coworkers. We also make them with persons to whom we are bound by racial, ethnic, or religious ties. And we often make them to people to whom we are bound only by a sense of our common humanity. We don't need a theory that explains why charitable behavior cannot proceed along sensible lines. We need a theory that explains the determinants of charitable behavior and that recognizes the powerful role that it can and has played in unregulated settings.

This practical ability to make interpersonal comparisons of utility is radically reduced when the *state* tries to make the reliable comparisons *for other people*. Government is a complex organization whose members have many different goals. Its lumbering structure and bureaucratic incentives block the reliable collection and processing of information. It responds slowly to changes in behavior by private individuals. It places individuals in broad categories to ease its self-created administrative burdens. It is subject to fierce and partisan politics. With all those difficulties, the superiority of voluntary transactions over coerced ones seems evident. The same amount of money distributed through one system does more good in the former system than the latter, which chews up huge portions of its revenues in administrative expenses and loses another significant proportion to fraud and abuse at every level of its operation. Of course, no system of market exchanges can help the newborn child left on the doorstep of a church or hospital. But the absence of voluntary *exchanges* does not prevent voluntary *assistance* to meet that need. All this is not to say that there are no differences between charitable gifts and commercial exchanges. Thus the common law reflects the sensible difference between these two types of transactions by holding that charitable promises—I will give you $10 tomorrow—are not enforceable, even though promises for future exchanges—I will sell you my desk for $10—are.[12] Yet, by the same token, it treats a *completed* gift as making the recipient the owner of the thing given.

HEALTH CARE AS A COLLECTIVE GOOD

Finding a positive right to health care in the difference between wealth and utility stresses the relationship between the individual donor and recipient by finding in that simple wealth transfer an increase in utility sufficient to justify the use of coercion. A second way of making the case for a positive right to health care starts from a different perspective and examines the relationship of the individual donor to the rest of society. As ably developed by Allen Buchanan,[13] the second part of the argument stresses the relationship between the charitable donor and other well-off individuals in society.

In essence Buchanan identifies an "assurance problem" that arises because those individuals who make charitable gifts cannot be sure that their equally well-endowed individuals will make similar contributions. In light of that insecurity, social actors are faced with one of two types of collective action problem. Under one scenario, each virtuous person thinks that his own contribution is insignificant unless others contribute to the common mission. So although he is willing to contribute to a worthy cause, he will not waste funds on a program doomed for failure. The creation of a decent minimum to health care overcomes that problem and allows each individual greater self-realization than could have been achieved in a regime when all individuals make their charitable decisions independent of what others do.

In the alternative scenario, we can posit a collective action problem in which cynical individuals decide not to make any charitable contributions at all, preferring instead to freeload off the contributions of their fellow citizens. We thus find the systematic underprovision of public goods that requires taxation for such matters as police protection and public roads. Once again, Buchanan's point is that the conscientious libertarian should recognize the need for a positive right to health care.

These arguments, while ingenious, do not carry the day. The first and most obvious point is that the widespread history of charitable activities, on matters that include health care and range far beyond it, belies the need for state coercion. To be sure, many individuals are reluctant to contribute to charitable causes, but voluntary institutions from religious organizations to friendly societies have long been able to nudge them along that path. Nothing says that a system of state coercion is better than a system of voluntary affiliation to elicit the levels of cooperation. And for most individuals, the entire sense of charitable mission and calling is surely lost when coercion replaces some mix of social cooperation and individual choice.

The second difficulty with this position is that it presupposes an odd motivation for charitable activity. I doubt that many people think of charitable efforts as being on a par with courts and police protection. The obvious benefit of charitable contributions are not rich individuals who are now spared the dangers of rebellion or the pangs of conscience. It is the individual who receives the contribution and whose material and spiritual life is improved by it. That connection can be severed even if others do not join in the effort, and, indeed, even if they are opposed to it. To be sure, all needy individuals do not benefit simply because some needy persons are assisted, but by the same token it is odd in the extreme to say that life-sustaining aid given to A doesn't help A because similar assistance has not been afforded to B. Small amounts of charity do small amounts of good. Individuals who want to help needy people don't need any assurance that others will follow their example. They do it because they believe that they are under a moral obligation to provide the assistance in question. And they can directly witness the good consequences of their individual deeds on their individual recipients.

Finally, even if we could identify some sort of public goods problem in the providing of charitable care, it hardly follows that the correct answer is a minimum right to health care. Under Buchanan's model, the free riders are those other well-to-do individuals who contribute nothing to actions that, by indirection at least, improve their own well-being. As that is the case, the indicated course of action is to bind them to contribute to the care provided. The free rider problem is overcome if all well-off individuals contribute even if not all needy individuals receive care. Corralling the reluctant parties can be done, moreover, without enormous complication by allowing charitable deduction for charitable goods and services, a mechanism that has long been in place under the tax laws. The gist of the deduction is that the government provides a matching grant, paid in effect from all other citizens, to those individuals who are prepared to spend their own resources in charitable endeavors. This approach will raise the hackles of the Social Darwinist who thinks that charitable care inevitably weakens the fiber of the population as a whole, rather than improving the fortunes of those in need. But for the vast majority of individuals who support the idea of charitable care in principle, it requires them to contribute pro rata. The ultimate distribution of authority thus leaves the power in the hands of those who make the gift, while expanding the pool of available funds.

IMPERFECT OBLIGATIONS

The public goods argument in the end does not fare any better than the previous argument that stressed the disjunction between utility and health. On balance, therefore, the common law theory of negative legal rights works better. That approach is compatible with the recognition of moral obligations, not enforceable as a matter of law, to make gifts of property or services to some persons in need. The legal position, moreover, was so well understood that these obligations were typically described as "imperfect" in the natural law tradition.[14] That somewhat obscure expression meant two things. First, it meant that no particular person had a personal right to insist on the benevolence of any other person. It was enough that wealthy people rendered assistance to some individuals or groups of their own choosing. Second, it meant that any person who did not receive help might protest morally, but he had no legal rights against his would-be benefactor. Thus, it was clearly permissible for donors to discriminate among objects of charity on the basis of religion, sex, or race if they so choose, although obviously they were not obliged to do so.[15] The imbalances of donors in some cases would frequently be offset in the long run by gifts of others: many people could quite consciously target those excluded by others. Yet the common law rules had no built-in gyroscope to right any imbalance, real or imagined. Rather that system sought to maximize total gifts to the needy, not to secure their ideal distribution. The chief technique that the common law used to achieve that goal was to remove the legal barriers that might have stood in the way of charitable assistance, by allowing for both private and institutional gifts. The judges did not require any certificates of need to open up a hospital, and they demanded no public statement of reasons as to why charitable efforts were directed in one direction and not in another. Once this charitable component is taken into account, the status of welfare rights therefore turns out to be less one of the ends desired, and more one of the means chosen to reach those ends.

The relevant issue, therefore, was not framed solely as one of good intentions, but also as one of how to implement these intentions. A state system on its face purports to guarantee its recipients the satisfaction of minimum needs. But the illusion of security that it creates is subject to constraints that even the state cannot control, for once demands outstrip resources, the painful process of contraction must take place. The common law system offers no grandiose guarantees that help will be forthcoming, but it relies on the decentralized efforts of private groups to fill the vital function. It is too easy to be mislead by the rhetoric of rights, when the issue is overall levels of performance in the long run. What reason is there to believe that the current system will be able to deliver the health care that it promises? It is not sufficient to set the aspirations of the legal system high; it is also necessary to reach the target. It is just at this level that the current structure is beginning to crumble, as the detailed analysis of the subsequent chapters painfully reveals.

CHAPTER 2

❖ ❖ ❖

Practical Obstacles to Positive Rights

DEFINITIONS AND DEGREES

Chapter 1 used the gap between utility and wealth to develop the case for charitable giving. However, the precarious nature of charitable giving leaves it as an unstable resting point in both the theoretical and political realms and thus creates a constant demand to convert imperfect moral obligations into enforceable legal ones. The obligations selected are not randomly chosen. In any complete system of welfare rights, food, clothing, and shelter go to the head of the list, but health surely does not fall far behind. Why not make this leap from the moral to the legal? The answer does dispute the proposition that health to all is a desired end. Rather the objection to this conversion rests on the more prosaic observation that *collective means* cannot achieve their stated ends. No single reason is conclusive, but, as a rough empirical matter, their combined weight in the end should be regarded as decisive.

The first question is one of definition and scope. In dealing with moral claims and social rights, problems of legal definition and enforcement are of no consequence. The entire edifice of charitable giving relies exclusively on a set of diffuse but durable cultural and social sanctions. A legal regime of imperfect charitable obligations is easy to catalogue: it does not require any public statement of *who* must contribute, *how much* must be contributed, or what *conditions*, if any, should be attached to any gifts. The donors decide those issues for themselves, without fear of legal sanction. Transforming social rights into legal ones now puts all issues of definition, implementation, and enforcement on the front burner. To see why invoking legal sanctions is so treacherous, recall the three universal imperatives facing any successful legal system: scarcity, self-interest, and enforceability.

SCARCITY

The legal entitlements must be geared for a world of scarcity, that is, for a world where some legitimate wants have to remain unsatisfied. The precise definition "legitimate wants" is always disputable, but it surely includes all wants with positive value to the recipient and no negative impact on anyone else. Good health usually meets that test. All of these wants can be satisfied simultaneously only when resources are abundant. They cannot be simultaneously satisfied when resources are scarce and the cost of creating rights are positive. The overall social level of production necessarily caps the amount of benefits that can be provided. The less wealth that is generated, the less wealth that can be redistributed. The social problem of coerced giving therefore is not solved simply by getting a stock of existing goods to persons in need. It also requires a set of rules to induce their production in the first place. These constraints on production cannot be ignored simply because public discourse describes health care as a "right" that should be respected independent of the market. What good is there in creating a set of positive rights that exceed the ability of any society to provide them? And what dangers lie in creating a set of positive rights that *reduce* the level of goods and services that are generated? Win/win transactions—that is, voluntary contracts—may leave people uneasy over the relative size of the gains taken by all of the players. Win/lose transactions enter into far more perilous waters. What confidence can anyone have that the new distributions in any real-world setting can offset the losses in total output that follow in the wake of government coercion?

A system of negative legal rights coupled with imperfect rights to charitable assistance does not face these problems. The basic rules of property, contract, and tort operate well no matter what the social resource level. They generate no negative sum games. Nor do these rules require forced transfers of goods and services that have not been produced. The older system has built-in internal consistency and social stability that cannot be matched by any rival positive system of welfare rights. The likelihood of individual deprivation may be higher under a common law system of negative rights—although even that is debatable.

What is not debatable is that any system of positive rights runs the risk of major long-term dislocations, as the current political travail over Medicare so clearly indicates. The effort to minimize risks to individuals within the system creates the risk of overload that increases the risk of overall system failure. Accordingly there is no easy way to comply with the Rawlsian maxim to adjust social institutions in ways that benefit first the least well off in society. What passes as redistribution to the poor within one generation may well end up as favoring the privileged of one generation at the expense of the young and the unborn.

SELF-INTEREST

Any legal system must deal with the self-interest of the people whose conduct it governs. Some people, however, will be out to beat the system, no matter how it is configured. We do not have to be an unthinking devotee of Thomas Hobbes or believe that all persons always act out of a narrow conception of individual self-interest: indeed the practice of charitable giving decisively refutes that view. But when the discussion turns from benevolence to coercion, our target population shifts: in the world of imperfect charitable obligations, the main task is to protect people who are interested in giving from threats and attacks by others. The form of restraint asked of selfish persons is no greater than the restraint demanded of them when they are not allowed to disrupt by force the voluntary exchanges by others. But the target population differs in a system of positive welfare rights. Now we must confront the opposition of those who do not give two hoots about anyone else and ask them to join in a charitable venture of which they want no part and to which they may be opposed in principle. The level of legal pressure to require their cooperation and sacrifice is, however, far greater than the level required to prevent aggressors from interfering with the gifts promised to third persons. In setting positive obligations, the state takes what others produce and thereby reduces their incentives to create wealth. With negative rights, we need only demand that they not take from others. Securing the compliance of unwilling persons is far easier in a regime of negative rights, because so much less is demanded of them.

The broad variation in the level of self-interest also takes its toll in dealing with the class of recipients. If only a tiny fraction of recipients are determined to beat the system, their behavior could so disadvantage the virtuous people who, of necessity, will find themselves compelled to imitate the worst characteristics of the bad players just to survive: "I will not cheat on the system if you do not cheat on the system" is a simple pact that cannot work if there are millions of players, some fraction of whom are certain to dishonor it by putting themselves first. Initially many people may be prepared to wait patiently in the queue so long as everyone else waits their turn. But the moment one person breaks to the head of the line, say, because of an ostensible unexpected emergency, someone else will do the same, in self-defense, of course. Was the stated emergency genuine or just a sham? Who can tell? When two people do it, a third will follow, and so on down the line until the entire queue unravels. A process of degeneration that starts with measured acts of self-conscious justification ends in a mad scramble for the door. The natural impulses to collective benevolence that are heard at the outset of any social program become quickly mute when the program is in operation.

ENFORCEABILITY

Any system of positive rights must be able to withstand the constant pounding in real-world settings, replete with its high transactions and error costs and its radical uncertainty about what is happening. It is often said that models of perfect competition work in certain unregulated financial or agricultural markets with their fungible commodities. But these classical assumptions do not begin to describe the netherworld of health care.[1] The claim is surely correct insofar as it insists that even knowledgeable consumers find it troublesome to price and evaluate health care services. But it is too facile to assume that these obstacles in collecting information and measuring outcomes throw us into the embrace of government regulation. The underlying imperfections do not stem solely from the method used to deliver services—the market—but inhere in the goods themselves. The informational gaps on price and quality that impede market operations do not magically disappear under regulation. It is still necessary to promulgate general rules, to guarantee their internal consistency, and to sensibly apply them to myriad hard cases. It is still necessary to hire physicians and staff, to purchase capital equipment, to lease buildings, to order supplies, and to monitor the quantity and quality of physician and nursing care. It is still necessary to admit students to medical school and to train them in their specialties. The choice in system design is never between perfect government and imperfect markets anymore than it is between perfect markets and plodding governments. The only issue is which form of delivery of health services minimizes the rough spots when both have evident weaknesses. And for any worry about self-interested business executives, an equal and opposite worry arises about self-interested or lackadaisical public officials.

In sum, the constraints of scarcity, self-interest, and enforceability plague any choice of system. The problems they pose are not artificial. Introducing these complications is not meant to simplify the choices by assuming that administrative costs are zero; or that all actors are risk neutral; or that actors have perfect knowledge of the probability of success of certain maneuvers; or that legislators and judges are well intentioned, well informed, and never make mistakes. Almost any system of rights yields the right social outcomes when these happy assumptions are satisfied. With that level of benevolence, we can move toward a world in which each person contributes according to his ability and each receives according to his need. But the level of selflessness and knowledge needed to make that maxim credible is never found in any broad social setting. The decisive test is not how a system of rights fares when the seas are calm; it is how that system fares when the seas become choppy. A system of positive rights is far harder to keep together in rough waters: owing to its elaborate construction, its hull is far more likely to run aground and break apart. It takes some wit to enforce contracts and to keep people from killing or maiming each other. It takes much more wit to force recalcitrant and self-interested parties into a single communal venture.

These obstacles make government coercion less successful than is often supposed given the extensive network of rights that must be precisely defined and enforced. But at no time does the overall resource constraint disappear because affirmative rights are created.[2] We could declare generally that each person had a right to an income of $1 million per year and forget about funding health care by decree in our new age of abundance. But the massive inflation that comes from having more dollars chase fewer resources would leave everyone worse off than before. In an environment with constant pressure to use expensive and heroic techniques in the treatment of well-nigh hopeless cases, how do we scale down ambitions to manageable levels? Not by giving everyone a right to health care on demand, which imposes intolerable burdens of overutilization.[3] Health care may well be "special" to some, but even if it is not rationed by price, it still must be rationed in some other way. Scarcity

and self-interest do not disappear just because market systems of allocation are rejected.

A more realistic approach is to declare that all persons are entitled
to receive equal amounts of health care, neither more or less. Yet it is hard
to see why such a proposal has anything to commend it. An equal
incomes policy offers the sure road to economic privation because of the
incredible rigidities of a planned economy, as the breakup of Soviet control over Eastern Europe shows. An equal right to an equal amount of
health care—if coherent at all—would impose a less draconian restraint,
but is hardly welcome in its own terms. The most productive people in
society would be required to wait in queues with the least productive,
even if they had the wherewithal to pay for their own care. Even the
Canadian system that refuses to allow people to buy their way out of the
national system does nothing to prevent them from traveling to Buffalo
for additional services. But where could Americans go if our system was
so restrained? Back to Canada? Down to Cuba?

EQUALITY THROUGH COERCION?

The principle has yet another defect. People do not need equal amounts
of health care. For some individuals with disabilities, a very large fraction
of income should be devoted to health care. But for those who have
escaped such a misfortune, a very different allocation of personal
resources makes far more sense. Placing all individuals into the same
straightjacket guarantees that some will make wasteful expenditures on
health and others will be left short. The equality constraint, when externally imposed, ignores relevant information available to all individuals.
The secret to personal success is to equalize net return from expenditures
at the margin, so that the last unit of wealth spent on health has no
greater (and no lesser) benefit to the individual decision maker than the
last unit spent on any substitute good or service. The equality constraint
is one sure way to flunk this test. So, by process of elimination, we return
to the issue of minimum standards on which Enthoven pitches his case.

The effort to articulate minimum standards, however, still gives rise
in one context to all the difficulties of knowledge and coordination that
have brought socialist economies to their knees. When persons make
voluntary gifts to others from their own resources, they compare the
value of what they transfer to the value of what they retain. When the

state coerces the transaction, it must decide, without knowing quite how, that differences in utility justify the forced transfer of wealth, even though this coercive transfer *reduces* the total amount of available wealth. It is easy to make the moral case for averting tragedy by talking about the cases of "extreme want" that everyone recognizes: indeed the classical writers used just that phrase in justifying their recognition of imperfect obligations.[4] Those extreme cases are surely the easiest for any system of private charity to identify and correct. It is far more doubtful whether any system of public coercion can respond to those cases without overshooting the mark and creating collateral disabilities of its own.

The precise calibration needed for a successful program of minimum standards is, however, difficult to obtain. Fine-tuning is not a realistic option. The political momentum of these programs is so massive that satisfaction of needs cannot be confined to the extreme cases thought to justify the coerced transfers in the first place. Instead, the eligibility requirements steadily erode. If the transfers could be based solely on some comparison between the wealth of the payers and the payees, it is highly unlikely that (if total wealth could be held constant) the utility of that wealth for the recipient would be less than it is for the transferor. But the political process often runs in very crude fashion and generates subsidies for tobacco, dairy products, grazing rights, water rights, zoning laws, and rich people in rent control apartments that defy any rationale of relative need as the basis for coerced transfers. And the huge transfer of medical services from young to old can hardly be justified as transfer from rich to poor. All too often those who benefit from the program are able to put forward as their public exemplar some poor person in need, however unrepresentative of the actual class of recipients that person may be. No matter where the benefit levels are set, someone can be found who will be unable to make do if any cuts are introduced. Thus programmatic extensions, once made, are always difficult to trim. There is no area in which stories of individual heartache could do more to shape, and to mis-shape, public policy.[5]

Matters are still more complex. Wealth transfers are always costly. The incentives of payers are impaired because they are not allowed to keep what they have produced. The incentives of recipients are impaired because they have less need to produce and more incentive to tax those who do. The administrative costs of the programs are positive, and the lobbying efforts to be a recipient or preferred supplier waste still more social resources. Finally, no program can precisely hit its target of taxing those who are more well off in order to help those who are not. Redistribution is a game that all can play. It is too easy to find federal programs (such as the increased taxation of social security payments) that treat $40,000 as rich, and other programs that treat $32,000 as poor.[6] Health will prove no exception to the rule that politics degrades all noble ambitions. Hence the relevant question is never whether an additional $100 means more to the poor than it does to the rich. Rather, it is whether $30, or $50, or some other figure means more to the poor than $100 means to the rich.

The upshot is that the state lacks the ability to design *and* implement a long-lived program of transfer payments that avoids these degenerative tendencies even after the conceptual barrier to interpersonal comparisons of utility is surmounted. Incomplete public knowledge and political corruption may not be necessary logical truths, but they provide a constant social drag sufficient to render the entire enterprise counterproductive. The more ambitious the social undertaking, the more powerful the obstacles. The issue is always one of comparative advantage: the goods that markets find it most difficult to supply are the goods that government will find most difficult to supply. The empirical objections to positive welfare rights cannot be overrun or ignored; it is a feat of blind optimism to assume that any political process is capable of translating the idea of minimum standards into a set of workable administrative norms, which must cover thousands of existing procedures, with new ones coming on line all the time. It is not enough to say, as Enthoven says, that "somehow" these can be overcome. It is necessary to explain in some detail how this can be done—if it can be done at all.

MINIMUM OR EQUAL STANDARDS?

The creation of minimum standards is, moreover, a far more daunting enterprise than its modest label might suggest. Someone must specify the minimum. Is it in wealth, which can be dissipated by fad or foolishness? Or should it be in goods and services, where food, clothing, shelter, education, and medical care come to the top of the standard list that can easily grow without restraint? These minimums could be set so low that reducing them by even a single calorie would lead to suffering or death. But minimum standards quickly transform themselves into "decent min-

imums" precisely to avoid these Malthusian overtones. Once disconnected from elemental survival, the standards creep toward ever higher minimum standards, notwithstanding the disruption of productive incentives
both for payers and recipients alike. The vast expansion in the overall level
of welfare rights has been well documented, and continues apace regardless of any and all efforts to curb it.[7]

Enthoven's articulation of the boundary line between mandatory
and luxury care, for example, is an illustration of the inexorable tendency.
A decent minimum means that this balance is heavily weighted to the
former: only cosmetic surgery or superior accommodations fall within
the class of luxury goods that can be safely left to the provision of market forces. There seems to be no middle ground between the two types of
goods, such as might be found if no person is allowed to receive care at
a level below that received by the person in the 25th percentile in the voluntary market. Instead the bottom is quickly brought up at least to the
level of the average; indeed from Enthoven's examples it appears that
very few instances of below-average medical care are tolerated. Nothing
is said here about quality differentials in necessary procedures, which in
principle could be tolerated only if minimum public standards were set
below average ones. The only allowable differences appear to be with
elective treatments and in the nonmedical components of hospital
stay—a tiny fraction of the overall problem. The line between minimum
standards and egalitarian outcomes disappears virtually at inception.[8]

The demand for a system of minimum rights also creates manifold
difficulties for figuring out how to equate marginal benefits and marginal costs, and the problem is endemic to any system of positive rights to
health care. Initially, there are no accurate prices for measuring costs, and
no observable metric for measuring benefits, and none for rationing services. Thus suppose the same procedure can be used to save the life of a
young woman or old one, otherwise equal in all respects, whereby it
yields a longer stream of benefits in the first case than in the second. Or
suppose that the same procedure can be used to save the lives of two men
of the same age, one of whom is a successful earner, and the other will be
a future burden on the system. In both cases, knowing who is helped
speaks volumes under any cost benefit analysis. Those who are able to
produce in the future or to enjoy the long-term benefits of care are the
persons who should receive it. Where markets are operative, the bidding
reflects these differences; and where private charity is provided, some

rough account of them will be made as well for even generous people are uneasy about spending their money in ways that they think useless or perhaps counterproductive. But state plans tend to operate in ways that help the needy today while reducing the resources available to health care tomorrow.[9]

MARKET AND SOCIAL INSURANCE

The effort to create a system of decent minimums involves yet another important structural cost—the conversion of an insurance industry from a competitive market capable of accepting or declining risk into a regulated utility required to take all comers regardless of condition at an equal price. Advocates for a right to health care, who draw a sharp distinction between *casualty* insurance supplied by markets and *social* insurance offered by government, often regard the conversion as a plus. The difference reflects in microcosm the broader differences between common law and welfare rights. Casualty insurance does not redistribute wealth. Instead it allows persons to even out their flow of wealth over different periods whether their luck is good or bad. The costs that are paid are thus offset by the increase in aggregate utility for the stream of payments that are made. The difference between these two conceptions of insurance is enormous because market insurance creates a set of win/win transactions, whereby all insureds obtain protection against sudden and unwanted fluctuations in income. Because the transaction yields an anticipated gain to each party and it thus will not be in the interest of any party to exit the system, the market will prove to be stable. Yet, by the same token, the market will provide no redistribution; coverage will not be universal, and greater risks will require higher premiums. Market insurance thus creates the same potential for exclusion as is found in other competitive markets.

Social insurance is designed to prevent insurers from "cherry picking" in order to assure universal coverage. The only way to avoid the risks of exclusion is to mandate the inclusion in the pool of those with inferior risk prospects. Social insurance builds in at the ground level a system of cross-subsidies across persons.[10] But simply because these cross-subsidies eliminate a cost of market insurance does not imply that they lack familiar costs of their own. Subsidies tend to lead to overconsumption of the subsidized goods and to underconsumption of the goods and services taxed to provide the subsidy. Those distortions remain, perhaps in heightened form, even in the area of health care. People adapt their behavior in thousands of small ways to changes in their external environment. Although it is impossible to identify in advance exactly what adaptations will take place in any individual case, some reduction in overall physical fitness will follow from the increased subsidies of health care. As the price of ill health goes down, the willingness of individuals to take health risks will increase. What is not apparent in individual cases and what may be masked by other trends (for example, better foods and medicines) will nonetheless take its toll. Nothing about the special nature of health care will spare us from this most ordinary and troubling of conclusions.

In addition, all systems of subsidies require extensive networks of coercion, first, to require companies to offer the insurance to high-risk customers, and second, to prevent low-risk customers from exiting the market. These tendencies are again always at work in every insurance market, and although it may not be possible to document them in any straightforward way, they are bound to increase as the level of cross-subsidy increases. The issue here is not just speculative, for it seems clear that at least some portion of the uninsured population consists of young adults who have decided that it is simply not worth their while to enter insurance pools with other individuals who have riskier health profiles than they do.[11]

The dangers of paternalism run still further and severely limit the kinds of contracts that firms can offer under any universal health system. All individuals have greater knowledge of their own health needs than do any potential suppliers of insurance. They can use that knowledge to signal insurers that they are low-risk individuals by choosing certain kinds of insurance coverage. The benefits flow in both directions because insurers will in turn tailor their policies to cater to low-risk customers. A policy with a large deductible or coinsurance feature is the probable outcome: individuals who expect low utilization of the services will migrate in that direction, whereas more intensive users will be reluctant to follow suit. The remaining pool of older insureds therefore require higher rates or greater subsidy to remain viable. This result could be countered by forbidding insurers to offer certain kinds of terms, but only at the price of preventing useful contractual innovations. That result could also be countered by requiring all citizens to become part of a single-payer system, without any exit rights at all, thereby revealing the heavily coercive and paternalist elements of the system, and creating a state monopoly with few incentives to control costs or prevent abuses by insureds.

The difficulties of both efforts at universal coverage are not known only as a matter of theory. The Clinton Health Security Act contained convoluted provisions to standardize coverage offered by different health plans in order to imprison all subscribers in a world of cross-subsidies.[12] The downward spiral of this approach is made manifest by what has happened with assigned risk pools for automobile insurance. The rates in the assigned risk pool must be kept low in order for its members to be able to buy the insurance. The resulting shortfall has to be made up out of general revenues or specialized charges on safer drivers. In California and New Jersey, the entire episode has run its course with huge deficits, political bickering, and massive administrative hearings, all because everyone is said to have some "right to drive"—but only at the expense of others.[13] The same risk is inherent in health plans.

THE FORFEITURE OF POSITIVE RIGHTS

Finally, the constant sore spots of forfeiture of rights and moral hazard raise equally unpleasant complications. In all systems of insurance, one central issue is to identify those actions by the insured that justify a termination of coverage. Forfeiture provisions are routinely inserted in commercial arrangements because simply offering insurance coverage will induce some people to take risks that they might not take if they were uninsured. Once insurance covers all or part of the losses, the private cost of misbehavior is reduced, so the likelihood of its occurrence increases, notwithstanding the larger social losses that ensue. Careful underwriting is needed to weed out high-risk individuals. For the policies that are written, denying coverage for suicide and willful destruction of property helps to counter the remaining risks.

The pressures on forfeiture provisions become more insistent in a system of minimum universal benefits because now the least desirable risks can no longer be excluded from the system. Foolish personal behavior (riding motorcycles without helmets, drinking, promiscuity, bad diet, ignoring medical treatment, and the like) now imposes risks on others.

Does the decent society continue to provide medical assistance to people who misbehave by acting as if their losses were caused by misfortune alone? Excluding bad actors from coverage raises the same moral dilemma that discredited the common law rules and ushered in a regime of positive welfare rights. Will the society that cannot let people die because of their inability to pay let them die because they have dissipated public resources instead of their own?

In principle, poverty could be treated more favorably than misconduct. Historically private charities made that distinction in a rough and ready way by extending greater assistance to the "deserving poor" while sharply rationing it to those who misbehaved.[14] But modern doubts about individual responsibility undermine this distinction both in theory and in practice. The source of need matters less if it matters at all. We assist all people who are in need whether through bad luck or bad habits. People who are neglectful of their own welfare may be excused because of the larger social injustices to which they have long been subject. No one can describe the complex skein of events that places individuals in need, so the safe political decision covers everyone for everything regardless, if only to avoid the scandal of turning away someone by mistake. No political system will be able to turn people away once the coverage is made universal.

The inability to cut people off from aid works its way back through the system. Suppose that some routine test could keep a diabetic from falling into shock. If that person is told that if these tests are not taken, no help will be given if his sugar levels become dangerously high, then the incentive to test is manifest. But if it is understood that no sanctions will be imposed at the second stage on account of misconduct at the first stage, the incentives to perform are reduced. The provider now must bear the costs of compliance at the earlier stage because it has to foot the bill when matters go awry. The individual now has a credible threat not to take routine health precautions. To be sure, the individual faces some limitation because no social guarantee of assistance can eliminate the risk of death or permanent injury. But even so, the odds shift in ways that make it more difficult for the government to secure the private cooperation of individuals at risk for illness, drug abuse, drunk driving, sexual promiscuity, and a whole host of other risky behaviors. This collective unwillingness to impose limits is no more successful in the public arena than it is in raising children. The social sanctions will unravel if carrots are used to shape behavior to the exclusion of sticks. At every stage, a set of expensive and intrusive public precautions will be used to replace a cheap and effective set of private actions. Even charities will have trouble enforcing their restraints on aid. Yet an impersonal state will only do worse because it cannot rely on the thousands of small, informal sanctions available to private parties. A regime of statutory minimum standards has substantial unacknowledged costs.

An instructive parallel can be drawn to the plight of the homeless. The dominant political impulse responds to the situation by spending public resources to provide decent housing and other social services. In response comes the timid suggestion that public support increases the number of homeless in the first place. The inevitable rejoinder is that no sensible person would ever opt for public support if otherwise capable of supporting himself. But that response overlooks one critical variable: the effect of government policies at the margin. Perhaps 99 percent of the population would be impervious to the incentives created by public assistance. But some portion of the population is teetering on the edge, and its behavior is likely to be altered in myriad unidentified ways, and for the worse. Providing increased care for today's homeless may induce friends and family members to toss out a difficult relative, thereby swelling the ranks of the homeless. Or it may tip the balance in a thousand other ways. No one knows the level of response—a 10 percent increase in homeless benefits need not provoke a 10 percent increase in the number of homeless. Yet we do know that between 1983 and 1988, the total number of homeless in shelters increased from 98,000 to 275,000, while the numbers of homeless on the street increased as well.[15] The desire to assist those in need must be set off against the risk of creating a new population of needy. Private charities have a better chance of finding that narrow window of opportunity.

The homeless problem therefore should alert us to the inescapable dilemma facing the articulation of any set of minimum standards: to make the minimum high enough to help those presently in need *necessarily* makes it high enough to induce once self-sufficient persons to receive aid. Doubling the benefits per person does far more than double total program costs. Additional people take advantage of the greater benefits; higher taxes on a smaller population base are needed to fund the burdens; and higher tax rates only force more people over the edge.

The parallels to health care should not be ignored. The rise in financial payoffs will unambiguously increase the demands for utilization under any system of comprehensive insurance with built-in cross-subsidies. Meeting these demands will place further burdens on the tax system and will crowd out other charitable and welfare activities—for example, education—that have also received public support (with very mixed effects indeed). We cannot even confidently predict that an increased investment in health care will lead to any systematic improvement in health. The overall decline in productive labor leads to reductions in nutrition and safety elsewhere in the system, and these translate into higher rates of accident and disease at earlier points in time. It is worth noting that even with the enormous increase in resources devoted to health care, life expectancies conditional on reaching old age have not increased as much as one might have expected.[16] The common perception of this issue is shaped by increases in life expectancy at birth, which in 1900 was around 48 years for men and 51 years for women. By 1970, at the dawn of the Medicare era, life expectancy at birth reached 68 for men and 75.6 for women—female life expectancy showed both a substantial overall increase and a greater relative increase. Those figures continued to move smartly upward so that by 1992, life expectancy was 72.3 years of age for men and 79.1 for women. But the overall tables suggest that most of the increase in life expectation comes from a reduction in death rates before individuals reach retirement age. Thus, for men who reached age 60, their life expectations were 14.4 in 1900 and 16.2 in 1970. For women the comparable figures increased from 15.2 in 1900 to 21 in 1970. But the advances in the post-Medicare era have not been dramatic either. For males age 65, life expectancy was 14.2 in 1979–1981 and 15.4 in 1992, notwithstanding the huge increases in the overall Medicare program. The comparable figures for women age 65 show about the same movement, from 18.4 in 1979–1981 to 19.2 in 1992. Nor is there any reason to believe that all, or even most, of the improvement came from end-of-life care, given the other improvements in diet and lifestyle over the same period.

The implications are well worth pondering. It could well be, therefore, that the effect of still greater public investment in health care is to reduce overall fitness and to increase the portion of people's lives that is spent under medical supervision. If so, the right to health care becomes completely counterproductive: the indirect increase in human suffering is left remediless as the apparent sources of suffering are fully dealt with. Starting from ground zero, why invite a system with these perverse effects? Why then yield to the special interest groups that generate them?

Given these fundamental constraints, the common law system of *negative* universal rights becomes more attractive relative to its modern alternatives. The negative system is internally stable regardless of the aggregate levels of wealth available at any given time. People start with their initial endowments in life, in liberty, and in wealth, and they may trade them for other goods they prefer. The trade itself is a private act that leaves, on both contracting parties, a risk of loss that cannot be shifted to strangers by either private lawsuit or public bailout. The system thereby encourages a high initial level of caution and prudence in making and performing contracts, which in turn *reduces* the level of mistake. But these lessons have largely been forgotten, so today we hear common laments about how a system so generous and well conceived could have gone so badly astray. We have witnessed the massive expansion of welfare, but we have not seen the contraction of poverty or even the equalization of incomes.[17] We have witnessed the huge expansion of health care, with similar poor results. These consequences did not just happen. They are the predictable long-term responses to a positive system of legal rights.

The subsequent chapters of Part One detail the perils of a regime of positive right in great detail. Chapter 3 addresses the question of the futility of medical treatment. Chapter 4 turns to the question of necessity. Chapter 5 speaks about the role of discrimination in the provision of health care, and Chapter 6 extends that analysis to examine the related questions of community rating and mandatory insurance coverage for pre-existing conditions. Finally, Chapters 7 and 8 address two comprehensive systems of guaranteed access: Medicare and the failed Clintoncare proposals.

CHAPTER 3

❖ ❖ ❖

Demanded Care:
An Exercise in Futility

A FINANCIAL AND CONCEPTUAL PROBLEM

Modern medical technology creates opportunities, sometimes unwelcome, for prolonging life. As a rough guess, most people in desperate straits do not want to be kept alive by extraordinary measures, even when others foot the bill. State payment for terminal care does not shield the dying patient from the physical assault on his person; nor does it insulate family members from the emotional drain of having to care for its dying member. These uncompensated costs often lead to requests to die in peace or for active euthanasia to relieve suffering. Yet if a small fraction of the population goes against the grain by insisting on "pulling out all the stops" to prolong life, the costs borne by others can quickly mount. The stakes get even higher when others demand expensive care before it is known whether the patient will live or die. A person, without fear of contradiction, could first demand extensive care for conditions that others might perceive as futile, only to switch fields later on and demand the right to end his life by active means.

End-of-life care comes in all forms. There is no quarrel that individuals should be able to receive, as a matter of course, palliative care that eases pain before death. All of the struggle, therefore, comes over those forms of treatment that are designed to improve a situation that others regard as hopeless. Interventions of this sort do not come cheaply, especially in intensive care units (ICUs), where a bed's cost per day is about three times that of operating a normal bed.[1] ICU beds are in constant use, often in futile cases, as demand rises to exhaust a subsidized supply. Crammed ICU facilities offer no evidence that prudent planning has deployed scarce resources where they are most needed. They only confirm the melancholy proposition that demand increases as price falls, independent of the social value of the services provided. No one doubts the value of ICU care to allow otherwise healthy individuals to weather a serious traumatic or acute disease. No one should question the right of any individual to spend the family inheritance on the last days of life if he so chooses. But the question of demanded care has an inextricable public component: should public funds—other people's money—be spent on care when the prognosis is hopeless and the treatment deemed futile?

So stated, the thorny question of demanded care lies at the intersection of two deeply held but inconsistent social values: an individual right to receive any needed treatment born of deep religious or moral conviction of the sanctity of life, and the independent professional medical judgment that futile treatment should cease.[2] I shall postpone until Part Two a discussion of whether the autonomy principle is sufficient to allow an individual to take his own life—alone or in cooperation with others. In this chapter I shall examine the converse challenge to the autonomy principle within a framework of positive rights: may a patient or his family secure public payment for futile treatment?

Helga Wanglie's husband refused to allow physicians to disconnect her life support systems even though at 86 years of age she had been in a permanent vegetative state for over a year, at an estimated cost between $800,000 and $1,000,000, expenses that were covered partly by Medicare and partly by her Medigap insurance.[3] Before lapsing into a coma, she reaffirmed her religious conviction in the absolute value of preserving life regardless of the cost, and she vowed to hang on until the good Lord called her.[4] The hospital board took the extraordinary step of allowing her physicians and nurses to sue to remove Mr. Wanglie as her guardian so that they could terminate care. They lost the suit, and Mrs. Wanglie died three days later.[5]

The justifiable desperation behind the lawsuit led to the wrong approach. The opposition to Mr. Wanglie's decision does not stem from his purported mistreatment of his wife or other neglect of his duties as guardian. If he wanted to spend his own money on futile treatment, his disgruntled physicians could withdraw in protest, and he could pay others to take their place. Mr. Wanglie did right by his wife in pressing his demands for financial support from Medicare and his Medigap insurer. Any grievance with Mr. Wanglie must come from these payers, not his spouse. An irate public could protest the waste of public funds, but it could hardly condemn the Wanglies personally for accepted benefits conferred upon them by law. Their Medigap insurer (and fellow policy holders) could protest, but only if the Wanglies demanded benefits not offered under contract. The Minnesota Court thus rightly refused to remove Mr. Wanglie from his preferred position. The difficulty with demanded care is not excessive familiar loyalty in times of crisis. It stems from the basic network of entitlements used to respond to a perennial social problem.

In the *Wanglie* case, the state seeks to meddle in family affairs to protect its own pocketbook. But the principles of autonomy that should protect individual choice of whether to live or die do not excuse an attack on the autonomy principle from the other end. More concretely, no person has any right to force other persons to contribute to his or her welfare, or even survival, against their own will. Demands of that sort are clearly out of place in a world that has only negative rights. But once positive rights of support are admitted into the legal pantheon, it is no longer possible to reject categorically claims of this sort. After all, some forms of government transfer payments are by definition permissible, and the only question is to identify which. The issue has led to an unending set of tensions because government taxes fund all kinds of subsidies and citizens object to paying for abortions,[6] homoerotic art,[7] or tobacco production. The opponents do not claim that these activities are illegal. They only say that they should not be forced by the political process to pay for the production of goods and services that they regard as too expensive for the price, or more forcefully, as antithetical to their own sense of right and wrong. None of these goods and services, moreover, are public goods that must be provided to all individuals if they are provided to some. Transfer payments to Mrs. Wanglie can be terminated while tax dollars continue to pay for defense and other necessary public services. Within the modern framework, an endless dispute has to take place which balances the perceived desirability of the activity against the costs, financial and moral, that are attached to it. In a society whose values are split as our own, no consensus is possible, either at the level of constitutional doctrine or political will. And the root of the difficulty lies not in the grubby particulars of each individual case, but in the carefree illusion that such questions can ever be resolved by discussion among persons with fundamentally different outlooks and orientation. In the end, therefore, the basic truth is that forced redistribution is a close cousin to forced association. Both confirm the basic point that a regime of positive rights in the name of patient autonomy is antithetical to any universal conception of individual autonomy.

The issue of demanded care, then, is a derivative of the larger dispute over positive right to health care. Once that claim is rejected, the futility debate comes clearly into focus. Anyone can spend his own resources on futile care, or purchase "futility insurance" to cover those expenses. But no one can spend a single dime of anyone else's money for that end any more than he could spend it for beneficial care. Neither useful nor futile care can be demanded as a right. The operative legal principle requires respect for separate persons, not for some sound collective assessment of the wisdom of a proposed course of treatment. Under this strict, and correct, application of the autonomy principle, futility drops out of the picture as a separate legal category. Perceptions of futility remain relevant only insofar as they influence the willingness of others to provide demanded care. Several reports have already announced that intensive care is futile for persons in a permanent vegetative state.[8] The effect of those pronouncements should not be to direct public funds, but to influence the expenditure of private parties, which can adopt exceptions to that rule in either direction as they see fit. Judgments about futility, however, should not become the opening wedge for a regulated, centralized economy.

Unfortunately, respect for *patient* autonomy has been transformed from an attack on paternalism or a requirement of informed consent into a weapon that allows some people to commandeer resources from others. Robert D. Truog, a neonatologist, sets out the basic position (which he then forcefully challenges) as follows: "It is commonly considered ethically unacceptable to remove one patient from life-sustaining therapy to make room for another. Just as respect for a patient's autonomy requires consent before *initiating therapy, so must we obtain consent before* withdrawing it."[9] But the odds of obtaining that consent are remote because the individual doctor assumes a role of patient advocate.

"In caring for an individual patient, the doctor must act solely as that patient's advocate, against the apparent interests of society as a whole, if necessary."[10] The upshot is that large quantities of care are demanded because the price is set below the social cost of its provision. As ever, perverse social incentives do not disappear in life-and-death situations.

The magnitude of these incentive effects, however, is often difficult to measure. The usual way to phrase the question is to ask what percentage of medical expenditures is spent within the last period of life, be it measured in days, weeks, months, or perhaps even a couple of years. The cost estimates usually take the form that "X percent of medical care goes for expenditures in the last Y days (or years) of life." The potential for last-period expenditures is enormous considering that an ICU on full throttle costs several thousand dollars per day per person, before adding in fees for special medical and hospital services. One early study examined the Medicare payments for nearly 20,000,000 individuals over the age of 67 who were enrolled in the program during 1978. Of that group, around 1,100,000 individuals died during the year, and this 5.9 percent of decedents accounted for some 28 percent of the medical expenditures within the system, with the remaining 94.1 percent accounting for 72 percent of the expenditures.[11] The same study reported higher utilization rates for Medicare decedents than for Medicare survivors: 92 percent of the decedents used medical services in the last year of life, and 80 percent had also used them the year before. For the survivors, the utilization rates were 58 percent in the last year and 55 percent in the year before.[12]

The multiple studies of last-period expenditures in the years that follow show, by and large, little deviation from the findings of the original study. On average, the studies continue to show that between 5 and 6 percent of the Medicare beneficiaries die in each year, and that the average expenditure on them is about 7 to 1, relative to persons who survive into the next period.[13] Further refinements show that the level of expenditures climbs sharply just before death so that 40 percent of the expenditures in the last year of life are concentrated in the last month of life. For 1988, the average Medicare expenditure in the year of death was $13,316, but other expenditures, most notably nursing home care, account for about another $16,000, making the total about $29,000 per person in the last year of life.[14] The total bill amounts to around 3 percent of the total health care bill, enough to constitute a difference but not a financial revolution.

Making sense of these numbers is far from easy. Cutting in the one direction is the observation that only after death can it be certain which expenditures were made in the last year of life. The element of uncertainty that pervades medical decisions is therefore bleached out of the findings that purport to demonstrate the excessive level of care. Yet here the counterargument is that, although prediction is never perfect, it is often highly reliable. Certain disease conditions are known to be terminal, especially in individuals of advanced age, so that arguments of uncertainty, although always relevant, are hardly decisive. The operative fact is that much of the uncertainty is not whether a person will die of a terminal condition, but when. Much of the end-of-life expenditure is therefore made on cases that are known, to a reasonable medical certainty, to be terminal, even if some irreducible element of philosophical doubt remains.

Cutting in the opposite direction is the likelihood that these figures understate the level of care that is lavished on some small portion of the population at the end of life. It is most unlikely that all decedents received equal amounts of care in the year of their death. Many people do not die in a hospital, so the end-of-life medical care is concentrated on a small fraction of those decedents: the reported bills for patients whose final illness is treated in a hospital average around $60,000 per person.[15] In addition, many people who die in one year had received extensive medical care in the previous year for a long-term chronic illness, so that looking only at the year of death understates social expenditures on terminal or otherwise futile cases. Some portion of the 72 percent of Medicare expenditures on survivors should be allocated to futile cases, and relatively little of the care administered in the year of death should be reclassified as being spent on routine care. The upshot is that these studies tend to underestimate the skew from heroic in-hospital measures. The only cautionary note is that people who die at home or in hospices still require some care; the health care bills at the end of life will not vanish even if all futile treatment could be eliminated.

The futility question also arises at the onset of life. The demand for neonatal intensive care units continues to rise, once again because the treatment for small infants with major disabilities is paid for by others. Robert Truog notes that oxygenation for newborn infants with respiratory failure succeeds within two weeks for 99 percent of the infant population if it will succeed at all. Yet desperate parents demand that treatment continue even when the odds of success drop quite literally to one in a million. Even then, the outcome may bring survival with serious brain damage. Yet, all the while, other newborns with far better prognoses may be denied access to the facilities that could save them.[16] No person behind a veil of ignorance, that is, without knowledge of whether he fills the first or second slot, would choose to protect the entitlement of the prior user. Yet, at the same time, no institutional rules provide, publicly and in advance, for the orderly transfer of ICU facilities from near-hopeless long shots to infants who stand to gain the most from them.

LONGEVITY AND QUALITY OF LIFE: GETTING THE BEST OF BOTH WORLDS

The problem of demanded care, for both old and young, is not a creature of poverty. Indeed, it may be the special preserve of the upper middle class, which possesses the access, talent, and determination to extract every possible benefit from a beleaguered medical bureaucracy. It is also an area with the potential for some major cost savings with, it is hoped, little diminution in the overall quality of life. How? The best approach backs away from the current system to see how voluntary and competitive insurance markets would handle the problem, putting to one side the question of solvency. In this setting, purchasers must make their judgments about needed care from the ex ante perspective, without knowing whether they face good fortune or ill. Putting the inquiry in this fashion exposes the weakness of the so-called ethical position that treats patient autonomy as decisive in the withdrawal of treatment just as it is in its initiation.[17] Under a contract model, however, initial consent remains indispensable to shield medical treatment from the charge of assault and battery.[18] The autonomy rules function best in setting boundaries between strangers. But once the treatment commences, strangers become trading partners who can set by contract the terms and conditions under which treatment will be continued or withdrawn, without the need for a second, fresh round of consent.

The implications of this model for life-sustaining treatment are hardly novel. Many standard long-term business arrangements contain clauses allowing one or the other side to withdraw on 30 days' *notice*, where notice, most emphatically, is not the same as consent. Consent gives the affected party a blockade position against any change in the status quo ante: it explains why Helga Wanglie remained on the ICU until she died. Notice gives no such power; instead, it recognizes and respects the unilateral power to withdraw and provides time for the other side to mitigate its losses by seeking alternative measures. The ex ante perspective thus forces the demands of the future into the present. Its power, moreover, is not limited to agreements made when a patient is admitted into an ICU. Generally speaking, the contracting mechanism works better the longer the gap between the time of contract and the occurrence of the events that trigger its obligations. The stronger our predictive knowledge of behavior, the longer a gap the parties can tolerate. The choice of optimal contracting time thus becomes a contest between knowledge and bias. Go back too far in time and the parties lack information for sensible decisions even if free from self-interest. But come too far forward in time and private knowledge (for example, whether we are well or ill) allows individuals to achieve results that are biased to their own interests, which can then be identified with particularity. The ideal time to contract is far enough forward to provide knowledge of the general behavioral patterns, but not so far forward to introduce bias. The more we know about these behavioral patterns, the further back in time we can move without losing the ability to analyze the basic challenges presented by certain repetitive situations.

In dealing with setting a constitution, it is often critical to think back to how matters should be organized in a state of nature; otherwise, one interest group or the other will be able to skew the political process in its own direction. Hence broad propositions about the level of individual self-interest and the uses and limitation of private property are required for the occasion. But for the more limited purpose of futile treatment, we need not peer back to the origin of all social institutions. It is sufficient to focus on the decisions that healthy people make in the prime of life. People know about the risk of fatal disease, but work behind the veil of ignorance on the question of whether and when the risk will materialize for them. That time therefore offers a sound benchmark for making decisions about individual utilization of heath care facilities. Intensive care for the last stages of life can be kept in perspective. The buyer no longer wants to figure out how to maximize the duration of life—or even some mix of the duration and quality of life—*after* a serious illness strikes. Instead the task is to maximize the present value of a person's future satisfaction in all states of the world, when sometimes death comes with a speed and certainty that precludes any medical intervention, and for which health insurance is, to pick a term, futile.

Given these constraints, how does any individual spend his limited wealth to maximize utility? Wealth committed in advance for care for use when sick or disabled is wealth no longer available for use when healthy. It cannot be used either for present consumption or for investment in human or physical capital. Wealth used to alleviate pain or cure disease *after* it strikes cannot be used to prevent their occurrence. Nor is it clear that wealth will buy similar increments in utility when a person is disabled as when he is well, when the class of useful expenditures shrinks: travel, athletics, and sociability may all be compromised by the physical and mental limitations imposed by disease or disability.[19] Spending enormous sums in caring for persons in a disabled state could produce relatively little personal advantage. Indeed, the damage rule in tort cases recognizes the diminishing marginal utility of wealth in cases of serious bodily impairment. Its general pronouncements assert that damages should put the injured party back in the position he enjoyed before the accident took place.[20] But sober minds quickly beat a hasty retreat from so grandiose a standard. "No rational being would change places with the injured man for an amount of gold that would fill the room of this court, yet no lawyer would contend that such is the legal measure of damages."[21] It is not surprising, therefore, that tort law uses another approach entirely to set damages. It identifies specific categories of damages—chiefly pain and suffering, lost income, and medical expenses—and seeks to quantify each one separately. Substantial sums can be awarded under these three categories, even though it is certain that they will fail to make anyone indifferent between their current injury (or death) and the received compensation.

The occasional disputes over demanded care in tort contexts force to the fore the basic conceptual question: how much money should any individual spend on his own care and well-being when it is certain in advance that no sum of money will bring him back to the pre-injury or pre-disease state of the world? Some strong evidence suggests that most people do not want to place all their eggs in one basket because first-party insurance typically pays far smaller sums than the tort law rewards. First-party insurance rarely compensates for pain and suffering and usually does not cover all lost wages. Nor need it cover all medical expenses, whether heroic or ineffective.[22] Armed with this general information, we can be confident that no person would ever spend all his own wealth on future health services. His insurance policy would not say "spare no efforts in my greatest hour of need." That policy would not follow the "rescue principle," that is, the strict injunction to prevent death and prolong life at any cost. Rather it is quite likely that the policy would focus first on the payment of medical bills, then on the recovery of some lost income, and only last on the pain and suffering that plays so large a role in tort cases. The price demanded from the insured for extensive coverage would require the excessive sacrifice of other things of value. Most people would not pay the price.

Should this approach be dismissed for assuming a level rational behavior unattainable on matters of health? No, and for several reasons. First, demands for end-of-life care constitute the quintessential rational response. When social costs fund individual benefits, why not make other people pay to vindicate your religious commitments or moral beliefs? The behavior is rational, given the opportunities and constraints.

Second, too often the question is posed as one that asks people to trade off length of life against the quality of life. But that tradeoff is less critical from the ex ante perspective. Most people would like to have both long life and good quality. Both are obtainable if they can make *binding* commitments when they purchase their health insurance. Most people want to maximize the length of days and defer the time when the quality of life declines. Investing heavily in heroic measures after the onset of serious illness reduces the resources available for nutrition, exercise, and safety—activities that could increase health and thus forestall the ultimate day of reckoning. The reduced funds available when contingencies occur need not come at the expense of comfort; forswearing heroics and lengthy stays in the ICU should suffice.

So understood, the basic form of the choice is: (A) have an expected life of 80 years, or perhaps longer, with the last week in extreme conditions, but without the ICU treatment routinely available today, or (B) have an expected life of 78 years, with the last six months of heroics in an ICU. Faced with these constraints, who would pursue (even on religious grounds) a strategy that promises shorter life and longer period of pain? Collectively, however, we opt for choice B by providing end-of-life care without cost and by making it impossible (in the name of autonomy) for individuals to bind themselves by contracts from going back on their word when illness strikes. Some institutional firmness is desperately needed to resist the demands for care by persons who no longer reside behind the veil of ignorance.

This approach is not limited to situations in which all persons have sufficient resources to compete for health care on even terms. Why give the egalitarian vision so much weight for health care when it receives far less weight in other contexts? People buy vacation packages, homes, and food keyed to their level of wealth. These different purchases lead to differences both in longevity and quality of life. Such differences must be accepted in order to avoid the underproduction of goods and services that arise when people do not get paid for what they produce or do not pay for what they consume. We do not need to redress the inequalities of wealth to encourage people to make early decisions of the level of health care they want to buy. Even if we did, a system of cash transfer payments or progressive taxation addresses the wealth problem directly without upsetting long-term insurance decision. But with or without transfer payments, instilling prudence cannot be done so long as social resources are used to purchase time in an ICU but not the more mundane goods and services that reduce or postpone the need for their use. We get what we pay for: less health and more crisis intervention.

SOCIAL RESPONSES TO FUTILITY

DEFINING FUTILITY

The basic problem lies in identifying those cases where excessive treatment should be halted by voluntary or, if necessary, coercive means. The futility principle is pressed into service to isolate the easy cases for discontinuing treatment without making any delicate cost/benefit judgment. A case with *no* hope for improvement produces zero net benefits at some positive cost.[23] Why operate if the consequence is certain death on the operating table? Anyone can do a cost/benefit analysis when there are no benefits.

But search as we may, there are few easy cases. The treatment/no treatment choice raises an all-or-nothing issue, which people are reluctant to reject simply by discounting the "benefits" of expensive therapies in light of the slender probabilities of their success. Instead of cutting off treatment exactly at the margin, they instinctively want to err on the side of continuing treatment in cases of genuine doubt. The desire to find some safe harbor translates into focusing on the likelihood of some improvement rather than on estimating its anticipated magnitude. The endless uncertainties in interesting cases always hold out some small hope, if not of cure, then of hanging on. Fact skepticism then quickly swells into a philosophical despair about making the concept of "futility" operational at all. "In short, the problem with futility is that its promise of objectivity can rarely be fulfilled. The rapid advance of the language of futility into the jargon of bioethics should be followed by an equally rapid retreat."[24] This counsel of despair shapes serious discussion even as serious stabs are made to isolate those easy cases where publicly funded treatment can be terminated without patient consent, be it with neonatal care, terminal cancer, or AIDS cases.

We can identify four distinct approaches to the question of demanded care. The first approach stresses voluntaristic solutions that induce patients to request a cessation of treatment by living wills or durable powers of attorney. The second approach also relies on individual evaluations, by seeking to precommit individuals by contract to limit their amount of care in end-of-life situations. The third proposal makes institutional judgments about futility based on the anticipated success of certain classes of treatment. The final approach goes to the opposite extreme and seeks to prevent futile care provided by using global budgets to reduce the flow of resources into ICU or similar types of care.

No one can oppose, in principle, the initial emphasis on living wills and durable powers of attorney, but we can suspect that they will not prove to help much. My own preference is to adopt some mix of the second and the fourth practices. If technically sound, the second could provide a viable contract solution to today's insoluble political dilemma. But, to the extent that contract solutions become riddled with holes, a system of global ICU budgets might provide some modest help. But even here the journey is all uphill, given our long tradition of first defining entitlements and then searching for budgetary support. Suitably sobered, it is time to look at these four approaches in some greater detail.

ADVANCE DIRECTIVES, LIVING WILLS, AND DURABLE POWERS OF ATTORNEY

One way to minimize the risks of futile care is to confer on someone else the power to stop treatment after the patient has lapsed into a coma or has otherwise become incompetent to manage his own affairs. In principle, advance directives allow a patient to direct his final care much as a will directs the devolution of his property after death. But these are couched as conditional commands made by individuals who have little knowledge of how they will respond in a set of extreme circumstances that they may have observed, but in all likelihood have not experienced. The risk of the approach is that sentiments will change and no one will be confident that the old directive fits the new circumstances when the individual is no longer available to state his wishes. It is often too hard to use a rigid plan to control a dynamic future. Living wills and durable powers of attorney abandon the effort to make decisions in advance of circumstances. They seek to fill the void in authority by creating an orderly succession of decision power during life by selecting the right people in whom to vest the power of attorney.

In practice, both of these devices are often disregarded by physicians who think that the imperative to preserve life (and fill ICU beds?) takes precedence over a patient's right to refuse treatment, however expressed.[25] Perhaps for that reason, we can find little evidence to show that these procedures reduce the level of expenditures on final illness, and some figures suggest higher expenditure levels for persons who have issued advanced directives (for example, DNR orders) than for those who did not.[26] Perhaps physicians take additional care to keep these patients from the brink before the DNR order would have to be obeyed. The expenditures after cardiac arrest may be lower, but the expenditures to avoid that arrest could well be larger, producing an overall wash. Alternatively individuals charged to use their own best judgment to represent an unconscious could believe their duty requires them to err on the side of continued treatment, especially when someone else foots the bill. Improved facilitation of advance directives and durable powers of attorneys are not likely to alter the demanded care equation by very much.[27]

CONTRACTUAL PRECOMMITMENT

A second attack on end-of-life expenditures seeks to force individuals to precommit themselves to the termination of medical care. In this system, no one makes decisions about treatment by looking at the progression of a particular disease. From pneumonia to diabetes, diseases come in all sizes, shapes, and combinations, breaking any apparent linkage between the type of disease and the futility of treatment. What is needed is some common measure that cuts across diverse, separate conditions. The best candidate for that task seems to be the APACHE III test.[28] APACHE stands for Acute Physiology, Age, Chronic Health Evaluation.[29]

Three types of variables influence the success of last-ditch emergency procedures. One is the short-term stress: the acute phase of the case. A second is age: the older the patient, the more difficult it is to bounce back. The third is basic health, captured by a "chronic health evaluations." The variables in APACHE III, the third iteration of the basic tests, selects from quantitative measures of standard physiological dimensions: pulse, blood pressure, temperature, respiratory rates, hematocrit (percentage of red blood cells in blood), white blood count, urine output, creatinine, sodium, glucose, albumin, billirubin, and BUN (bound urea nitrogen). The power of the index depends on the choice of variables and the assignments of their relative weights good for normal and most critically, extreme cases. The output is an index number that, when used in conjunction with the basic disease condition, is translatable into a prediction of survival.

The present APACHE scale runs from 0 to 160+. The probability of death is close to zero when the index is 0; it increases first gradually, then more rapidly, and then slows down again in the upper ranges where death in hospital becomes highly likely. On average, the death rates in hospital for APACHE 120 equal 90 percent; by APACHE 140, they are over 95 percent, and by APACHE 160, death verges on moral certainty. Yet even these estimates may underestimate the futility of given treatment because the index does not capture the length or quality of life after release from the hospital. With these pronounced disabilities the prospect of readmission or death within a short time seems highly likely, especially for older patients.

The physicians who developed the APACHE test have shown commendable caution about its use. The test is defended as a tool of global policy to aid in the classification and treatment of disease. It is not recommended for its making decisions in particular cases. As is so common in medical circles, information is a good, but coercion, even with prior consent, is a bad. Its designers have no intention to change the current division of power between patients and physicians, but they hope that additional information will lead patients and their families to discontinue treatment when the odds of recovery become small. Only in rare settings requiring triage might APACHE III function as a neutral decider of who gets treatment when no person has pride of place. At most, there is only a hint that the test could override patient's wish to stop treatment as futile.[30]

It is in principle an open question of whether to use the APACHE III test more aggressively in rationing care than its inventors advocate. Why not? Surely, we can dismiss the global objection that it is immoral to use imperfect data to make social decisions about the deployment of public or private resources. Imperfect information rightly poses difficulties for any intelligent decision making, but to insist on perfect information is to demand institutional paralysis. It is dangerous to despise or dismiss reliable information that combats wasteful and counterproductive social practices simply because it is not perfect. We should resist any tendency to duck hard questions of principle by pretending that the data is never adequate to assist in making hard choices. APACHE III should be welcomed if it helps rationalize the system. The mistakes that it introduces should not be treated as a veto against its use. They should be compared in frequency and severity with the mistakes that are avoided.

Although this global objection against APACHE III fails, other less dramatic problems remain. What level of dollar savings can be obtained from aggressively using the test? If the only reliable cutoff point for terminating treatment were APACHE 160, when hospital death rates are over 95 percent, why bother to test if the target population will die within 24 hours? Yet if the test cuts end-of-life costs only at APACHE 120, when the probability of death in hospital hovers around 90 percent, who decides whether the sacrifice of 10 percent chance of survival is worthwhile when that judgment depends in part of prognosis for future well-being—is there brain damage, loss of sensation, and so on? It is not within the province of any lawyer to give definitive answers to these social questions, but perhaps it is worth sketching a way to think about them.

The first step in this process is to establish by agreement a set of guidelines that indicate when treatment ceases. Here the relevant information could be presented to an individual or plan in tabular form. Column A contains the APACHE III ratings, corrected for various types of disorder, and the probability of death in hospital. Column B contains a schedule of additional premiums for increasing APACHE III insurance by fixed-point intervals from APACHE 0 to APACHE 10, and so on down the line to APACHE 120, 125, 130, . . . , 160. These explicit tables are meant to force honest ex ante revelations on consumers as to their willingness to purchase health insurance increments, judged by its impact on their survivability.

This dramatic information could be supplemented by a further breakdown that reveals the source of the increment. One column could indicate the number of days spent in hospitals or the number of days in ICU before death at each APACHE III level. Special information could be provided about the cost of care for persons in a coma or a permanent vegetative state. Still additional figures could indicate the expected length of survival and quality of life for the fraction of the population that leaves hospital. This information could be updated regularly, and individuals could then shift the levels of health care purchased based on the revised information. The reliability of the test could be disclosed, which becomes fairly high, especially as we move to serious cases. Thus, in speaking about APACHE III, its creators write (without any intention to endorse this program) as follows: "The overall predictive accuracy of the first-day APACHE III equation was such that, within 24 hours of ICU admission, 95 percent of ICU admissions could be given a risk estimation for hospital death that was within three percent of that actually observed."[31] Needless to say, any insurance contract need not specify a termination of coverage on the strength of a single test. It could easily require that the number be exceeded on two or more successive days; that independent third parties inspect the result, or whatever other device seems appropriate.

The attractiveness of this system lies in its ability to force everyone to run comparisons at the time of their initial purchase. Its success depends on the ability to hold customers to their promises thereafter when they may have strong religious and personal reasons for regret. But these are not cases where they have made a pact with the devil or a potential murderer. These are cases where the question is how much additional care does the individual want to purchase, in light of his knowledge about the future. The case for holding individuals to their bargains is that they passed by the option to buy the most expansive coverage in the world. Their decision to forgo thus becomes conclusive evidence that they valued the additional cash in hand more than they valued the protection it could have afforded, assuming it was needed at all, sometime later. Once these purchase decisions have been made, hospitals and other health care providers could project their anticipated demand for ICUs and scale back their operations accordingly if the demand to treat the chronic conditions of old age turns out to be weak. Updating the information avoids any centralized determination of some idealized measure of proper ICU. The APACHE avoids the objection that can be rightly lodged against the British system, namely, that its state-run determinations are too stingy, because capitation fees induce physicians and hospitals to skimp on care. So why not give it a chance, at least on an experimental basis, no matter what the reluctance of its creators?

Simply showing that the test generates sound incentives hardly suffices to secure its adoption in a voluntary market. It is one thing to promote a test in learned articles, and quite another to make it the focal point of who lives and who dies. At the very least, therefore, using the test contractually depends critically on the reproducibility of the APACHE III data, for matters will be complicated mightily if test scores could vary with the time of day or with food and medicines administered before the test is run. Stable test results in noncontractual settings advance the case but hardly settle the matter because it is an open question of whether test outcomes remain stable when so much turns on them. But it seems likely that the APACHE 130 insurance becomes unglued if the test yields 140 in the morning and 120 in the afternoon. When should the test be administered? Who should administer it? How many times should it be run? Do insurance companies get to redo the tests? Perhaps the soft underbelly of enforcement will wholly negate any beneficial effect that an honest calibration of preferences could provide. Revelations of test irregularities in just one case could discredit the test politically no matter how successful its overall performance is.

The present commitment to patient autonomy may condemn any rationing effort, be it through APACHE III or any other scheme. Thus, it is therefore odd to consider how this test could be extended from private contract to the public provision of health once we think about health care in a world of positive rights. But, on the off chance that APACHE III gains a foothold, it is useful to sketch out a plausible path of extension. The first point is that every patient must be forced to choose between some other good they care for and critical care at the end of life, even if they have no resources of their own to place on the table. That result could be accomplished by granting them a health care budget for some definite period of time for various types of medical services, supplemented perhaps by their own private payments. The information on APACHE III tests could then be supplied to allow individuals to choose the mix of medical services within the budget constraint. Extensive treatment for ongoing diseases leads to a reduced commitment for end-of-life care. As with contracts in the voluntary market, the coverage limitations must be *strictly* enforced after the fact, making overall public confidence in the system critical to its success. But if the choices are allowed to bind, the law could blend individual choice with public funding, much as a voucher system allows parents to use state funds to pay for private education. To be sure, this system is heir to all the ills implicit in any affirmative right to health care, but it might allow explicit decentralized choices to rationalize the overall structure in a way that Medicare, for example, cannot.

I suspect that the resistance to APACHE III will be great on a combination of technical, administrative, and moral grounds. But even if it cannot be deployed to deal with futile care in demanded care situations, perhaps cruder, but simpler, tests could take its place. Thus one rule might limit ICU stays to two weeks after entering into a permanent vegetative state for people not prepared to pay for the privilege. Other rules might ration ICU time by age. Similar rules might prevent expensive neonatal heroics for newborns by denying treatment at public expense to babies weighing under, say, 750 grams. These proposals are easier to state and apply than APACHE III, but they lack its range and scope. It should be a sign of despair that the overuse of patient autonomy has rendered these tests stillborn. The willingness to commit to any form of contractual solutions exacts its toll here as it does in other areas.

TREATMENT SUCCESS

The medical profession today seems to have little interest in the precommitment strategies just discussed. Instead of relying on private preferences to determine when treatment ceases, some effort is made to set the "objective" conditions that allow physicians to conclude that treatment is futile. Schneiderman, Jecker, and Jonson, for example, begin their analysis by denying that patient autonomy should block a public review of patient care expenditures. Thereafter they search for some "objective" measure of the true state of affairs, relative to the "subjective" hopes of physician and patients. Recognizing the dangers of making systematic judgments about individual cases, their program consolidates findings across cases to fashion quantitative standards: "when physicians conclude (either through personal experience, experiences shared with colleagues, or consideration of reported empirical data) that in the last 100 cases, a medical treatment has been useless, they should regard that treatment as futile."[32]

A clean slate of no positive responses does not guarantee that the next case will not prove the exception to the rule. But at least physicians can be confident, with a confidence of 95 percent, that the treatment has at most a 3 percent likelihood of success, and perhaps less. But can this test be made operative? How do physicians decide which cases should be grouped in the same class, so as to count against the target? Is it enough for all cases to have the same disease, or must they also have the same causal agent, the same prior course of treatment?[33] Slice the salami thin enough, and it becomes well-nigh impossible to accumulate 100 consecutive similar cases. Each case becomes an adventure in a world in which futility is banished. And if, by some miracle, physicians report improvement in only one or two of these cases, the scheme may be scuttled even if the case itself was misdiagnosed. Similarly this standard does not set out an appropriate response if treatment helped prior to the last run of 100 cases. Why ignore early successes and look only to part of the whole data set? Their test does not resolve the philosophical doubt about the next case, any more than does an APACHE III score of 160. Once again, unless we are prepared to tolerate some errors of premature cessation of treatment, the unhappy conclusion is that treatment is never (really) futile. Once again we are back at square one.

GLOBAL BUDGETS

An alternative approach to futility abandons individual choice in favor of systematic coercion. Global budgets set at the center certain expenditure limits for ICU and similar care and then allow the physicians and hospitals to allocate those funds as they see fit. The pressures on resources should induce some form of sensible institutional triage, leading physicians and hospitals to deny care in hopeless cases and to allow trivial injuries to cure themselves. Constrained by budgets, physicians will avoid the familiar heroics for which they can no longer receive dollar-for-dollar compensation. De facto, they may decide to use APACHE tests to curtail the levels of intensive care in order to meet their budget targets. Utilization levels will shrink without anyone quite knowing how it all happened. The budget constraints force internal allocations to bleed out less meritorious cases.

Some evidence suggests that this method can work. In ordinary times, the ICUs constitute perhaps 15 percent of American hospital beds, which differs markedly from the British practice that devotes only 1 percent of its beds to ICU care.[34] The British solution sidesteps the question of who gets the ICU beds, reducing supply to levels that require hard physician choices, which tend over time to direct resources to the patients who need them most.[35] One study of intensive care at the Massachusetts General Hospital reported that physicians faced with an unanticipated shortage of ICU nurses adopted an informal rationing system to weed out cardiac cases admitted primarily for observation and monitoring. Instead they reserved ICU facilities mainly for current or anticipated acute episodes.[36] The global restraints reduced ICU admissions by 22 percent and led to shorter stays. The percentage of admitted cases with heart attacks rose from 31 to 45 percent, with no increase in overall mortality. These results could not have been obtained with a first-come, first-served allocation system, for then the percentage of cardiac cases would not have increased. Rather the global constraints created local incentives—hard to articulate, but easy to observe—that altered admission and treatment patterns to save costs without impairing overall effectiveness. What is needed is evidence that a return to full ICU staffing led to a restoration of the prior profligate practices. For why should hospitals keep expensive beds idle when paid by piecework?

The experience in the Massachusetts General ER shows both the strength and weaknesses of global budgets. These work by inducing the decentralized decision making at the local level, much like competitive markets. But competitive markets do not operate off central budgets set by political institutions. The critical difficulty with global budgets comes from the opposite direction, for without the interposition of market prices, who sets the budget limits? The difference between British and American ICU utilization rates may be stark. But which system picked the right numbers, or indeed, how can two systems pick such divergent numbers? Both the British and American approaches could be wrong, but they cannot both be correct. We could have too many ICU beds and the British too few. Our system could well allocate too much money to patient care, and their capitation system too little.

Unfortunately nothing in the physician and patient responses at the hospital level will indicate which global budgets are correctly set. Instead both systems must rely on a political process that is prey to many of the biases evident in the present system. Physicians may exaggerate the indispensability of their services in pleading for extensive investments in end-of-life care. Other groups will push programs for education or welfare, and no one can know who is right or wrong, or why. The global administrative cap does not generate any useful evidence about aggregate demand for medical types of services. In the United States at least, there may be insufficient resolve to keep to budgets that impose restrictions on ICU utilization. In a world of imperfect choices, this might be the best that can be done. In the end, however, global budgets work only as well as the political consensus that lies behind them. The tide of patient autonomy may be strong enough to sweep all else aside. We pay collective lip service to the ideal of cost containment in cases of medical futility. In so many other contexts, we allow insurance polices to be written that exclude certain events from coverage and allow individuals in need to go without compensation. But in this context, our collective actions speak louder than our collective words: by refusing to allow failure in individual cases, we do our best to bring about failure on a grand scale.

CHAPTER 4

Necessity and Indigent Care:
The Right to Say No

My initial attack on the positive rights to health care was undertaken abstractly, without any attention to the particulars of present policy. Chapter 3's analysis of the futility question marked the transition from theory to practice by showing in one context how the theory of positive rights runs awry in a particular setting. Those mishaps were not, however, isolated events. This chapter deals with the state's use of its licensing and contracting powers to secure services for some segment of the public, most notably indigent persons and Medicare recipients and often for emergency care, for which they lack the ability to pay.

These developments are at odds with the basic autonomy model. That model allows all individuals and all voluntary associations to choose their trading partners and to refuse to deal with others for good reason, bad reason, or no reason at all. The controversial status of "the right to refuse" is also important because it supplies the link between health and civil rights. In the area of civil rights, the paradigmatic wrong is that of the white person who refuses to hire a black person solely out of invidious prejudice. In the health case, the paradigm case is the refusal to treat a poor person who would otherwise die. In both settings, informal sanctions are always thought unequal to deal with even the most egregious cases. And in both settings, this new conception of wrong quickly extends beyond the core cases that fueled the new legal initiatives. The antidiscrimination laws can be used to cover sex, age, disability, sexual orientation, and political persuasion. Yet these same fluid conceptions of wrong easily tolerate both public and private discrimination against whites, against men, against young people under special justifications—diversity, affirmative action—that coexist uneasily with the general antidiscrimination norm. Next discrimination is measured by consequences and not by intention, and the consequences never show the perfect levels of proportionality that are posited in theory. To bring about those results, the antidiscrimination principle by degrees becomes so transformed that it often works to sponsor the very forms of discrimination that it is supposed to curtail. The original wrongs are the ones most reviled, but least encountered.

The same expansion of government power is evident in the area of health care. Because individuals and institutions are denied the categorical right to refuse to provide treatment in any particular case, that refusal must meet some independent standard of public justification. The center of gravity thus shifts by degrees from suppliers of health care to regulators of health care. This chapter traces that evolution in three stages. The first part examines the basic common law norm. The second part asks whether that right to refuse must yield to the state power to license physicians and hospitals. The third part examines the use of federal power to limit physician and hospital power to choose patients and to set fees.

THE COMMON LAW EVOLUTION

The common law guaranteed all ordinary individuals the right to choose their trading partners. From that general proposition it was an easy inference that an ordinary supplier of goods or services could refuse to deal with any individuals who were unable to pay the stipulated fee. Yet the rule goes still further and allows all individuals, including physicians and hospitals, to refuse to provide medical services even to individuals ready, able, and willing to pay their standard medical fees. In *Hurley v. Eddingfield*, the defendant, a licensed physician, refused to treat a long-time patient who had sent a messenger with payment urgently requesting his services.[1] The patient was violently ill, and his messenger stated that the patient could not procure any other medical services was turning to the defendant for assistance. The defendant refused to come, and the court held that he was within his rights. Nor—a point to which I shall return—did the requirement of a state license to practice medicine change the outcome. "The [licensing] act is a preventive, not a compulsive, measure. In obtaining the state's license (permission) to practice medicine, the state does not require, and the licensee does not engage, that he will practice at all or on other terms than he may choose to accept."[2]

Hurley addressed the obligations of an individual physician, not those of a hospital or other charitable institution. And it noted that cases involving common carriers were off the mark. Indeed that difference did matter. With common carriers, the Indiana court, in a case decided the same year as *Hurley*, vigorously stressed the exacting public nature of the service obligation.[3] But for institutions not endowed with state monopoly power or the state power of eminent domain, the rule of choice remained unchanged, given the scarcity of available resources and the dominance of individual autonomy. The two Massachusetts cases quoted in the Introduction bear repetition on the central point. "A party has a right to select and determine with whom he will contract, and cannot have another person thrust upon him without his consent"[4] was how the proposition was put in a commercial case. Charitable institutions played by the same rules. *McDonald v. Massachusetts General Hospital* did not waver in stating the general proposition: "Nor does the fact that the trustees, through their agents, are themselves to determine who are to be the immediate objects of the charity, and that no person has individually a right to demand admission to its benefits, alter its character [as a public charity]. All cannot participate in its benefits; the trustees are those to whom is confided the duty of selecting those who shall enjoy them, and prescribing the terms upon which they shall do so."[5] The remedy for any breach of trust lay "in the superintending power" of the court to act, on petition of the attorney general, to ensure that the resources are devoted to charitable purposes for which the organization was formed. The decision thus treated charitable obligations as imperfect: no individual could force a charitable institution to provide him with care.[6]

Over time, this right to exclude has been subject to systematic attack, both through the evolution of private law and the state's assertion of its licensing power. One line of criticism invokes revisionist contract principles to give individual patients a right of action. In *Wilmington General Hospital v. Manlove*[7] the court held liable a private hospital that had undertaken to render emergency care to the general public.[8] "[L]iability on the part of a hospital may be predicated on the refusal of service to a patient in case of an unmistakable emergency, if the patient has relied on a well-established custom of the hospital to render aid in such a case."[9] The patient who had come to one hospital was not required to conduct a long and possibly futile search for other care.

This contractual approach suffers the same weakness of all efforts to forge a future obligation from a past practice. The reliance argument was a strained effort to overcome the evident intention of the hospital *not* to create legal relations to bind itself to charitable care. Its past practice may help people to make intelligent estimates of the probability that their needs will be tended to, but it hardly *binds* the hospital to supply its services free of charge. Why infer this one-sided obligation in an autonomy-based world? Contracts typically create benefits to both sides, and the hospital does not gain when its past acts of generosity are converted into future sources of legal liability. There are enormous practical benefits to being able to announce standing policies without being legally forced to adhere to them. If *Manlove* was correct, all charitable hospitals had long been subject to extensive legal obligations of which they were ignorant.

The contrived creation of a binding obligation to provide care is not only wrong in principle, it is also ineffective in practice, in light of the anticipated response. *Manlove* does not claim that the right to refuse service is void against public policy. Rather it accepts the legitimacy of the contract form and then burrows away at it from within by implying obligations that go against the manifest intention of the party it seeks to bind. The institutional counterattack is to shatter any ostensible expectation created by past practice and silence—thereby making a clear statement of policy that preserves the hospital's right to turn away any given patient at the door. To be sure, some ambiguity remains if that policy is first articulated when a patient arrives at the hospital doorstep, but a hospital under *Manlove* can take systematic public steps to preserve the right to reject patients at will. It can add statements at the bottom of its advertisements and post them on its doors. It can instruct physicians and ambulances of its practices. At the end of the day, no diffuse claim of customary reliance can trump an explicit contractual term that provides to the contrary. The hospital that publicly reserves its right to refuse service has not waived that right by conduct or past practice. The odd question is why any court would want to put an institution to the burden of making clear what the public at large already knew. It is not surprising that

Manlove's contractual strategy remained a minority position in the battle over required service—one quickly overtaken by events and far more aggressive legal strategies.

THE STATE LICENSING POWER

The next push to create a right to emergency room care relied on an amalgam of legislative and judicial action. In *Guerrero v. Copper Queen Hospital,*[10] the court inferred the duty to provide emergency care to indigent patients from the state's general legislative policy that "a General Hospital must maintain facilities to provide emergency care."[11] It then took this general command one step further and held that the duty to provide care was owed not only to state or county residents, but also to illegal aliens from Mexico. In one decision, the court took two leaps with a single bound. Having first inferred a statutory duty to provide care without compensation, it then refused to carve out an exception for illegal aliens because "this condition was equally obvious to the legislators, and they chose not to make an exception in the law."[12]

Guerrero may well rest on an incorrect reading of the statute, but the point is of little consequence here. The larger issue of principle it raises cannot be easily evaded. For purposes of analysis, therefore, let us assume that explicit statutory language conditioned the issuance of a license on the willingness of the hospital to provide indigent care. At the heart of the dispute is the scope of the state's licensing power, which had received so narrow an interpretation in *Hurley.* May the state use its power to license hospitals not just to prevent fraud and insure competence but to identify a class of individuals entitled to receive uncompensated care? As a first approximation, it is easier to impose these obligations on hospitals than on individual physicians, who receive some sympathy for being impressed haphazardly into service against their will. Hospitals operate through organized programs, which can be structured to minimize the exposure of any individual physician to sudden swings in their legal fortunes. The duty to provide ER or uncompensated care can be factored into the underlying contract of service, introducing some measure of individual stability for institutional obligations.

Even after these allowances are made, *Guerrero* is, in the end, still misguided. The earlier, more limited conception of licensing found in *Hurley* remains the preferred point of view for individuals and institutions alike. The power to require the provision of indigent care is said to rest on the power of the state to license hospitals, or physicians, in the first place. But from where does that power come?[13] To answer that question, we must first demystify state power. The state is not an entity endowed with special powers; it is entitled simply to work its will by fiat on the individuals subject to its power. The state should not be thought of as a person with independent rights and duties. Rather, the state, like a corporation, should be regarded as a complex nexus of relations governing the affairs of citizens. Both state and corporation act through agents and for the benefit of the individuals, be they the citizens or the shareholders whom they represent. In day-to-day matters, the state responds to the demands of its various constituents, and its rights do not rise in any obvious way above those of the individuals whom it represents in any given transaction.

In a world of limited government, the state's power to license cannot be simply exercised at will. People have a strong right to enter into whatever calling or occupation they choose as part and parcel of their ordinary rights of self-determination, a point that itself has received some strong constitutional affirmation.[14] If so, the state cannot burden with taxes and conditions an occupational choice that it could not subject to an outright ban. To allow that tactic to succeed is to permit government to act by indirection when the direct route has been blocked. It is for just that reason that the protection of freedom of speech is not limited to direct actions of state censorship. All efforts to attack speech by taxation, regulation, or the creation of new forms of liability rule are subject to parallel scrutiny. In particular, the power to issue licenses has always been subject to close constitutional review, lest censorship of speech be introduced through the back door.[15]

State licenses work similar limitations on occupational freedom and should be subjected to a similar skeptical eye. To make sure that these licenses do not run roughshod over individual choice, the state's power to deny a license must be justified solely by reference to the same ends that allow the state to sanction discrete acts by some (potentially licensed) party. The state may prohibit, before the fact, only that conduct whose outcome it can punish after the fact. The license power must be directed to the same ends as criminal prosecutions and private damage actions. It exercises a collective power in advance because no individual has the incentive to enjoin future conduct that is more likely to harm someone else. Who would seek to enjoin another driver from using the freeway because of the remote possibility that he might be hurt? Licensing pools this injunctive function into the hands of the state and, by overcoming the free-rider and coordination problem, exercises some modest ability to stop some wrongful conduct before it occurs. Yet by acting in advance, the licensing power also creates the risk of over-breadth: the absence of a license can block lawful as well as unlawful actions, which is why the power should be exercised sparingly to curb the potential for abuse. The power to issue a license does not make the state a co-owner of the labor of the persons or voluntary institutions whose conduct it regulates.

Physicians and hospitals are no exception to the general rule. A physician could maim any one of a thousand patients. None of these individuals has a strong enough private incentive to enjoin threatened harm that is far more likely to fall on others. Nor can large groups of iso-lated individuals pool their resources by agreement in order to take the needed steps. The costs of identifying the relevant parties, of assessing and collecting their contributions, are just too great, especially when some people are happy to sit idly by and reap the benefits of an injunc-tion obtained through the effort of others. Under an optimistic formu-lation, state action, funded by taxation, can overcome these coordination problems. The upshot is not a total ban, but a system of licenses that sets the terms and conditions under which people can engage in certain activities. No one thinks that a system of licenses is robust enough in and of itself to eliminate the need for damage actions or fines after the fact—one a private, the other a public response. By the same token, licensing can no longer be condemned as intrinsically corrupt on a priori grounds. No new ends are undertaken by the state, and all persons share in the benefits of preventing the harms in question. And licensing is perfectly compatible with allowing, after injury occurs, individual law suits to redress individual injuries. After harm occurs, the victim has all the right incentives to sue, so there is no longer any collective action to justify fur-ther state intervention.

This optimistic formulation assumes a neat dovetailing of public systems of licensing with private rights of action for the mishaps that manage to slip through the net. Generally speaking, this system works well. But government licensing is not immune from the usual pressures for expansion in government programs. *Guerrero*, for example, repre-sents using the licensing power for an impermissible set of ends. Begin with the assumption that, independent of its licensing power, the state could not compel individuals or institutions to render health care to other persons in need; just this assumption was made in *Guerrero* itself. If so, granting the license cannot be conditioned on the willingness of individuals or institutions to undertake those additional obligations. Stated otherwise, the license may be used to enforce a set of existing obligations that are imperfectly remedied by damage actions: it could, for example, be conditioned on a showing that hospital safety conditions meet certain minimum levels. But that license cannot be withheld unless a private institution is willing to undertake a vast new network of service obligations. The question for redistribution does not become any easier for the state under its licensing power than it would without that power. The state unilaterally imposes its license requirement without the consent of the individuals it regulates. That power cannot be used as the first stage of a two-stage process to achieve ends—the limitation of individual and institutional self-control—that could not be done in a single, and candid, step.

Unfortunately courts have viewed the use of the licensing power with far greater sympathy in cases of medical licensing than in speech cases. For example, *Massachusetts Medical Society v. Dukakis* allowed Massachusetts to condition the power of individuals to practice medicine on their willingness to waive their right to "balance billing,"[16] that is, to collect for Medicare recipients amounts in excess of the Medicare compensation levels for specified procedures.[17] The court held that physicians can always abandon their profession or refuse to treat Medicare patients if they do not want to comply with the condition. Hence, we are assured, they are not compelled to act against their own will. Yet this condition is not imposed by the party to the grant, but by the state solely through its licensing capacity. Its power to do so is no greater (but no less) than its power to impose a system of price controls of physician's fees generally, wholly without regard to the licensing power. Nor is the scheme saved because physicians still retain some scrap of choice after the condition is attached to the license. We might as well say that licensing poses no threat to speech because individual publishers can simply shut down their presses, or that gunmen should escape punishment because they happily give their victims a choice between their money or their lives. The physician is entitled to remain in the profession and to charge patients what they are willing to pay. What is needed, but was not supplied, was an explanation as to why any physician should be asked to choose between those two valuable rights.

This point is especially important because these new limitations on billing procedures upset the long-term investments in human capital so necessary for embarking on a medical career. Most physicians face high exit costs from their profession because they must abandon a large portion of their human capital. The ability to make lifecycle investments depends on the stability of the legal framework in which people must make choices. It is as though the state could first require a public utility to construct expensive new facilities specific to a particular use, and then refuse it the power to set rates that provide it with sufficient revenue to cover, not only their future costs of operation, but their original sunk costs.[18] It is not only physicians, but also the public at large, that loses from any radical shift in social expectations.

Similarly, the announcement effects of the new policy introduce a new level of uncertainty that complicates the investment decisions of new physicians. The licensing condition thus imposes a dual risk of expropriation of labor from present physicians and the disincentive to invest in labor by future physicians. The same difficulty applies to investments in human capital, where the state has, if anything, less justification for intervention because individual physicians or groups lack any semblance of monopoly power. A legislative ban on balance billing via the licensing power should be regarded as unconstitutional taking as a matter of first principle, although the current judicial approach to these issues virtually foreordains a different result.

FEDERAL MEDICARE CONDITIONS

State licensing power imposes relatively few limitations on the right of hospitals and physicians to set their own policies on admissions and fees. The federal restraints tied to participation in Medicare cut more deeply. Because the federal government does not license physicians, it has to look elsewhere for its power, and ironically it finds its mandate in a robust appeal to the principle of freedom of contract. No individual or institution is required to participate in Medicare, so any participation operates as a waiver of their common law right to refuse to deal. Medicare price controls thus emerged unscathed from a takings challenge. "It is well established that government price regulation does not constitute a taking of property where the regulated group is not required to participate in the regulated industry. . . . In the instant case, appellants are not required to treat Medicare patients, and the temporary freeze is therefore not a taking within the meaning of the Fifth Amendment."[19] With those words, the court upheld a federally imposed 15-month freeze on Medicare reimbursements.

The difficulty with this passage lies in its failure to ask the prior question: where does the federal government acquire its money for Medicare payments in the first place? The statutory language communicates the sense of voluntary participation by its enrollees by announcing that the Medicare program is "for aged and disabled individuals who elect to enroll under such program, to be financed from premium payments by enrollees together with contributions from funds appropriated by the Federal Government."[20] But the elective nature of the program is belied by the last clause, for the federal "contributions" hardly come from voluntary sources. To be sure, by statute the "Federal Supplementary Medical Insurance Trust Fund" is empowered to receive "gifts and bequests"—pious window-dressing at once charming, disingenuous, and wholly misleading. The key figure is the sizable and ever-increasing contribution from general revenues.[21] The fraction of payments from premiums paid dropped from 50 percent at its inception to less than 30 percent today, off a far larger base. Who could turn down this voluntary assistance and take their chances on an alternative private insurance program without tax subsidy?

Within this institutional framework, claims of physician voluntariness myopically ignore the system of taxes and subsidies that make government the sole primary provider of medical services to persons over age 65 and to disabled persons. Any bargains made with this entity should not be viewed with the same degree of deference as those that emerge from a competitive market because no private hospital or physician could circumvent government regulations and deal directly with Medicare enrollees. The tax subsidy to Medicare enrollees puts the government in a monopoly position against Medicare physicians. If any case calls for a hard judicial look to see if government bargains are illicit extractions, this is it. In the abstract, we cannot say how this federal discretion over prices will be exercised. But it is the height of irony that courts that have remained ever so alert to the dangers of monopoly power by private parties, even when they do business with the government,[22] are wholly indifferent to potential abuses of state power by uncritically accepting its claim of voluntary physician acceptance.

So fortunes under Medicare have turned. A program that lavished great prosperity on physicians in one generation squeezes them far harder in the next: to paraphrase Gerald Ford, hospitals and physicians have learned to their sorrow that the government powerful enough to give you all you want is powerful enough to take away all you have. Perhaps a profession that has feasted for a generation must learn to fast, with scant consolation to its younger members who never supped at the government table. But those not privy to the program must protest the destabilization in long-term planning brought about by repeated changes in government policy. The dispute is not merely a question of who wins and who loses a fee dispute. It goes to the stability of the system as a whole, which is compromised when government negotiates from a monopoly position that confers enormous discretion on its key officials.

EMTALA: NO REFUSAL FOR EMERGENCY CARE

The Medicare dollar has also been the linchpin of the federal effort to force physicians to treat certain classes of patients under the Emergency Medical Treatment and Active Labor Act (EMTALA).[23] EMTALA applies to any "participating hospital," that is, a hospital that has signed a long-term contract for providing services to Medicare patients,[24] which is to say virtually all major hospitals. As part of the price for participating in Medicare, EMTALA requires hospitals to provide services free of charge, to all persons, whether or not enrolled in Medicare, who need emergency treatment or who are in active labor. The bundled consent linking EMTALA to Medicare reimbursement is no small detail because it eliminates any federal obligation to compensate any hospitals, public or private, for costs specifically incurred in meeting EMTALA obligations.

EMTALA's carefully articulated framework covers the hospital/ patient relationship from arrival to discharge or death. The basic statutory obligation is triggered whenever "any individual comes . . . to the emergency department and a request is made [for appropriate treatment]."[25] The statute does not impose obligations to see patients seeking merely primary or urgent care that falls short of emergency care, which leaves hospitals some measure of autonomy for the less serious, and less onerous, portions of their business. For cases that cross the emergency threshold, however, the hospital "must provide an appropriate medical screening examination within the capability of the hospital's emergency department"[26] to determine whether a medical emergency exists. If that emergency medical condition exists, the hospital by law

> must provide either—
> (A) within the staff and facilities available to the hospital, for such further medical examination and such treatment as may be required to stabilize the medical condition, or
> (B) transfer of the individual to another medical facility in accordance with subsection (C) of this section.[27]

Subsection C then provides that the transfer may not be undertaken unless the patient or his guardian has provided informed consent, or "(ii) a physician . . . has signed a certification that, based upon the information available at the time of transfer, the medical benefits reasonably expected from the provision of appropriate medical treatment at another medical facility outweigh the increased risks to the individual and, in the case of labor, to the unborn child from effecting that transfer."[28] The statute also allows individuals to refuse either treatment or transfer, but only after suitable disclosure of the relevant risks and benefits of these options.[29] Elsewhere the statute specifies the detailed conditions for an "appropriate transfer," that is, one requiring the transferring hospital to minimize risk to the patient or, when appropriate, to an unborn child, and to ensure that the receiving institution has the space and personnel to treat the transferred patient and is willing to accept that responsibility.[30]

The statute also imposes heavy sanctions for violating these obligations. Any physician who "negligently violates" the obligations with respect to transfer and signs a certificate for transfer which he "knew or should have known" did not promise benefits in excess of risks may be fined up to $50,000, and similar penalties apply if he "misrepresents" material data about a patient.[31] A "gross and flagrant" violation opens the hospital up to a suspension of its privileges to participate in Medicare.[32] For hospitals, the sanctions for "negligently" violating the statute include fines up to $50,000 ($25,000 for hospitals with fewer than 100 beds) and potential suspension from the Medicare program, all at the discretion of the Secretary of HHS or his delegate.[33] This linkage between EMTALA and Medicare is odd if only because only a small fraction of the EMTALA cases are Medicare patients. Only the ease of sanction, not the organic connection between the two programs, dictates the result. Wholly apart from Medicare, EMTALA also allows for private damage actions and equitable relief against the hospital for "personal harm as a direct result" of the hospital's violation of the statute,[34] a provision which has (correctly) been construed *not* to authorize ordinary actions for medical malpractice against a hospital for noncompliance with the section.[35] In addition, any other hospital forced to incur financial obligations because of the hospital's breach of duty may recover those costs from the offending hospital.[36] Finally, the statute includes commonsense definitions for emergency medical condition, serious injury, transfer, and stabilization.[37]

EMTALA's complex structure represents a systematic statutory rejection of the common law rule that allowed hospitals and physicians to decide whom to treat and why. EMTALA was crafted in response to many graphic incidents of uninsured individuals who were either "dumped" to public institutions, or who died because they were otherwise refused care.[38] The prior evidence in support of EMTALA was both systematic and anecdotal. One study examined transfers to public hospitals from private institutions in the years before the passage of EMTALA and found that they steadily increased.[39] Thus the number of transfers to Cook County Hospital in Chicago rose from 1294 in 1980 to 2906 in 1981, to 4368 in 1982, and to 6769 in 1983. The same study revealed that in a sample of 467 transfers during the last two months of 1983, 87 percent of the patients were transferred because they lacked health insurance; of these, about 22 percent received intensive care within 24 hours of their arrival. Nearly 10 percent of patients died after transfer, about $2\frac{1}{2}$ times the death rate for those not transferred. Transfer delayed treatment by about 5 hours, thereby increasing the risk of death. The guidelines of the Chicago Hospital Council make safety of the patient the primary objective in transfer, but this sample suggested that this norm was honored more in the breach than in the observance. The financial burden of these transfers was not inconsiderable, and the authors estimated that about 12 percent of the Cook County Hospital annual budget was spent on providing care to transferred patients, for a total of about $24 million, of which only 15 percent could be recovered from other sources.

The anecdotal evidence presented to the Senate Hearing was every bit as dramatic.

> Terry Takewell was a young diabetic. Gasping for breath, he was taken by ambulance to the only local hospital in Fayette County, Tennessee. Takewell was not treated, but instead was carried out the door by a hospital administrator and set on the edge of the parking lot. He was picked up by neighbors and brought home. He died the next day. Terry had no insurance and owed the hospital a lot of money.[40]

The hearings did not contain any rebuttal or explanation from the Methodist Hospital of Somerville, whose conduct was under scrutiny.

EMTALA reversed the common law outcome in these cases. Once again, the statute proved impervious to constitutional challenge because both hospitals and physicians participate in Medicare. At first blush, EMTALA is all gain and no pain, which accounts for the passionate support it has in academic circles, notwithstanding quibbles at the edges.[41]

Despite this formidable consensus, EMTALA is an institutional mistake whose intended benefits are more than offset by its hidden costs. One obvious question is, how serious is the problem it addresses? Beware of the power of anecdote to drive public policy. Terry Takewell's story deserves some further scrutiny. The case was not chosen at random, but was selected carefully from perhaps thousands of possible cases for the House Hearing by the late Congressman Theodore Weiss, long an ardent promoter of EMTALA. Yet the official summary was incomplete, judging from the newspaper stories reproduced in the House Hearings.[42] The hospital administrators denied the gist of the tale, claiming that Takewell had been examined and was not in a life-threatening condition when turned away from the hospital. He had also received indigent care about a dozen times in the previous few years and had proved an uncooperative patient who had refused to sign any standard consent forms. The hospital annually donated about $700,000 in free medical service. Also undiscussed was Takewell's conduct in the days and weeks prior to his last arrival at the hospital. Did he abide by the restrictions on diet and behavior incumbent on severe diabetics? The full picture should raise a moment's uneasiness of formulating public policy on anecdotal evidence not subject to cross-examination.

Similar doubts creep in about the systematic studies on transfer. Public hospitals incur heavy costs when they receive transfers, but private hospitals incur costs when no transfers are made. Indeed, in one sense, the willingness to order patient transfers raises only one side of problem. The companion question to the Cook County dumping study is whether Cook County or the state of Illinois is willing to allocate general revenues to pay for indigent care. If so, it could reimburse the private hospitals for their expenses. Once the financial obligation is clarified, the public authorities could make the further decision whether a high- or a low-cost provider of medical care is needed in a particular case. It may thus increase risks by transferring one patient to free up more money for others under the general budget cap. The problem of scarcity cannot be wished away by a plea for greater budgets beyond the taxing capacities of the local governments.

To understand EMTALA, therefore, we must go beyond the dramatic incidents of a single transfer to a broader understanding of its long-term institutional consequences. In this connection, we cannot assume that the only changes wrought by EMTALA are intended, with everything else unchanged. Nor should we assume that the consequences of the statute are likely to be small because it generates relatively little litigation, or because it is possible to imagine a set of obligations that are still more stringent than those the statute imposes.[43] It is critical to estimate the day-to-day impact of the statutory scheme. In so doing, we must remember that no aggressive and complex legislative program has only benign or intended consequences. A 1991 GAO study reports that caring for emergency cases places heavy burdens on hospital physicians and staff and often forces the postponement of scheduled, cash-paying surgeries.[44]

Once EMTALA limits the freedom of a hospital to ration care inside its ER, the hospital's adaptive responses will take place earlier in the cycle. The chink in EMTALA's armor is that its obligations are not absolute, but conditional. It applies only to hospitals that "have an emergency department," and these obligations are set "within the staff and facilities" available to that hospital.

The existence or size of ER facilities and staff, however, are not fixed by legislative fiat or divine command. Hospitals can reduce their statutory exposure by shrinking their ER capacity or closing it altogether.

Sooner or later, the budget constraint will force one result or the other. Neither action violates EMTALA, but both reduce the total level of ER services available for sick people, both for those who can and cannot pay for treatment. The sponsors of EMTALA may have thought that no hospital would "dare" to cut off its nose to spite its face, but metaphors of this sort do not control major policy decision on the deployment of resources. Nonprofit institutions cannot afford to run big losses.

These concerns seem to have been borne out by the patterns that have emerged after the passage of EMTALA and, in part, because of it. It is surely sobering for a *defender* of EMTALA to juxtapose two different stories: first, Terry Takewell left to die on the hospital steps, and second, the decision to maintain these facilities at all. Thus the 1991 GAO study carries the sobering title "Trauma Care: Life Saving System Threatened by Unreimbursed Costs and Other Factors."[45] Its key findings make the basic point. "Nationwide, about 60 trauma centers have closed in the past 5 years leaving about 370 designated to provide trauma care. Major urban areas are particularly hard hit."[46] And "[o]f the 35 trauma centers GAO reviewed, 15 have closed—12 primarily because of financial losses."[47] These trauma centers are especially important because their intake involves gunshot wounds, automobile accidents, and other major injuries. They are expensive to run and vital to the chances of patient survival. The GAO study does not attribute all the dislocation to EMTALA, but it does explicitly conclude that EMTALA, although not cited by name, is a dominant driver of the overall financial crunch, which has its greatest impact on trauma centers located in inner-cities.[48]

The picture has not improved since 1991. Newspaper reports from Los Angeles bemoan the decision "to close urgent care ERs at all county public clinics and reduce outpatient services by 35 percent at the remaining six public hospitals," in the face of increased demands for access and use.[49] As of 1992, the number of trauma centers in Los Angeles has gone from 20 to 9.[50] The same story reports that "Chicago has problems of its own. In mid-January 1992, six hospitals were forced to stop accepting ambulance patients because of ED (emergency department) overcrowding. . . . Chicago, like other cities, has also seen a decline in the number of trauma centers; of an original 10 city and near-suburban hospitals with designated trauma centers, four have dropped out of the network."

One of those hospitals was the University of Chicago system. It is perhaps instructive to recount what happened and why. The culprit is regulation of which EMTALA is a part, but only a part. EMTALA only requires hospitals to accept patients for emergency treatment. But EMTALA does not require hospitals to join the ambulance networks that feed patients into hospitals. Those initiatives are carried out at the local level, under the supervision of city government. Before the 1988 break-down of the network, the 10 Chicago hospitals worked out among them-selves a protocol for directing traffic to those ERs with the greatest available bed capacity, even if not the closest to the point of pickup. The network agreement responded to both considerations of benefit and cost. Often the most expensive admissions to an ER take place in the early morning hours on a weekend, when drinking, fighting, and reckless driving often take place. But the fluctuation in admissions between days is large. To outfit several emergency rooms in each trauma center is very expensive, and to assemble backup teams takes both time and money and imposes emotional wear and tear on staff. It makes little sense to mobilize a third or fourth team at one hospital when an idle team is wait-ing at a second. The additional time in transportation is offset, perhaps entirely, by the reduced waiting time after arrival at the second hospital.

Geography also played a role. Chicago is a long, thin, city along Lake Michigan, and many of its traumatic injuries occur on the South Side. For those accidents, the University of Chicago, south of County Hospital, is often the closest hospital. On average, its patient intake and financial exposure can both be reduced by a diversion policy that sends some ambulances to the nearest hospital with open and available units— a maneuver that both reduces and equalizes cost. The then Health Commissioner of the City of Chicago vetoed this diversion system and required the nearest hospital in the network to take all cases, period. It then dared the University to pull out of the network, which it did because of the prohibitive cost. That decision was made in 1988, and the University Hospitals remain out of the network today. A small compro-mise by the City could have kept the network in tact. Instead its aggres-sive pattern of regulation produced the all-or-nothing choice from which "none" was chosen, to the detriment of all concerned.

The point here can be generalized. Since the passage of EMTALA, the total number of ER facilities (including the critical trauma units) has declined substantially: more than 700 hospitals have ceased services because of overcrowding.[51] In other institutions, the rationing has been achieved by limiting the kind of equipment, the number of doctors, and the number of available ER beds. Notwithstanding this contraction, the number of visits to the ER since 1965 has about tripled from 30 million to 92 million, far outstripping population growth during the same period. It is pointless to pile on further anecdotes to confirm the distress and chaos of the current situation, which by any objective measure is far worse than it was a decade ago.

No matter where we look, the overall situation has all the features of an overheated market that cries out for internal restraint: extreme rationing on its supply side and queues on the demand side. Thus one recent study found that only 51 percent of patients admitted into an ER had problems that were assessed prospectively as requiring urgent care.[52] The remaining 49 percent of admitted cases were classified as nonurgent. A second study found that 32 percent of the visits were nonurgent, 26 percent were semiurgent, and 42 percent were urgent.[53] The estimates of the additional costs imposed by inappropriate ER use has been estimated at between $5 billion and $14 billion.[54] As might be expected, the chief explanation for resorting to the ER stems from the lack of access to ordinary primary care, and it seems that the costs of hospitalization for patients admitted through the ER are, for persons with comparable diagnoses, higher than those for persons who are admitted by other means.[55].

Any mystery associated with ER use dissolves once we cease treating health care as "special." The usual laws of supply and demand have more to say about the problem than any glorification of the intractable problems of health care delivery. Part of the problem, no doubt, stems from the high costs of receiving primary care through other means, which induces resorting to the ER, which has both lower costs to the individuals and higher costs to the overall system—one standard consequence of building subsidies into the system. The same imbalance occurs when the government sets maximum prices for tomatoes: there are too few tomatoes and long lines to purchase them. Remove the price constraints and supply and demand will slowly work themselves back into balance—at least if consumers and producers are confident that a second round of intervention does not loom just over the horizon. The return to equilibrium can, with stable political conditions, also happen in health care. One part of the solution, therefore, is to lower the costs of achieving primary care through other means. The rise of cheap and efficient systems of health care, chiefly through health maintenance organizations, should help in this direction. The situation could be improved further by removing legal and regulatory barriers, such as those that relate to liability and mandatory packages of minimum services, that drive up the cost of delivering health care.

The problem can also be attacked from the other side by imposing some charges on the use of emergency room facilities. A recent study of emergency room utilization in the Kaiser-Permanente Medical Care Program examined the effect of a small copayment on the utilization of emergency room care between 1992 and 1993.[56] The number of patients, matched in relevant demographic respects was large: over 30,000 in the experimental group; and nearly 100,000 in two control groups. The effect of the copayment was exactly what standard economic theory, with no allowance for the unique status of health, would predict. The copayment reduced utilization by about 15 percent in the period of a year, with the decline concentrated in those patients whose conditions were not likely to present a serious emergency condition. In reviewing the data, the authors found "there was no suggestion of excess adverse events in the copayment group," and they concluded that their study confirmed the results of earlier work in the field that "the selective use of relatively small copayments can safely reduce inappropriate use of the emergency department among people who are employed and covered by health insurance."[57]

The lesson should not be lost in an excess of sentimentalism. Ordinary businesses do not close their doors or limit their output because they have too much business. They close or downsize because they have too little business. But in the emergency room context, regulation often leads to that dangerous result. The excess business is in part forced on the hospitals by EMTALA and other regulations that impose duties without covering their correlative costs. The increased volume magnifies the amounts of an unrecoverable loss, which become ever harder to bear as insurance carriers bleed out the hidden subsidies long used to prop up Medicaid, Medicare, and other uninsured patients.[58] Medicine illustrates the wisdom of the old garment industry joke: no one makes up in volume what is lost on each transaction. To minimize losses, hospitals constrain available space when they cannot limit admissions—another instance of the mortal peril of beneficent regulation.

Today demand increases continue unabated because no price or other governance mechanism forces people to reveal their honest preferences. The patient's private calculation asks only whether the wait is worth the service, which it often is when prices are kept artificially below a market clearing price, and perhaps at zero. In the end, many people find that the vindication of their legal rights translates into the same poor ER service available to everyone else: chronic delays, harried emergency room physicians, and overcrowding, all getting worse.[59] Patients can wait six hours or more to be seen in the ER, and some significant fraction, perhaps between 10 and 15 percent of the total, leave the ER without being seen. A substantial fraction of these are admitted shortly afterwards, often for serious conditions.[60] Some people may die in full possession of their rights under EMTALA simply because no care was available at the institution of their choice. Should these nameless cases be mentioned in a Congressional Hearing orchestrated to expand the scope of positive rights?

With this unhappy picture of chaotic and crowded emergency rooms, we might think that compliance with EMTALA is widespread. But EMTALA has been berated as a paper tiger,[61] and some evidence suggests that patients are refused care and transferred out of facilities, perhaps in large numbers, despite the major legal risks *if* the hospital gets caught. There are no reliable studies of the rates of transfer out of emergency room since the passage of EMTALA, but one study guesses that some 250,000 illegal transfers have taken place, a total far less than 1 percent of millions of ER cases.[62] But suppose all of these transfers were prosecuted to the full extent of the law—that hospitals were caught and assessed the statutory fines of perhaps $50,000 per case, exposed to a raft of private actions, and subject to discipline and removal from Medicare. The entire operation would shut down. The threat of enforcement that seems credible in an individual case is not sustainable if pursued systematically. Underenforcement should not be understood simply as an unfortunate byproduct of a high-minded scheme. Instead underenforcement has to be built, albeit cynically, into the program at the front end for it to survive. The budgetary constraints under which hospitals labor, although dismissed as largely irrelevant at the passage of EMTALA, turn out to be all consuming in shaping its administration.

Underenforcement has another inevitable consequence. The constant stream of violations creates a substantial risk of selective prosecution of hospitals and physicians. Indeed, the merits of the individual case are often quite beside the point. One-well publicized news story can inflict enormous reputational injuries on an institution, guilty or innocent. At an administrative hearing, a hospital could raise any one of several defenses to administrative action under EMTALA. It can claim that the patient consented to transfer, that an alternative institution was in a position to supply the patient with superior care, or that the patient appeared stabilized before transfer, even if the subsequent events falsified that original prediction. But what institution would be brave enough to contest these issues down to the wire, even if correct, in the face of a government threat to suspend Medicare payments. The high set of statutory penalties frustrates any consistent patterns of government enforcement. In some cases, it will breed indifference; in others, it will breed excessive zeal. But, in the long haul, the inconsistent patterns will breed public cynicism and distrust of big government.

But, wait, there is more. EMTALA makes no effort to equalize the uncompensated burdens across hospitals with ERs. Nor (as with the question of ambulance diversion in Chicago) does it provide any statutory mechanism to facilitate cooperative ventures among hospitals who seek to even out the utilization levels across ERs. To be sure, diverting a single transfer could increase the costs of treating this patient, while substantially reducing the cost of treating the *next* patient in the system. On balance, if the expected gain to the second patient exceeds the expected loss to the first, the initial diversion should be blessed both by government and by potential patients who do not yet know their place in the queue. But diversion requires transfers over the objection of patients at the head of the queue—perhaps one who bypassed nearer facilities to go to a tertiary care institution. As such, all equalization plans could require following policies that conflict with EMTALA. EMTALA does not allow hospitals with ERs to husband resources for anticipated use. Instead, patients receive the untrammeled right to target any specific institution for emergency care, without regard to the stability and balance of the system as a whole. Willy-nilly, it imposes substantially disparate financial burdens on different local institutions within the same region, without equalizing burdens, which in turn drives those institutions nearest the fire line toward the shutdowns that have become common in recent years.

EMTALA also denies hospitals control over their caseload even when patient dumping is nowhere in evidence. The current case law under EMTALA takes the obvious position that "stabilization means stabilization," no matter what the costs and benefits in any individual case. In the *Matter of Baby K*,[63] one federal appeals court held that a hospital that admits an anencephalic infant through its ER is obliged to stabilize its condition at its own expense at the insistence of its mother, even when its own ethical protocols regard further treatment as inappropriate for all patients, regardless of their ability to pay. Baby K was dutifully stabilized in intensive care immediately after birth and on three separate occasions afterwards when taken by her mother into the ER. The judicial response was both correct and abject: "It is beyond the limits of our judicial function to address the moral or ethical propriety of providing emergency stabilizing medical treatment to anencephalic infants."[64] The plain language of the statute controls, and only Congress can alter it, if and when it returns to the issue. A statute designed to meet the ostensible evils of patient dumping introduces an overbreadth problem for which no effective countermeasures are available. Treating Baby K hardly counts as a preferred use of public funds.

Finally, EMTALA never faces up to the danger of moral hazard and dangerous behavior. Some individuals eligible for treatment under EMTALA have taken excessive risks because they know that some of their costs are borne by others. The GAO study makes it all too clear that a huge portion of the business of trauma centers is penetrating injury (for example, gunshot wounds); blunt trauma (for example, automobile accidents); and many of these cases are associated with drug use.[65] But in the face of this mounting evidence, today's attitude makes an uneasy choice between two unsound philosophical attitudes. The first states that additional amounts of ER care do not increase individual misbehavior, but only respond to harms that should be treated, as it were, as acts of God. The second says that such increases are possible, but they are likely to be small, and morally irrelevant in any event.

The net effect of this basic stance is to turn a blind eye to the mix of ER cases, especially in the inner-city. Relatively few arrivals are struck by lightning or hit by falling bricks. The bulk of the admissions relates to drugs, alcohol, firearms and the like. Thus the dumping studies only reflect the severity of the social situation; they do not dwell long on its source. Often the evidence is given anecdotally, usually orally, with no attribution. But they speak to self-inflicted harm, as with diabetic patients who do not test their blood sugar levels. One published account—from the *Wall Street Journal* no less[66]—hints at the problem of an addict who infects herself through heroin use after being hospitalized with bacterial endocarditis—a life-threatening condition that attacks the heart valves, Yet on release, she refuses drug treatment and reinfects herself, requiring another round of hospitalization at public expense. That same article tells of another Vietnam veteran whose disability stipend of $1,200 per month is spent to purchase cocaine and alcohol. He readmits himself to the VA when his funds are exhausted, only to check out on receipt of his next check—several times a year. Similar stories are told of expectant mothers who arrive at the ER without medical records in a state of weakened health attributable to bad habits generally, or to the excessive consumption of drugs or alcohol, or both. EMTALA protects them all.

So what is to be done? One possibility is to create a conservatorship to limit the power of chronic abusers to spend their various benefits. But that restraint requires patient consent and may expose the treating physician or other guardian to physical risk.[67] More to the point, we need not finesse the problem but should face the structural questions head on. A sensible response to the question of emergency care will only be forthcoming when the power to make decisions is decentralized. As far as government is concerned, any hospital should be able to "just say no" to any patient, without giving reasons for its decisions.

But within the institution, how should that awesome power be exercised? I doubt that many would choose to refuse care to first time offenders, but their own internal budgets will induce them to impose unreviewable sanctions against chronic offenders. Unfortunately the current law makes it impossible for a hospital to treat drug addicts or alcoholics just once, or even twice, with this stern warning: there is no treatment next time, period—no matter what their personal consequences, including death. To the question, "you cannot let them die, can you?" we have to avoid the reflexive answer, no. To restore long-term stability to the system of emergency care, the answer has to be "yes, we can sometimes." That threat becomes credible only if it is acted on at least once. Otherwise, as soon as that ultimate threat ceases to be credible, any lesser threat loses its credibility as well. How can you tell an individual that you will fine him if he does not take his medicine or do his exercises? He says no and you have to take him in. How can you tell an individual that he will have to wait longer for care when he knows you will have to pay the additional costs of his treatment out of your own pocket? Faced with this perverse set of incentives, any hospital is forced to treat individual derelictions much as it would treat its own because it bears the financial costs if matters go worse. We have created a peculiar inversion whereby a hospital has to beg the patient to take routine health precautions, not only for his own benefit, but also to minimize the hospital's financial exposure.

Allowing institutions to stand tough permits them to break this cycle and to increase the effectiveness of their own indigent care. We need to adopt a policy of calling the bluff of those who say "you can't let us." But the purpose is not to make people die, although it is certain that some will. It is to minimize unnecessary deaths by broadcasting far and wide the consequences of self-destructive conduct that often results in death in any event. If taken to heart, an unmistakable warning will increase survival rates beyond what any desperate treatment could do and reduce the financial drain on hospitals and taxpayers as well. And it will make better care available for individuals who suffer serious injury through no fault of their own. Yet no matter how imperative it is for hospitals to hang tough, matters will grind to a halt if everyone knows in advance that the hospital that says no faces horrendous liability and ceaseless denunciation. Absent the political will to cut people off, we get what we pay for: more of the self-destructive conduct. EMTALA is part of the problem, not its cure. Only when hospitals can say no and make it stick will the cycle be broken. No educational or altruistic exhortation will do that job.

The overall picture should by now be clear. The right question to ask of EMTALA is whether over time it will increase the number of lives saved, or more properly, raise them to a level that justifies the public expenditures. Looking only at its obvious successes, the answer seem yes. But these victories are offset by EMTALA's hidden systemwide costs. Price controls generally create excessive demand and long queues; they cause existing firms to leave the industry; they make it unattractive for new firms to enter the industry; they increase the risks of selective prosecution; they reduce the incentives of consumers to reduce risk and improve health; they prevent cooperative ventures by regulated firms. Health may be "special" relative to other goods, but every single bad feature of price controls and forced association comes back to haunt the legal system that pays no heed to the peril they present. The question is not whether hospitals should admit indigent patients who lack the ability to pay. Of course they should—lots of them. Rather the question is whether hospitals should have the power to admit or exclude potential patients or turn that prerogative over to a federal government utterly unable to manage its vast resources. The received wisdom and current law both answer yes, but the correct answer is no. The refusal to deal lies at the ability to form and organize voluntary organizations. Collectively we must learn to let others, acting individually, just say no.

CHAPTER 5

❖ ❖ ❖

Wealth and Disability

FROM REFUSAL TO DISCRIMINATION

Canonically the principle of freedom of association embraces for all individuals both the right to associate and the right not to associate. Those two extremes are also sufficient to allow each person to determine the terms and conditions on which to associate with others. Because A may decide to do business with B while refusing to do business with C, it follows that C cannot complain if A offers to do business with both, albeit on different terms. The control over association allows everyone to discriminate in the terms and conditions they offer to people with whom they are willing to trade. In a world that prizes freedom of association, the word "discrimination" carries only positive connotations: to "discriminate" refers to the ability to make the fine or keen distinctions between persons or things.[1] The discriminating person pursues desirable associations and shuns undesirable ones.

The principle of discrimination carries with it, however, a more ominous connotation. Even before the Civil Rights movement gained force, discrimination was often condemned as a dangerous social practice when used to expand the influence and control of monopoly power. Governments often possess that monopoly power, and when they exercise it to give some right to A that they deny to its competitor B, the attitude toward discrimination rightly changes. The entire structure of American federalism would, for example, be unrecognizable if states were routinely allowed to discriminate in favor of their domestic corporations at the expense of their out-of-state rivals.[2] Discrimination by private firms that possess monopoly power is also suspect, given distortions that take place when some parties are favored over others.[3]

In dealing with discrimination in health care, discriminatory practices by private firms with monopoly power is not on the table. Rather the types of discrimination at issue here are those practiced by private firms operating within a competitive environment, as is typical for much of the health care industry. In this connection, the Civil Rights movement has largely driven the principle of freedom of association from the field by denying the term "discrimination" its once positive connotations. Discrimination, as it is now understood, treats "invidious" as its unspoken predicate. This new social mindset links the noun "discrimination" with the pejorative "discriminatory," and it transforms the adjective "discriminating" from a positive to a negative sense. This new standard usage signals a sharp departure from the original sense of "civil rights," which had nothing to do with private discrimination and everything to do with civil capacity. In its nineteenth-century usage, civil rights (as opposed to political rights, like voting) secured to all persons the rights to contract, marry, own property, make wills, testify in court, sue, and be sued. That conception was strongly anchored in the tradition of negative rights—rights that were necessarily violated when any person was denied civil capacity for reasons of race or sex. It is easy to take these rights for granted now that they are no longer challenged, but their recognition was the result of a hard-fought struggle to end the formal and explicit subordination of black slaves and all women.

The Civil Rights Act of 1964 ratified the change in intellectual direction: no longer was civil capacity for all persons the sole object of a regime of civil rights. Instead its target was private discrimination, chiefly by employers, but by easy extension to landlords, universities, banks, and insurance companies. Hence the central provision of Title VII makes it a wrong for any employer "to fail or refuse to hire or to discharge any individual, or otherwise discriminate against any individual with respect to compensation, terms, conditions, or privileges of employment, because of such individual's race, color, religion, sex or national origin."[4] The provision is selective in its application—employees are not bound—and explicitly rejects the principle of freedom of association for competitive markets as well as for monopolistic ones. The Act tends to undercut the distinction between public institutions, which were bound under classical theory by a nondiscrimination obligation, and private institutions, which in a competitive setting were not.

The Act's explicit linkage of "to refuse to hire" with "otherwise discriminate" marks the culmination of the new strategy. If you cannot refuse to offer a person a job because of race or sex, you cannot adopt the subterfuge of offering a job on unacceptable terms. It would have been economic suicide for the state to require every firm to hire the first person who comes through the door on the same terms as the most qualified applicant. So the strategy of state control is narrowed. The law does not to require contracts to be made, but it does prohibit discrimination on certain stated grounds: race, color, religion, sex, or national origin. Once the antidiscrimination seed is planted, the tree will grow.[5] The forbidden grounds of discrimination have since expanded to include age and disability, and increasingly sexual preference. Yet these forms of discrimination do not carry the same level of disapprobation: age and race are very different propositions, to say the least, as the former was universally practiced when the latter was made illegal. But political pressures tend to blind legislators to these social differences. Indeed the current rules contain an odd reversal in that they impose *greater* sanctions for age discrimination than race discrimination, in the form of double damages for "willful discrimination."[6]

The expansion of liability took place as well along a second frontier. The original Civil Rights Act was color-blind in its intent and language; its application has been anything but. Starting in the 1970s, Supreme Court interpretations of the Act have carved out blanket exemptions for "protected classes"—most notably racial minorities and women—in whose favor discrimination is routinely allowed or encouraged under the rubric of diversity or affirmative action.[7] Yet when applied for the benefit of these protected classes, the law has been remorseless in its application. Proof of intent—fairly implied by the Act's phrase "because of"—has yielded to proof by statistical inference in the absence of intent; and the so-called bona fide occupational qualification has been narrowed so that it survives only in cases of strict necessity. An Act once touted as a mild and moderate remedy for the ills of institutional discrimination has become, through its departures from its original design, a dominant constraint on the operation of labor markets.

This expansionist pattern replicates itself in the field of health. Breach the autonomy wall, and there is no stopping point in regulating refusals to deal. Discrimination must be tackled as well to prevent circumvention of the original provision. To be sure, the forbidden grounds of discrimination in health do not perfectly track the employment cases. Race and sex discrimination may lurk in some individual cases or in specialized areas—for example, who should be the proper subjects for clinical tests,[8] or what are the proper rules for organ transplants[9]—but overall the categories of race and sex do not loom as large as they do in employment or education. Instead the key categories tend to be wealth, as it relates to the ability to pay for services rendered, or medical condition or disability, which relates to the incidence of risk, in individual cases. In both contexts, once the wall surrounding associational freedom has been torn down, the antidiscrimination norm quickly exerts its coercive force.

I believe that the modern carryover of the antidiscrimination law into the area of health care is a mistake similar in content to the basic mistakes of equating private discrimination in competitive markets with the state's denial of civil capacity to all its citizens. In health markets, like employment markets, the forms of discrimination offer rational responses to serious social problems. They have survived for so long because of their inherent ability to ration care and to stabilize market institutions. To be sure, we can identify some cases in which these practices prove irrational or unjust (the charges are not the same), but no single counterexample should be allowed to torpedo any general regime, especially when the legislative remedies for market discrimination spawn more difficulties than they eliminate. As happens in other contexts, legislation against discrimination falters on questions of proportion and degree. It treats the aberrant case as the standard case and regulates the latter as though it had the moral stigma of the former. To function well, the discrimination laws subject broad categories of behavior to uniform commands, ignoring subtle variations that can, and often are, picked up in the field by workers who are acutely aware of both the dangers of discrimination and the necessity for its use.

This chapter deals with two manifestations of the discrimination issue, namely, whether the level of care should vary either with wealth or with medical disability or status. Chapter 6 attacks the problem in another guise by asking whether insurance companies and other health care providers can use differential risk to discriminate in the rates charged to various classes of customers, or whether they must adopt, as is now frequently proposed, community rating systems that disregard these risk differentials. More concretely, may insurance contracts exclude coverage or increase premiums for pre-existing conditions, including those attributable to genetic defect or disease?

WEALTH DISCRIMINATION

Understanding discrimination in health cases often takes its cue from larger social questions. Earlier I argued that a variety of practical reasons blocked the creation of positive entitlements to health care, however defined.[10] In one sense, setting that level of minimum health care depends in part on the total level of resources available within society. And lest we pay too much attention to the distributional questions that shape the modern debate, it should be stressed again and again that the surest way to improve the welfare of the citizenry at large is to increase the aggregate levels of wealth. This approach reminds us that an "overreaction to very small risks impedes the kind of technological progress that has historically brought dramatic improvements in both health and material well-being."[11] It also should remind us that the surest path to improved longevity rests not on the provision of health care as such, but in the overall increase in social wealth, which has a direct payoff in reduced mortality rates. One study of mortality rates in the United States estimates that each 1 percent increase in income reduced the levels of mortality by 0.05.[12] And the increase in longevity in the United States grew more rapidly from 1900 to 1970 (at a rate of around 0.8 percent per year) than it has since 1970, when that rate has slowed to 0.3 percent per year.[13] The effort to guarantee minimum rights to health care does not have the payoff we hope.

Another way of attacking the inequalities in health care is to forsake the language of substantive minimums and to invoke the antidiscrimination principle in its stead. If we believe that wealth and income should be equally distributed in society to all persons, it becomes easy to defend a system that mandates the equal distribution of health care resources, regardless of the ability to pay.[14] In one sense, the egalitarian principle is less intrusive than the minimum standard because it prescribes no floor on health care, but only prohibits the preservation of differences. Yet, in another sense, it is far more restrictive than the minimum floor because it limits what some people can spend on themselves by what they are willing to spend on others. But whether more or less intrusive than a regime of minimum health care rights, the egalitarian premise leaves many questions unanswered. A world in which two people have equal incomes and different states of health is one of enormous inequality. The difficulty for the egalitarian regime is to decide whether it wants to equalize the distribution of satisfaction across persons, no matter how difficult the questions of implementation, or whether it stops at the more modest goal of equalizing wealth generally, or the resources devoted to health care in particular.[15] This conflict within the walls has no easy resolution, for no amount of resources can reverse major misfortune, cure chronic diseases, or forestall death. The equalization of end-states, however desirable in principle, imagines an ideal that no social system can obtain. The egalitarian who backs off from that grandiose objective has not proved unfaithful to his principles. He simply has recognized that the legal order cannot overcome natural constraints.

The most common formulation of the egalitarian ideal skirts these difficulties by holding that everyone has a right to health care regardless of ability to pay. The major question is: Why is this principle appropriate for health care when it has been rejected for vacation homes and fast cars? The incentive arguments that allow the creation of wealth differentials in the first place operate with life and death expenditures as well as with ordinary consumption choices. Indeed most rich people regard the ability to seek out the finest medical care worldwide as one of the blessings of their wealth and would doubtless sacrifice the second home before forgoing the good health care. Nonetheless the ethical insistence on dispensing health care without regard to wealth lay at the root of the defunct Clinton Health Security Act. Although its detailed substantive provisions have been long buried, its aspiration of universal access, comprehensive benefits, and equality continue to hold broad appeal, even when, taken together, they lead to the familiar socialist maxim—from each according to his ability (to pay), to each according to his need (for medical treatment)—in the limited domain of health.[16] The intellectual challenge for that position is to find the alchemy that blends ordinary markets for goods and services with preferred government distributions of health care. This modern alchemy cannot work any more than Isaac Newton's.

The first difficulty rests on the simple proposition that health depends on far more than health care alone. Indeed its most powerful determinants over time come from elsewhere. Caloric intake and diet, education levels, lifestyle, and living conditions also make a critical difference, and these are directly correlated with income and wealth, individual and societal. To secure equal outcomes in the domain of health, it is not enough to secure equal access to health care. It would be necessary also to equalize all the opportunities of life, which is far too costly to do.

Individual health also depends on public infrastructure to control water purity, air pollution, and sewage disposal. Although these projects are typically funded through general revenues, they are not parceled out equally to all citizens. So long as local patterns of residence are influenced by wealth, the public goods received by given individuals will vary with these local influences, often substantially. As a basic rule of thumb, any group in society usually taxes itself so that, on the margin, the quality of its public goods is roughly comparable to the quality of the private goods its members purchase. So stated, public infrastructure will emerge when people can keep water clean in their own homes; environmental protection will gain public support only when homes can be kept free of waste and debris. It will hardly do for any society to indulge in expensive pollution control projects that take food out of the mouths of its hungry citizens. And it seems pointless to provide manicured public gardens for people who lived under cracked roofs.

It seems evident, therefore, that both the public and private services outside the health care system vary widely by wealth, and that the health of the citizenry varies with these expenditures long before the first dollar is spent on health care. Equalizing expenditures on health depends on far more than making adjustments *after* people enter the health care system. Rather, it becomes imperative to take into account the expenditures that they make, voluntarily or collectively, to avoid entering the system. Yet only by making *greater* direct public expenditures on health for the poor and less affluent can we try to equalize overall health care expenditures across all persons. Indeed even that venture could come up short because the differences in health attributable to income could be so great that *no* skew of health care expenditures could offset the outside imbalances. Equal health expenditures on rich and poor alike would not equalize health. However, the costs of equalization in terms of lost production would be so great that everyone would suffer.

The successful effort to prohibit discrimination by wealth also frustrates any goal of intergenerational equity. That problem cannot be addressed solely by looking at the static question of how to divvy up health care without regard to wealth *today*. A comprehensive view should ask how today's health care allocations influence the available levels of health care a *generation* from now. One working hypothesis of intergenerational fairness requires the present generation to leave the next generation its equal measure of wealth and material resources, so that persons deciding behind a veil of ignorance would be indifferent to whether they were born today or tomorrow. "Each generation must not only preserve the gains of culture and civilization, and maintain intact those just institutions that they have established, but it must also put aside in each period of time a suitable amount of real capital appreciation."[17] Historically the ordinary rules of negative liberty have ensured levels of growth that have allowed successive generations to far outstrip this goal. But any prohibition on discrimination by wealth compromises this goal and mortgages future unborn persons in order to satisfy the demands of the needy in the present generation.[18]

To see why, assume one patient pool of ten individuals each earning $100,000 a year and a second patient pool of ten individuals who earn nothing and require $20,000 per year of public support. Let us further assume that equal treatment requires that equal expenditures be made on different persons with the same prognosis of success, regardless of their ability to pay. Assume further that all twenty people have the serious condition for which a fixed budget of $20,000 is available. If we spend $1,000 on each person, each has a 50 percent chance of survival. If we allow individuals to spend their own wealth on their own health care, those ten individuals (to take an extreme case) each have an 80 percent chance of survival, whereas the other ten surely die. The number of expected lives in the first generation thus is reduced from ten to eight.

Some people may dismiss that result as indefensible on moral grounds, but even those with egalitarian impulses should be concerned about the long-term implications of that decision. Thus if the ten rich people are allowed to allocate their health expenditures to themselves, the population in the next generation will have eight productive individuals instead of five productive and five unproductive persons. The egalitarian policy therefore imposes a social gain that sees the elimination of some $300,000 in future income and the increase in public support payments of $100,000, a $400,000 annual reduction in annual wealth from the world in which the five persons with $100,000 incomes survive. That wealth reduction plays out in the second generation by reducing the overall level of health and the total amount of resources available for health care for the higher number of people who will need it.

The refusal to allow wealth to be a determinant of health care expenditures thus prejudices the rich and poor of the second generation for the benefit of the poor of the first generation. The stark allocation just proposed for the first generation will, and should, be softened in practice by charitable care, which in part responds to the difference between utility and wealth. Medical assistance is not, and should not be, an all-or-nothing set of choices. But allowing wealth to matter is likely to do far better in the long run than any policy that insists on allocating health care without regard to the ability to pay. To repeat, any effort to redistribute from rich to poor in the present generation necessarily entails the redistribution from the future to the present generation in violation of the veil of ignorance norm. If the cycle is allowed to continue, the size of the base can be expected to shrink over each period in which the game is played. Some discrimination by wealth in providing goods and services is far more conducive to a long-term sustainable base. What is unethical about considering these systematic concerns is, frankly, a mystery. We do it all the time to ensure sustainable yields from common pool resources such as fisheries. Why, then, do we ignore the issue of future generations in dealing with the desirability of egalitarian treatments?

The argument here is not that we should ignore all claims for compassionate redistribution today. It is that we should not legislate on the matter, but rather make accommodations at the field level, knowing it will sometimes misfire. By the same token, it is wholly indefensible to attack as immoral the common practice of having medical residents perform their initial operations on charitable cases, albeit the outcomes are on average likely to be less successful than when experienced surgeons operate. Clearly we cannot exhaust the talents of the ablest surgeons by requiring them to perform all cases; nor could we train the next generation of surgeons unless younger surgeons gain experience in dealing with live patients, if only to learn from their mistakes. Of course, provision should be (and is) made for senior parties to supervise in some cases and be on call in others in case of trouble. But once again these arrangements should be locally designed and should not subject any hospital to external penalties because the ability to pay is used to allocate medical services.

One ethical imperative that competes with other ethical considerations affords no basis for a massive government mandate to ignore the role of wealth in the allocation of health care.

DISABILITY: THE OREGON MEDICAID EXPERIMENT

Disability is often asserted as another ground on which it is forbidden to ration health care. But, as with wealth, that assertion fails before a comprehensive overview. The basic problem is neatly highlighted by Oregon's plan for allocating its state Medicaid budget.[19] The prior Oregon practice extended virtually full coverage for all types of procedures to the 231,000 persons then on the Medicaid rolls. The state's choice was whether to extend coverage to an additional 131,000 low-income individuals by excluding certain types of procedures from the program. To form its list, state officials held extensive open community meetings as well as sessions with experts. At the end of the day, its revised list contained some 709 condition-treatment pairs, which it then placed in rank-order for their overall medical effectiveness. A sample from the overall list follows:

RANK	PROCEDURE
2	MEDICAL TREATMENT FOR TUBERCULOSIS
158	MEDICAL TREATMENT FOR AIDS
366	LIVER TRANSPLANT FOR CIRRHOSIS PATIENTS (NO ALCOHOL INVOLVEMENT)
510	SPINA BIFIDA
583	CERVICAL DISK DISORDERS
600	BREAST RECONSTRUCTION FOLLOWING MASTECTOMY
690	LIVER TRANSPLANT FOR CIRRHOSIS PATIENTS (ALCOHOL-INDUCED CIRRHOSIS)
702	MEDICAL TREATMENT FOR AIDS IN THE LAST MONTH OF LIFE
708	LIFE SUPPORT FOR LOW BIRTH WEIGHT (UNDER 500 GRAMS) BABIES

Given its resource base, Oregon planned to fund procedures 1 through 586, but not those ranked below it.

Just looking at a few items on the list should create an enduring sense of wonderment. How can any informed cost/benefit judgment rest on the limited information used to generate the list? So much depends on the severity of the disease, the psychology and cooperativeness of the patient, overall health, family support, and the like. Nor is there any reason to suppose that all individuals would rank the same perils in the same order. Responses to breast reconstruction, for example, doubtless vary enormously across women, and for good reason. The point here is not to criticize the Oregon Medicaid approach. It surely represents a more concerted effort to use resources wisely than most state allocation schemes, and its limitations are inherent in any process that substitutes generalized survey data for the more concrete and complete knowledge that particular actors generate in market settings.

For these purposes, however, the issue is not why or how the basic index was constructed, but its unfortunate collision with the Americans with Disabilities Act,[20] which led Louis Sullivan, then Secretary of HHS, to reject it.[21] No specific provision of the ADA was cited, but the proposal was faulted because "it was based in substantial part of the premise that the value of the life of a person with a disability is less than the value of the life of a person without a disability."[22] That conclusion rested in part on the methodology used to construct the list, which rested "on certain community values," including "quality of life" and "ability to function." "These two values attach weight on 'restored' health and functional 'independence' and thus expressly value a person without disability more highly than a person with a disability in the allocation of medical treatment."[23] The letter then listed several possible sources of discrimination that were of concern—the lower treatment for alcoholic cirrhosis of the liver from nonalcoholic; and the low ranking for treatment of infants with very low birth weights.

How any of these concerns tie into the language of the ADA was left unexplained in Sullivan's memorandum, but for these purposes, it hardly matters. The larger lesson rests on the window that the particulars of this dispute offers on the larger question of discrimination in the distribution of health care, be it by government or by private charity. Should the state or a private donor take into account the impact of individual disability either prior to or subsequent to treatment? At one level, the discussion here echoes the treatment of discrimination by wealth. Choosing how to spend resources is not simply a contest between two persons, A and B. That choice also influences the sustainable level of treatment that can be supplied over the long haul. If A can be made healthy when B cannot, the resources available for treatment in the next generation will be greater than otherwise. Improvident health care expenditures today preclude wise expenditures tomorrow.

Even if the choice is confined to the current generation, the ADA approach should be rejected insofar as it refuses to take into account the net benefit promised by certain treatments to the extent that these might be influenced by individual levels of disability. To focus sensibly on this question, it is useful to examine three separate variations of a common theme. The first involves an individual who starts with a severe disability that can be eliminated by medical treatment. The disability is impending blindness and the proposed treatment is cataract surgery, with a very low cost and a high probability of success. Cases in this class offer reasons for discriminating *in favor of* the disabled person. Because the patient started at such a low ebb, the increase in expected utility will reach its greatest extent. The state or private party that wanted to maximize net positive changes in utility would propel these cases to the head of the queue.

In other cases, that same criterion of anticipated gains in utility sends other disability cases to the rear of the queue. Suppose that A is in a permanent vegetative state and now needs an emergency appendectomy to survive. The operation is certain to succeed. Should it be performed or should the patient be allowed to die? So long as life is regarded as sacred, the transformation from death to life has an infinite, or at least incommensurate, utility. But once that vegetative state is regarded as impoverished, we should dismiss as idle any claim of a real increase in the patient's utility. To see the conflict, assume that conditions of scarcity require us to perform *either* the appendectomy on a person in a permanent vegetative state or on a person who is otherwise in normal health. Do we really want to say that the only acceptable results are to do both, to do neither, or to flip a coin? Would any parent of two such children authorize, or even allow, the appendectomy on the child in the permanent vegetative state? If so, why should the ADA decree that evaluation of proposed treatment should always disregard the level of personal enjoyment made possible by its success? The cure in one case returns an individual to productive life; in the other, it increases the total financial and social drain. Why does any antidiscrimination principle force us to be blind to the differences between these two polar opposites? It is not clear whether the ADA would require equal treatment in this case. But if it did, it offers yet another case for its prompt repeal—or, failing that, for a clarifying amendment.

The extreme case, however, does not solve all the problems in the middle. Our instincts once again become clouded if asked to choose between two individuals in need of an appendectomy, one who has lost a limb and the other who has not. In this case, someone could still prefer to restore to health the person with the full complement of limbs on the grounds that the net increase of utility is greater after the fact. But that judgment does not carry even a tiny fraction of the conviction as the similar judgment in the previous case. All people have a unique set of potentials and disabilities, and no one is very good at estimating interpersonal comparisons of utility once we venture beyond the easy cases. The amputee might well have a strength of character and achievement that makes him the envy of others. But once again the stirring denial of the relevance of disability in that case might not persuade most people to fund an operation on a quadriplegic, a terminal AIDS patient, or a victim of Alzheimer's disease, instead of on a person with the potential to resume a normal life.

The only safe conclusion from these countless examples is that the ADA's antidiscrimination norm is wrong to mount a categorical defense of the proposition that the value of the life of a person with a disability is no less than the value of the life of a person without a disability. Some powerful moral instincts do cut in this direction, but we should resist the temptation to give them dogmatic expression in law. In those cases where the instincts are strongest, the practices will follow, even without the law. We can preserve the sensible cases without the risk of excessive regulation. The Oregon proposition rested on the modest proposition that the present condition and anticipated improvement of a patient could tip the balance in favor of an otherwise healthy person. Most people are uneasy about these matters for all the right reasons. It is the certitude of the statute that falsely assumes a simple answer to a complex question.

The HHS rejection of the original Oregon Medicaid proposal raises other questions that do admit of easier answers. Should the program be allowed to use weight to decide which premature babies receive care? Weight is often the best proxy for the success of premature infants. Care given to a two-pound baby at birth could produce a healthy infant; far more care on a one-pound baby might at best produce a child whose life will be crippled by disabilities. No one could object to concerned parents spending their own wealth on a longshot venture, but some level of discrimination, based on probable outcomes, seems welcome, if not necessary, in the expenditure of public funds. The ADA defines a disability as "a physical and mental impairment that substantially limits one or more of the major life activities of such individual." Why then cannot we look to outcomes to decide that certain treatments should be forgone? In its denial of the obvious, the ADA pushes its own logic to a bizarre conclusion. Many parents have rejected heroic treatments for their own infants (even at their own expense) when the prognosis of success was too low to justify torturing everyone concerned. Why the ADA should deny these judgments is hard to fathom. Caring for the needy is itself a form of social investment, which should not be made without regard to its intangible returns. It *is* a form of *justified* discrimination to treat people who can be helped extensively relative to those who cannot be helped at all. But it is also a form of *justified* discrimination that should escape the condemnation that lay at the root of the HHS position.

❖   ❖   ❖

CHAPTER 6

Community Rating and
Pre-existing Conditions

RISK CLASSIFICATIONS

It is an odd commentary on our times that the most common criticism of unregulated private insurance markets is their tendency to match the premium charged the customer with the risk assumed by the carrier. That outcome is achieved by separating insureds into categories that roughly mirror their anticipated costs to the carrier. The insurance company that lumps disparate individuals into a single risk classification invites its own economic ruination. The high-risk individuals within the group will stay because they enjoy a deal better than they can find elsewhere. The low-risk individuals will quickly migrate to rival carriers who charge them lower premiums commensurate with their lower expected losses. Left with high-risk insureds and a blended premium rate, the original insurer is destined for insolvency unless it learns to classify risks as well as its rivals. Yet when risks are accurately priced, both high- and low-risk customers tend to stay put unless a more efficient insurer can service the line at some lower cost. Correct risk classification allows the insurance market to reach a stable equilibrium.

Perfection in classification, however, is neither required nor advisable to maintain this state of affairs. Because no insurance company has, or can gather at reasonable cost, all the information relevant to determining the risk to given individuals, rough classifications are enough to preserve the market equilibrium. No wise insurer will strive to form tiny subclasses populated by virtually identical individuals because it is unwise to spend a fortune on medical examinations and background tests in the vain hope of eliminating all wobble—that is, implicit cross-subsidies—from the system. Any workable risk classification system allows some individuals to use private knowledge to squeeze into a too favorable risk category. But the size of these potential gains are likely to be contained by simple but robust tests—by age, sex, or prior medical history—that block these abuses. The successful insurer therefore fights a two-front war. First, it works to deter its rivals from cherry picking its best risks by keeping their prices low. Second, it works to prevent too many insureds from insinuating their way into a too favorable rate class. Over the long haul, a competitive insurance system rewards the firms that make correct risk assessments *and* the individuals who present good risk profiles. As with all competitive industries, market pressures bleed out cross-subsidies between customers.

The constant attacks on market insurance all stem from its success in preventing this redistribution of wealth from healthy to sick customers. Thus, in context, no one can trot out the usual suspects for market regulation, namely, that insurance carriers and their insureds systematically misperceive or mis-price their risk. The familiar villains of asymmetrical or imperfect information and widespread insurer or customer irrationality, when present, lead to capricious outcomes, which unregulated markets assiduously try to avoid. It is a sign of their success that the chorus of complaints here is directed to the converse result: the limited information that insurance companies collect in open markets is *too* accurate and therefore prevents those with the greatest need from getting someone else in the insurance pool to pay for their health insurance. The social argument reduces to the single proposition that it is appropriate for healthier people to pay the health insurance premiums for sicker ones as though that program of redistribution had no attendant costs. But making the insurance industry leaner and more efficient pushes hard in the opposite direction. Efficiency means more accurate risk classification at lower administrative cost. Efficient markets bleed out redistribution; they do not foster it. Only regulation can do that.

One way that regulation can bring about redistribution is to prevent the insurer from collecting the information necessary for setting rates. Once again the argument misses its mark. Notwithstanding the familiar charges of the exploitive position of insurance companies in competitive markets, the real business risks run in the opposite direction.

The insurer has no market power to dictate price, but individual customers possess something more valuable than any insurer's fleeting claim of market power: private knowledge over personal medical risks. If allowed to keep that information private, they will happily purchase insurance at bargain rates. The risk of asymmetrical information is rife in insurance markets, and it is a risk that falls to the firms.

Not surprisingly, the common law of insurance has long sought to counter that risk by requiring insureds to make full disclosure of all material information. As early as 1828, Judge Bayley wrote: "I think that in all cases of insurance, whether on ships, house or lives, the underwriter should be informed of every material circumstance within the knowledge of the assured; and that the proper question is, whether any particular circumstance was in fact material, not whether the party believed it to be so."[1] The duty, as codified by statute, is stated with special strictness for marine insurance: "the assured must disclose to the insurer, before the contract is concluded, every material circumstance which is known to the assured, and the assured is deemed to know every circumstance which, in the ordinary course of business, ought to be known by him. If the assured fails to make such disclosure, the insurer may avoid the contract."[2]

The traditional legal view thus rightly regarded the mischief maker as the potential insured, not the insurer. Redistribution through insurance amounts therefore—no more and no less—to a turnaround in world view, complete with a new cast of potential villains. This clash between efficiency and redistribution in insurance markets comes to a head over two issues. One is grand and abstract, and the other has a narrower focus but is of such enormous practical importance that has been made a centerpiece of the health care debate in the aftermath of the Clintoncare debacle. The larger issue is that of community rating, and the smaller one is that of pre-existing medical conditions, that is, known disabilities of an individual who has sought health insurance, either individually or as part of some group plan. It is useful to take up these issues in sequence.

COMMUNITY RATING

A system of "community rating" limits the permissible grounds for risk classification by an insurer. Restrictions of this sort are already in place in other lines of insurance. State insurance codes commonly limit the

classification schemes for automobile insurance. California bars classification by territory, by sex, and by age, while allowing experience rating
based on individual accident history. With health insurance, the same
pressure for uniform policy coverage has taken hold as well: age and sex
are more frequently regarded as irrelevant characteristics, notwithstanding their predictive value. Territory may be taken into account in setting
community rates, but although the claims experience is tolerated for bad
drivers, it is firmly out of bounds with health. To hold otherwise is to
concede the relevance of prior medical history and thus to defeat the
desired level of coverage.

Whatever their difference on particulars, community rating systems for both automobile and health insurance are basically meant to
block the risk classifications that private insurers use to constrain wealth
redistribution. An extreme proposal of this form was contained in
Clinton's Health Security Act, which championed a community rating
system tied only to family size and geographical area.[3] The present New
York law, although narrower in scope, requires community rating, but
only for the sale of policies to individuals or to groups of between 3 and
50 individuals.[4] For those regulated transactions, it is illegal for the insurer to take into account, age, sex, health status, or occupation. Open
enrollment is a staple of the basic program: any individual, group member, or dependent "must be accepted at all times throughout the year for
any hospital and/or medical coverage offered by the insurer to individuals or small groups."[5] Other statutes of equally recent vintage follow the
same line.[6] Still others have adopted modified versions of community
rating plans that allow some, but not all, factors on the list to set premiums. Thus the New Jersey statute disregards age, sex, occupation, and
geographical location, but it takes into account health status.[7] Florida's
modified community rating system takes into account the "eligible
employee's and eligible dependents' gender, age, family composition,
tobacco use, or geographical location."[8]

The pure forms of community rating interfere far more powerfully with the ordinary underwriting practices than do the modified forms.
Any comprehensive assessment of these statutes would require a detailed
examination of how each variation works out in practice. For these purposes, however, it is most instructive to look to a standard form of community rating in order to assess its effects. The New York statute was

passed in 1993, and the early evidence confirms that its mandate creates the predicted cross-subsidies. The American Academy of Actuaries reports that "the young would subsidize the old, males would subsidize females at most ages, the healthy would subsidize the sick and the poor may subsidize the wealthy, since young people generally earn less income than older people."[9] Before the passage of the statute, going rates varied four- to sixfold for persons from age 20 to 64.[10] Under the statute, premium compression reduced top premiums by about 20 percent for 9 percent of the insured groups and 18 percent of the insured individuals. At the other end, 21 percent of the groups and 30 percent of the individuals received rate increases of up to 20 percent, with 5 percent over 100 percent. Many insureds dropped out of the pool altogether. Within a year of the program's operation, for example, the median age of policy holders under one insurer (Mutual of Omaha) rose by 3.5 years from 41.5 to 45 years old.[11] Nonetheless New York State Commissioner of Insurance Salvatore R. Curiale pronounced the program a success because of the protection it gave to individuals with bad claims histories seeking renewal.[12] Those forced to pick up the tab had a different view.

Standing alone, testimonials either way count for little because they are endemic to all subsidy situations. The ultimate test must look at the overall effects of the program. It is an undeniable good to help individuals in need. But, as the general theory indicates, coercive regimes that create positive rights contain substantial hidden costs that impair their effectiveness. First, the New York subsidy plan undercuts any rate distinction between employed and unemployed workers. Because firms can no longer capture the gains from keeping their workers in trim by taking aggressive health measures, they are less likely to insist on exercise, diet, or smoking restrictions.[13] To be sure, some incentives remain because the firms can still benefit from the improved productivity that good health brings to its work force, but even so, at the margin, the statute dulls this desirable effect. The sheer magnitude of the cross-subsidy—estimated at 44 billion dollars per year nationwide—not only reduces the profitability of the regulated firms, but also increases the rate of unemployment.[14] As the cost of keeping workers rises, some of them will be let go.

Community rating also alters the dominant patterns of individual behavior for the worse. Cross-subsidies necessarily allow everyone to pass off some part of the costs of their own risky behavior onto other persons.

Accordingly everyone is more likely to engage in riskier activities, whether driving faster or eating richer foods. The countless facets of life in which care is reduced make it very costly for a firm to monitor individual behavior. Overall the deterioration in care levels across the pool of insureds is a classic illustration of the prisoner's dilemma. Everyone takes less care than is ideal. Everyone undertakes riskier activities. The redistributive impulse brings in its wake higher overall system costs.

The long-term implications of community rating are also unnerving. A system of community rating cannot survive if all insurers must cover their insured risks solely from the premiums they collect. Yet the community rating system denies the insurer the right to refuse to write demanded coverage in an individual case simply because the premium does not cover the risk. Whether by design or by chance, some plans will be more heavily subscribed by individuals, perhaps because of the greater expertise in handling specific disabilities or diseases. Yet now an insurer develops expertise at its peril. Faced with the influx of high-risk patients, these specialized firms will go bankrupt if denied transfer payments from rival firms with superior books of business, or from the public treasury. Stated otherwise, the traditional pattern of risk-adjusted pricing must be preserved *as between* insurance carriers to keep the system running on an even keel in the long run.[15] The New York statute responds to this difficulty by allowing the Commissioner of Insurance "to promulgate regulations to assure an orderly implementation and ongoing operation of the open enrollment and community rating" systems established under the statute.[16] However, it offers no guidance on how to achieve that laudable objective. The battles over regulations necessarily drain off valuable resources that would be better devoted to patient care.

Nor do we have any reason to believe that community rating can operate within the previous systemwide budget constraints, such as they were. Compliance costs are not trivial and must be covered either from premiums or general revenues. The general fitness of members of the insurable pool is likely to deteriorate somewhat with cross-subsidies because of the reduced incentives for good health. In addition, calibrating any needed transfer payments between insurers will tax the political system when low-risk individuals are exiting the pool and high-risk individuals are clamoring to get in. The long-term prognosis is for systemwide instability. The short-term protection for high-risk individuals comes at an undisclosed systemwide price, part of which is paid by the intended beneficiaries of the program.

By what right are they kept in the program? One reason might be to counter the risk that some fraction of these low-risk individuals may choose to opt out in the belief that they will receive care in the event of extreme illness whether or not they purchased insurance. Thus one defense of universal coverage takes this form: "These free-riding individuals impose an external cost on others when they become ill and shift the costs of their care to others. They should be required to finance their care by obtaining the minimally required health insurance."[17] Yet the other, unspoken alternative is *not* to supply that care in time of necessity at public expense. If so, the alleged external cost disappears, even if some people die or are injured. Yet if that bad outcome happens more than once or twice, the inability to obtain the care in time of need will lead many young adults to think twice before going without health insurance—which they could purchase at low rates in a market not permeated by paternalism, coercion, and cross-subsidy. Social Darwinism is a bit too unfashionable in modern circles of thought. The constant collective unwillingness to bear the consequences of one's own decision only postpones the day when the well runs dry.

Coercion, then, is too often taken for granted. Yet, ironically, it is unclear whether the coercive strategy will work. Once low-risk persons are not allowed to switch, they will fight any expansions in insurance coverage. Or they might leave nonetheless, not by withdrawing from the plan while remaining within the state, but by leaving the state. Once coverage is mandatory, exit is the preferred option if the implicit tax from community rating overrides the benefits from staying put. For states with small boundaries, this exit option is serious both for the individual and the firm. A plant in the Boston area relocates to New Hampshire. An Illinois factory opens a branch in Indiana. Individual workers migrate across state boundaries. Worse still, in-migration of new firms and workers is deterred by the implicit tax. The size of these effects is hard to estimate, but don't think that they are necessarily small. State after state—California, Illinois, and New York to name three—worry about the impact on job creation of high payroll taxes for workers' compensation. The exit option effectively controls the level of state income taxation and has worked to knock out the estate tax. Don't think that it cannot happen here.

PRE-EXISTING CONDITIONS

ON THE FRONT BURNER

The question of pre-existing conditions closely relates to the issue of community rating. The two were linked together, for example, in the 1993 Clinton Health Security Act, which sought to ban both the exclusion of pre-existing conditions and the imposition of waiting periods before coverage took effect.[18]

Indeed, the recent passage of the Health Insurance Portability and Accountability Act (HIPAA) of 1996[19] deals with just this topic. The measure had received broad support on both sides of the political aisle. Its prolonged stay in political limbo turned solely over whether to couple its introduction with tax-deductible Medical Savings Accounts (MSAs), which give a tax subsidy for private savings to provide for future health care risks.[20]

These insurance reforms all gain their appeal from their apparent ability to increase both access to, and security of, long-term health coverage in a private market setting, even in the absence of any provider monopoly that might justify some form of common carrier regulation. It is ironic that Congress is now happy to introduce this major system of federal regulation on a grand scale while it balks at introducing the MSA programs on anything other than a highly limited experimental basis, even after some private employers have reported solid success using the concept. Some part of the appeal of mandated coverage lies in the uncritical belief that this exercise of government power does not displace or heavily regulate the provision of health care, as it did under Clinton's Health Security Act. Rather, the sanguine view is that government only guarantees the continued access of all individuals to health care in a private market, a far more modest form of interference.

The attractiveness of the new scheme depends implicitly on the distinction between direct government administration and indirect government regulation of health care markets. But that distinction is not, and should not be, regarded as categorical in either theory or practice. All forms of regulation limit the power of individuals to choose their associates and thus trench upon the right to exclude, one of the key incidents of ownership. Regulation over prices and association is both in theory and in fact an assertion of partial government ownership over private firms. The distinction between the operation and regulation approaches is of degree, not of kind. Creeping regulation blends into ownership. The absence of a clear demarcation between the one strategy and the other should counsel caution before starting down the regulatory path. On any view, therefore, these complex proposals require some close examination of their own, but before that can be usefully undertaken, I will first define the nature of the underlying problem and why it prompts so much frustration and debate.

THE MARKET RESPONSE

Suppose a ship sank at sea on January 1, 1997. On February 1, 1997, would its owner be allowed to purchase insurance against that known loss at rates that presupposed that the boat was still in productive use? Not unless the coverage equals the value of the loss, which is no insurance at all. A similar issue arises with pre-existing conditions. Here it may well be that they have not given rise to actual loss, but in some cases it is only a matter of time before they do so. In others, the future loss may not be certain, but the risk is surely heightened. In an unregulated market, insurers strive mightily to avoid making wagers that they have already lost or are sure to lose. The only question that they face is how best to prevent these risks from filling their book of business.

In an unregulated market, one standard response is for insurers to insist on full disclosure of all conditions that materially affect risk. In that setting, moreover, the firm does not have to rely solely on disclosure to protect its vital interests. To better protect itself (and its low-risk customers), the insurer could run its own tests to identify these conditions and to exclude from coverage individuals with serious conditions such as AIDS and Huntington's disease. In addition, it could protect itself by contract against having to pay for risks that had materialized before the purchase of the ostensible insurance coverage.[21] This provision guards against the obvious risk that a person will enroll in a heath plan on day one and then schedule major surgery for day two. But the standard clause also covers all situations in which a dangerous condition has been identified in any way within a 12-month interval prior to the effective coverage date. In the absence of legislation, clauses of this sort are generally held to deny coverage when symptoms are evident before the policy period, even though the precise diagnosis is only made afterwards.[22] Yet even here, some courts have allowed the principle to fray at the edges by applying the principle of contra proferentem—construe any ambiguous term in an insurance policy against the insured—to permit juries to award coverage on the shaky ground that treatment cannot be "for" a condition unless and until the correct diagnosis has already been made.[23] Similarly, most courts will enforce a waiver of the pre-existing conditions clause against an insurer, which can happen if the employee had full coverage from a prior employer.[24] No matter how these close cases are decided, it is critical to note that the standard clause is intended to *expand* the scope of coverage. Even for persons with pre-existing conditions, coverage under the standard clause is never denied for conditions that were asymptomatic and otherwise unknown when the contract took effect. In those cases, the moral hazard of insured misbehavior is not nearly so acute, so the insurer can profit by extending the coverage on fair rates. The purpose of the pre-existing condition clause is to insure the minimum conditions for contractual stability: namely, that all those parties to the contract are left better off ex ante than they were before.

This contractual exclusion of pre-existing conditions has been attacked on a number of grounds. One ground is that this rule makes insurance unavailable to certain key insureds, namely, those with the highest risk profile. But this objection misunderstands what is meant by availability of insurance. That charge has a certain cogency if insurers band together to restrict the competitive sale of the insurance product. And it certainly applies when the government decrees that certain forms of insurance should not be sold at all. But it is quite another thing to say that insurance is not available when there is no risk to insure in the first place, for now the fault, if such there be, lies not with the insurance market, but with the underlying social problem.

Suppose that it is known for certain that I will incur an obligation of $100,000 five years from now. That loss is important to me, but it is uninsurable no matter how many insurance companies operate in the market. No insurance policy will be written unless it promises gains to both the insurer and the insured. So long as the loss is certain to happen, there is no risk to insure. Any nominal "insurance" sold at market rates will simply be a prepayment plan, discounted down to present value, say, $70,000, in order to cover the anticipated loss. No matter how many firms are in the market, none will agree to cover the loss for less than that sum. The absence of the risk transforms the insurance company into a banker that borrows $70,000 to pay on a promise to pay $100,000 in five years.

Now suppose that this five-year obligation will with certainty lie in the range of $100,000 to $200,000. This is an insurable risk, but the premium rate includes a *fixed* premium of $70,000 for the guaranteed payment, plus some figure for the variable loss, a premium that would hover around $35,000 if the expected total payment on the appointed day was $150,000. Stated otherwise, insurance is possible only over the variance in expected outcomes. The example just given therefore is a combination of a loan to the insurance company plus an insurance contract. The individual who only wants insurance will only pay, as a first approximation, a $35,000 premium for a policy that contains a $100,000 deductible and a $100,000 limit. He will be unable to procure any insurance coverage for that first element of loss, even in a competitive market.

Many health expenditures have this characteristic. The effort to buy long-term nursing care has components of prepayment and genuine insurance. Thus the combined payment must be very high, and many individuals will simply prefer to save for the future on their own or through some form of tax-free annuity. The absence of a vibrant market for future nursing care is not a market failure. It is in part a recognition of the limited variation in future outcomes, coupled with a material risk that the early coverage will be purchased by the individuals more likely to use it.

Pre-existing conditions raise similar issues. Insurance is not available to cover these conditions because of the lack of variation in the underlying risk. No matter how competitive the market, the transaction is part prepayment and part insurance and should be priced accordingly. It is, however, wholly incorrect to suppose that some market failure justifies government intervention. Rightly understood, insurance availability is not an issue in this context, as it would be if a number of distinct sellers conspired to restrain sales in violation of the antitrust law. To the contrary, the key problem is the known shortage of wealth of the parties who face these certain losses or high levels of risk. If they do not have the wealth to cover the losses, they will not have the wealth to cover the risks.

CHERRY PICKING

Paul Starr, one of the most articulate architects of the Clinton plan has also attacked the restrictive coverage of pre-existing conditions as an unjustified "cherry pick" of the best risks.[25] In fact, the contractual logic operates the other way. No company ever makes a dime from the insurance policies it does not write. It only makes money from sales whose costs are lower than the premium received. The insurer loses an opportunity for profit if it excludes a person from coverage because of one condition. At some risk, it can make a profit by writing coverage on other risks to the person. Under the standard agreements, any person with the AIDS virus or Huntington's disease *can* still receive health insurance for an automobile accident or appendicitis. Providing partial coverage of persons with pre-existing conditions does not constrict the reach of the market; it extends that reach by offering limited protection to persons who otherwise would be wholly uninsurable.

Paradoxically, cherry picking will occur precisely because insurers are forced to cover pre-existing conditions at a standard premium. Because the insurer can no longer vary price, it has two choices. First, it could exit the market altogether, which it will do if the losing contracts are too onerous. Alternatively, it could remain in the market and seek to cut its losses by excluding by hook or by crook high-risk persons from coverage. Yet once the insurance carrier is allowed to adjust its premium levels, that incentive disappears. Now its self-interest could aggressively try to cover as many market segments as possible, *provided* that it knows that its contractual limitations will be fully enforced. But if the contractual protections are compromised, as by the intermittent application of a contra proferentem rule (under which ambiguous language is construed against an insurer), the insurer will once again find reasons for abandoning the market altogether, to the great detriment of its shareholders, employees, and low-risk customers.

BEHAVIORAL MODIFICATIONS

The standard criticisms of the present contractual regime also ignore the perverse incentives for individual risk management created by mandating coverage for pre-existing conditions. When pre-existing conditions can be excluded, potential insureds have a strong incentive to engage in prudent conduct from an early age, whether or not they purchase health insurance at that time. Individuals with no disability may gamble on staying healthy while going bare. Their plan is to save on premiums while young and to purchase the insurance at attractive rates with a clean bill of health later on. Alternatively they can purchase insurance while healthy to lock in protection against a not-yet-existing condition, thereby mooting the pre-existing condition problem. In the abstract, it is hard to decide which path promises the better result. Both, however, are more desirable than ignoring risks to future health with the knowledge that insurance (albeit of a very special kind) is always available no matter what happens in the interim. Prohibit the exclusion of pre-existing conditions and taking greater health risks becomes a more viable strategy. Any needed health insurance can be purchased just before the adverse consequences come home to roost—a private gain and a social loss.

In addition, as was the case with community rating, mandated coverage is likely to increase the frequency and severity of pre-existing conditions by some indeterminate amount. The standard moral hazard remains in place. In this new environment, individuals will prefer to bear the small fraction of the increased costs of insurance protection relative to the far larger fraction (close to 1) of the costs of accident and disease prevention that would otherwise fall their way. Thus, if insurance costs $100 and prevention costs $80, the rational self-insured individual will prefer to self-insure and save $20. But if he can purchase insurance at a pooled rate of $70, his private incentives change. He will now buy insurance at a net social loss of $20. Because prevention costs are not limited to medical services, they cannot be similarly socialized (so as reduce their total to $56, so that the ratio of insurance to prevention is unchanged) without inviting state domination of all aspects of human life. Accordingly we should expect some higher utilization of health services when pre-existing conditions are covered than when they are not. It is hard to guess exactly what the increase will be, but if conditions associated with drugs and alcohol abuse are included on the list, as they were in the general Clinton health plan,[26] the effects could be huge, not small. In this setting, too, the conflict between redistribution and production is not eliminated; it is just obscured.

GENETIC DISCRIMINATION

The objections to the insurer exclusion of pre-existing conditions often points to the distinctive problems of genetic discrimination. Genetic discrimination is usually defined as "discrimination directed against an individual or family based solely on an apparent or perceived genetic variation from the 'normal' human genotype."[27] There are some important quibbles with this definition. The use of "solely" in this context is probably too restrictive in light of the broader definitions of discrimination in employment and other contexts, which make discrimination unlawful if it is one of the substantial factors underlying a given decision. Putting 'normal' in quotation marks is yet another effort to undercut the soundness of the market practices by acting as though the stated grounds for distinction are themselves suspect. But for our purposes, the uneasiness is not with the marginal difficulties in defining and applying the concept; rather, it is with the operation of the basic rule in the context of the core cases to which it applies.

Straight-out cases of genetic discrimination should raise no special issues in principle.[28] The case for or against cross-subsides is in general no greater here than in any other area, so long as we accept that A's need, no matter how great, is never a source of B's legal (as opposed to moral or charitable) obligation. Nonetheless, the subject is often thought to be an urgent illustration of the inequities of excluding coverage for pre-existing conditions for two related reasons. First, because these characteristics are inherited, they are less likely to be influenced by behavior and more likely to form part of the background for any given disease, often through no fault of the insured individual. Second, modern testing in principle allows both individuals and insurers to identify these conditions in advance of illness far more reliably than was possible by piecing together scattered bits of family genetic histories.

True to form, the hostility toward market insurance and private discrimination reaches its academic zenith in the view that insurers should be precluded from using these genetic tests to set rates or determine coverage. More forcefully perhaps than with other pre-existing conditions, genetic discrimination is said to stigmatize certain individuals and to dignify the base and irrational prejudices that others harbor against people born with certain inescapable disabilities.[29] The entire thought progression shows how completely the theory of social insurance replaces the traditional norm of required disclosure with a new norm of protected concealment. This new development has yet to take complete control in practice, and it should not. The status quo should be preserved and protected.

To see the magnitude of the proposed policy shift, we should ask what happens when the common law norm of full disclosure is applied to these concealed medical risks. Today routine tests allow for the reliable identification of the AIDS virus and for Huntington's disease[30]—one inherited and the other not. Wholly apart from insurance matters, many individuals face the wrenching decision of whether or not to be tested for a genetic condition that could turn out to be fatal. Taken as a matter of individual choice, the subject is one that the collective we should not attempt to influence one way or the other. It is a hard choice to know whether the possibility of a clean bill of health is strong enough to override the fear that the tests will communicate a death sentence at some uncertain future date.

Yet the most controversial issues in genetic testing involve the relationship between the person with the affliction and other institutions. Here the common proposals insist that testing be voluntary and that all results be kept confidential, out of the hands of the organizations and groups with whom that person might choose to do business.[31] That rule is fine for the individual tester, but once again it imposes external costs on others. Without the disclosure norm, some individuals (in part out of desperation and fear) will privately test for these diseases. If they test positive, they can then purchase large amounts of health (and life) insurance at standard rates and thus reap an enormous windfall from the general population. If the tests are negative, they can decline to purchase insurance or buy less. The stakes are large and the potential for selection bias enormous. In the long run, the practice could impose serious losses, if not bankruptcy, on the insurance industry if it must pay for the increased disabilities for which it cannot collect premiums.

These incentive and moral hazard arguments are not irrelevant to genetic defects. Even though these condition are certain to manifest themselves, an individual could heavily influence the time at which a latent condition will turn active. Consider, for example, the relationship between diet and diabetes or between exercise and heart disease. The timing and severity of most genetic risks remain subject to individual control. Even for those risks that are not, should individuals have legal claims against others who are in no sense responsible for their conditions? Should the fellow workers of a given employee be required to provide the subsidy for that employee's deadly diseases? And how should the size of any such subsidy be determined? Any case for redistribution must impose a societal obligation, not one directed exclusively at the workers within a given firm. It is difficult to fashion any moral case for holding healthy individuals to greater obligations simply because they share the same employer as a group of highly susceptible individuals.

By the same token, we can anticipate fierce resistance to the candid assumption of any public obligation to provide health insurance for persons with pre-existing conditions. A system of regulation loads the subsidy onto a set of insurance companies. The public pays only indirectly, by a reduction in tax receipts from the regulated insurers. Shareholders pick up the rest of the obligation. The identical subsidy could be funded out of general tax revenues. It only requires the government to pay insurers a sum that makes it worth their while to insure high-risk patients with known conditions at standard market rates. But this outcome will not happen at the federal level, given our eternal preoccupation with annual deficits, driven in substantial measure by runaway medical expenses. It is even less likely to happen at the state level, where the pressures to run redistribution off budget are, if anything, stronger than at the federal level. Not only does regulation generally shift costs from taxpayers generally to insurers, employers, and fellow employees, but regulation also ships a part of the cost out of state—a temptation that local voters and local politicians find it impossible to resist. Simply requiring all redistribution to be funded from general revenues offers no panacea to the question of government redistribution. It has done little to halt the massive growth of Medicare at the federal level. In this context, it is at least a start because it might supply some reality check on the public appetite for redistribution by more closely aligning the people who support the program with those who must pay for it. In a more sober constitutional environment, off-budget redistribution would be off limits, but not in our legal system. The problem of redistribution through regulation is hardly unique to health insurance. It arises, for example, with rent control programs, which, with barely a murmur of constitutional protest, impose the burden of this ill-conceived subsidy on the landlord instead of the public at large.[32] Those pressures are every bit as great in the health area. We can be confident that regulation will dominate over taxation in this area precisely because it is the covert and inefficient means of redistribution.

THREE'S COMPANY

The downside of requiring health insurance to cover pre-existing conditions should by now be evident, but the flip side of the problem also deserves attention. It is often said that requiring coverage of these conditions is justified not only for redistributive purposes, but also to promote the efficiency the overall job market in ways that fragmented competitive firms cannot.[33] The problem—and it *is* a problem—can arise when unemployed persons cannot obtain jobs because of their known medical risks. It could simply arise from a change in insurance carrier without a change in employment. Most critically, it also arises when employed persons cannot take a better job because of the forfeiture of current insurance for pre-existing conditions.

The ideal scenarios in these cases are not hard to outline. In the first case, it is better for people to be on the payroll than not. In the second case, it is better for the new insurer to assume the same risks as the prior carrier. In the third case, it is better for the worker to take a new job. Overall, it is worth promoting the free mobility of labor and the free substitution of insurance carriers—the very goals frustrated by any employee-based system of mandated health insurance.

It is, however, a mistake to posit any causal relationship between contractual freedom in health insurance and unwanted rigidity in labor markets. In the first case, excluding health coverage for pre-existing conditions does not prevent people from entering the work force. As noted earlier, it helps them to enter, albeit with partial coverage. To the extent that they are better off with a job and some insurance than with no job and no insurance, excluding coverage imposes no real barrier to entry into the labor force. A complication arises only if unemployed individuals, on taking a job, lose more comprehensive health benefits supplied to them under Medicaid. This situation is no different from one where high welfare benefits deter persons from taking low-paying jobs. In both cases, the unfortunate incentive effects should be chalked up as another hidden cost of a welfare system, with its inherent tendency to induce unemployment. It is not attributable to markets as such.

The situation is more complicated when a second insurance carrier is asked to take over the coverage of the prior insured. But even here, a market solution is possible if it makes economic sense for the second insurer takes over the contingent liabilities of the previous carrier. The premium for that added risk need not come from the insured, but it could be paid by the current carrier, which is now excused from liability for these pre-existing conditions. So long as the second carrier is in a better position to monitor the risk, everyone should win.

The third situation—where workers shift jobs—is at once the most important and the most ticklish. The initial reaction should be one of puzzlement: why is there any problem at all? The limitations on insuring pre-existing conditions are commonplace in insurance contracts, but these would not survive in an unregulated environment if the inefficiency is as pronounced as the critics urge. So long as the illness does not get worse with the job shift, the job shift produces an overall net benefit that the employee should be able to share with both his present and his future employer. This transaction presents no obvious externalities or informational barriers, so what then explains the present market rigidities? A first stab at an answer is that the new hiring only makes sense for the second firm if it does not have to assume the costs of treating the new employee's known condition. If the new job promises additional productivity gains of $5,000 but costs the new employer $10,000 in higher insurance, the deal will fall through. Socially, however, the $10,000 loss to the second firm is offset by the $10,000 gain to the present employer who would be released from its health obligation if the employee quits. Socially the shift still makes sense.

So why doesn't the switch take place? More concretely, because transaction costs are low, why not arrange for a three-cornered deal where the present employer (or its insurer) agrees to pay the prospective employer (or its insurer) a fixed sum of money for that second firm to assume the potential liabilities of the current insurer. That transaction will require both firms to estimate the anticipated costs of honoring existing obligations. But cost calculations of that sort are not normally insuperable: even today firms must often set reserves against such contingent liabilities. If so, a market response could allow the job shift without incurring all the costs of regulation. To be sure, the assignment may be risky before the patient settles on a course of treatment of a known condition: the second insurer will fear that the employee has already opted for the most expensive form of treatment, for which it will have to exact full compensation. Nor is it likely that the assumption of liability will make sense where intensive treatment is indicated. Individuals who are undergoing active chemotherapy are not likely to assume the added burdens of a new job. But in many cases of serious but stable conditions, some assumption of liability should be possible.

Another way to look at the transaction is for the employee to purchase insurance against future disability in his *initial* insurance contract.[34] The basic plan calls for an initial purchase price with two components: the cost of care for the initial period, and an additional sum—call it a severance payment—sufficient to fund the purchase of a second insurance policy for the next period in the event that some dangerous condition is detected during the initial policy period. That severance payment can then be spent to renew the policy with the original carrier at the higher rate of insurance or to purchase a new policy from a different carrier covering another employer. It is not necessary for the original carrier to specialize in high-risk insureds, but it is necessary for some organized market to make accurate risk classifications for persons with identifiable conditions: there must be a secondary market, for example, for persons who are HIV positive or at risk for the onset of diabetes within the next period. That market also must feature unregulated rates because if its prices are kept below their true cost, the scheme will break down. The severance payment will be large enough to cover the regulated price, but the employee in the second period will find no insurer who will write the risk at a loss. Thus, suppose the severance payment equals $1,000 when the cost of insurance for the known condition is $1,500. No second-tier insurer will enter that market for the glory of assuming a $500 loss. The system is only viable, therefore, if the initial severance payment is set equal to the anticipated cost of coverage in the second-tier market, or $1,500.

This long-term market has not yet emerged, even though it is a common commercial practice for one insurer to pay. An excess carrier may receive a substantial payment from the primary carrier to assume the risk of environmental or product liability. One possible culprit may be regulation. Long-term contracts are required, but some statutes forbid insurance contracts whose duration is more than a single year.[35] Insurers could well fear that the government will then alter the terms of severance or renewal. One scenario is that the obligation will be treated as binding on the insurer, but not on the employer, who can be awarded a refund on that portion of the premium that covers the reinsurance risk. A decision of that sort could transform a long-term contract into the familiar heads-I-win-tails-you-lose proposition, which would lead to an evaporation of the market. To combat that risk, all relevant jurisdictions must reaffirm the sanctity of the original contract, which is not an easy task in an age in which the presumption of freedom of contract operates at a low ebb.

The more optimistic explanation is that these contracts do not appear because of high transaction costs. If so, the original judgment that the market is inefficient must be modified. It may well be inefficient relative to some ideal standard, as is all government activity. Rather, the current situation with reduced job mobility is efficient in the weaker, but socially relevant, sense in that the costs of correcting a market imbalance are higher than the cost of that imbalance itself. But even if this transaction cost story is correct, it hardly follows that regulation should force transactions that do not make sense for the parties. The refusal to allow firms to limit the coverage that they supply to workers will reduce their willingness to hire unknown workers and in its own way can hamper the very job mobility that it seeks to promote. As ever, the costs of regulation are hidden and hard to quantify. And once again they are real.

STATUTORY INTERVENTIONS

State Law Words of protest notwithstanding, pre-existing conditions have become a more common target for regulation at the state level. Thus the 1993 New York insurance law reform illustrates the difficult and uncertain course that has to be followed. The Clinton health plan, for all its length and complexity, was far too short for responding to the perils of either community rating or pre-existing conditions.

The basic purpose of the New York statute is to permit potential insureds to obtain coverage for a pre-existing condition from a new insurance carrier, which must accept the individual and family dependents that fall into a coverage group. But unlike the Clinton program, the New York legislation did not stop with the simple categorical requirement of coverage. It introduced complex mechanisms to protect the solvency of insurers under the new requirements. That statute does not cover individuals seeking individual coverage, where the risks of self-selection are too high, but it does cover any individual who applies for groups between 3 and 50 persons.[36] The first version of the statute provided that coverage had to be made available under the second policy so long as the coverage dovetailed with the first policy. The statute did not take into account the possibility that the coverage provisions of that second policy might supply benefits more generous than the policy it replaced, and thus it created a clear invitation for individuals to shift coverage to increase benefits levels or to acquire new coverage when older limits were exhausted.

In time, a statutory modification cured the first of these problems by requiring that the second policy be issued only on terms substantially similar to those of previous policy,[37] without explicitly addressing the problem of exhaustion of limitations. In addition, the New York statute allows an insured at most a basic 12-month waiting period before acquiring the new coverage.[38] But it also promptly credits against that waiting period any length of time that the insured had coverage under the previous policy (including any waiting period before that coverage was granted), so long as the gap between policies does not exceed 60 days. These rules apply even if the insured had received medical attention for the identical problem under the last policy.[39] A special section was added to the statute to require the issuance of "non-cancelable disability insurance" to women whose breast cancer had been diagnosed more than three years prior to her application, so long as her physician certifies that the cancer has not recurred.[40] Finally, the statute contains global provisions designed to allow the superintendent to promulgate regulations that promote insurance stability with both open enrollment and community rating.[41] The bottom line: any person with continuous coverage for the previous 12 months will have no interruption in coverage with the change in jobs.

This statute itself imposes a complex administrative apparatus, complete with a system of rate regulation, designed to control the very forces that it has unleashed. It is far from clear that its layers of countermeasures adequately blunt the opportunities for strategic shifts that arise when coverage cannot be refused. The simple objection is that the statute requires firms to take risks whose expected costs are far higher than the premium in question, and then it trusts that they will make up the shortfall from the rest of their book of business, which is itself subject to erosion from price competition. The size of the losses imposed depends on the effectiveness of the waiting periods and on the willingness to allow general rate increases to offset the particular shortfall. Yet even if insurance carriers survive the new spate of regulation, its wisdom is far from assured given the collateral dislocations that it brings about. As with other regimes of positive rights, the effort to place everyone in the lifeboat increases the risk that the lifeboat will sink.

Federal Law   The Americans with Disability Act[42] (ADA) also contains complex provisions squarely directed at inquiries and examinations directed toward the discovery of pre-existing conditions. The statutory tightrope stipulates that an employer "shall not conduct a medical examination or make inquiries of a job applicant as to whether such applicant is an individual with a disability or as to the nature and severity of such disability,"[43] but in the next breath allows "preemployment inquiries into the ability of the applicant to perform job-related functions,"[44] without explaining how the second task can be accomplished without violating the basic prohibition. Surely some employers will opt to make no inquiries at all, lest they run afoul of the law. But if all sources of information dry up, the costs of hiring all workers increases, to the detriment of sick and healthy alike.

It is also debatable whether the statutory prohibitions can wall off an employer from information about the disabilities of a prospective employee. In particular, the ADA does not address squarely the possibility that a healthy worker will volunteer complete information about his medical history precisely because he knows that an impaired rival cannot follow suit. If that becomes common practice, one unresolved question is whether the employer has made an "implied inquiry" given an evident unwillingness to hire persons who do not come forward with these declarations. Should the practice continue, an amended legal regime no doubt will become more coercive by prohibiting any *truthful* disclosures of good health as well. The circle of prohibition would thus grow from nondisclosure to required silence for the benefit of a third party. Once again the statute seeks to deny parties the information that is necessary for the operation of efficient markets.

The situation, however, is more complex because a disabled employee may want both to reveal and to conceal information, albeit for different purposes. The ADA thus partitions the use of medical information, making it unavailable at the initial hiring, while preserving it under wraps until needed for diagnosis and treatment. Accordingly no medical examination is allowed before employment is offered, but one may be required thereafter if two conditions are satisfied. First, the examination has to be conducted on all employees if it is to be conducted on any—nondiscrimination again.[45] It is as though we must drill an obligatory dry well to prospect for oil. This ADA provision thus satisfies the legal but not the economic definition of discrimination by sanctioning a system whose formal incidence is equal but which yields disparate economic returns. Second, the ADA now provides that the information gathered from the examination be placed in a confidential file, access to which is limited to cases where managers need to learn of necessary restrictions on employment or to discharge first aid and safety functions.[46] Otherwise the information remains dead to the employer on matters of job assignment, promotion, and transfer. The basic litmus test is to reveal the information if it benefits employee health or safety, but not otherwise.

It is questionable whether these strictures can achieve their stated end. For workers with patent defects, the question of concealment is quite impossible. Deaf, blind, and crippled persons cannot benefit from the provision that might prove of some assistance to diabetics and perhaps epileptics. And persons with latent but manageable defects might prefer to keep them hidden lest the wall break down such that the information is used covertly on matters of promotions and assignments. Leakage in the information bucket is likely in most situations to undermine the effectiveness of the scheme.

Yet even where the insurance market remains viable, this system of partial disclosure will induce firms to adopt other strategies to cut their losses so long as concealment is treated as an employee birthright and not an employer peril. First, we should expect to see a trend toward higher wage and salaried workers. When workers have better health and higher productivity, the employer wins both ways. Furthermore, more offices and plants will tend to locate at a distance from the inner city, where these risks (along with others) are perceived as greater. We should also see an intensification in the trend to substitute independent contractors for employees. The independent contractor works on a short-term basis for so many different employers that none is likely to bear the sting of the ADA. Social security supplies the necessary clue: the independent contractor pays his own, and the same legal regime applies for insurance and medical benefits as well. Lost in the undertow are healthy persons who have reduced opportunities for obtaining traditional health benefits. But no hard-pressed employer will take those consequences into account. Workers will be shed at the cost of some organizational efficiency in order to deflect the greater regulatory burden.

The remaining employees should likewise experience some downswing in the "neutral" insurance packages they receive. Because employers cannot exclude certain diseases and disabilities by name, they will cut back coverage across the board to control costs. Workers will suffer some reduction in wages (or smaller increases) to offset the ADA's mandated costs. Plans will be tailored to increase insurance copayments and deductibles and, most importantly, to place sharper limits on the amount of catastrophic coverage that is available. Once again, the costs will be split between employer and healthy coworkers. Finally, firms will continue to shift from investments in human capital to investments in plant, equipment, and other machinery, as the cost of labor increases relative to that of equipment. At this point, the ADA's prohibition against disability discrimination should be seen for what it is—an elaborate set of cross-subsidies that reduces the total level of social wealth as it transfers wealth between parties.

This entire system should provoke an uneasy social response. The usual refrain about employment markets is that they function poorly because of the imperfect information that each side has about the intentions and capabilities of the others. For that ailment, the appropriate remedy is a *disclosure* statute that neutralizes the games so frequently played when parties have imperfect and asymmetrical information. But the ADA marches labor and insurance law in exactly the opposite direction by making information a near-forbidden commodity. It is at most only a tad harsh to say that the ADA licenses concealment of information that one party knows the other party will regard as material. From that melancholy observation, it is but a short leap to the obvious tension between the distributional goals of the ADA and the common law prohibition against fraud, which has long covered concealment and many cases of nondisclosure.

There is surely something amiss in yet another system of positive rights whose implementation comes at so high a cost. An alternative approach would allow the employer freely to demand the information and require the state to pay some additional sum of money to compensate the employer for the disability in question, much as the state can pay insurance companies to cover at standard rates the additional risks for high-risk populations. The obvious disadvantage of the compensation system is the inability to price the dislocations to the firm that has to hire workers with disabilities. Some losses to productivity are direct and perhaps easily measurable, but many derive from impediments that disabled workers impose on coworkers, or from the special but "reasonable" accommodations in plant and equipment now required by statute.

The unworkable nature of this compensation formula should lead us to rethink the use of coercive techniques to respond to workplace disabilities.[47] A simpler and more sensible approach combines subsidy with markets by substituting the carrot for the stick. Now the state makes grants to firms for making their premises handicap accessible and for hiring specified numbers and types of disabled workers. This grant alternative tends to concentrate disabled workers in a few firms and thus runs against the mainstream objectives of many ADA supporters. But their passion is driven by the sense that their rights cannot be compromised by the costs imposed on other individuals. Yet here the demands are constrained by scarcity, and the size of the budget, as set by the political system, can determine the number of grants and hence the concentration of disabled workers. The object is to create "transparent budgets" so that the public gains more reliable information on the size of the subsidies it creates than it does from a regulatory program whose full cost is concealed under the rhetoric of rights. The choice between hidden and public subsidies, between hidden and public taxes, is central to the operation of a responsible democracy, even one committed to redistribution. The difficulty with these programs, however, has not led to a lack of innovation in this area, as the recent Clinton administration initiatives reveal.

The Second Clinton Initiative   Notwithstanding the decidedly mixed performance at the state level, "portable" coverage for pre-existing conditions has retained its political allure even after the demise of the 1993 Clinton Health Security Act, discussed at length in Chapter 8. The scope of this new proposed federal intrusion should be evident even from a short and incomplete summary of the contents of the newly minted Health Insurance Portability and Accountability Act (HIPAA), whose central operative provision states, in no uncertain terms, that no insurer to a group health plan can choose to decline coverage or set rates for the plan or its members based on health status, medical condition, claims experience, receipt of health care, medical history, evidence of insurability (including conditions arising out of medical violence) or disability of a participant or beneficiary."[48] Elements relevant to the accurate pricing of risk are thus systematically excluded from view.

The initial contract would not, of course, guarantee permanent coverage, so HIPAA also requires that all coverage be renewed except for a limited class of reasons, such as nonpayment of premium, that is non-correlated with the risks assumed by the insured or the profitability of the account in previous years.[49] Likewise, a program that requires any insurer to take new groups indefinitely is not sustainable, so HIPAA also contains provisions that guarantee availability of coverage to all small groups within the state unless the insurer can show that it did not have the financial capacity to shoulder the additional burdens.[50] The obvious import is to make sure that decisions to take or to reject business are without discrimination on any of the many grounds forbidden in the earlier part of HIPAA. To make those provisions stick, HIPAA then notes that once a firm decides to withdraw from this market (as it well might), it must wait five years before it can once again market group health plans in any state where the firm has decided not to keep or renew its portfolio of business.[51] No strategic withdrawals would be allowed.

Similar restrictions apply to the portability of individual coverage between health plans. Once again the fundamental provision states that any individual who was once a member of a group health plan would be entitled to receive individual coverage without regard to that person's health status, medical condition, claims experience, receipt of health care, medical history, evidence of insurability, or disability.[52] By analogy to rules for group health coverage, full insurance also must be offered to individuals who have previously been enrolled in a health plan for the previous 12 months.[53] The pre-existing conditions of a new enrollee may be excluded from coverage for at most 12 months, and that period is reduced "by one month for each month in which the participant or beneficiary" has received coverage from some other employer.[54]

If all the theoretical arguments in favor of the voluntary response to pre-existing conditions are correct, this program is likely to create more dislocations than it causes for precisely the reasons identified earlier. The obvious gains from the program will be there: some individuals will be able to either obtain or keep coverage that they would otherwise be denied. And it is pointless to argue that any great social program could ever pass unless it created some net benefits for some portion of society. But it is important not to be carried away with the rhetoric of aspiration when it is clear that mandating access carries with it collateral consequences that are undesired by even the strongest proponents of the present program. We do have experience with other misadventures, some popular and some aborted, which reflect on the larger social enterprise of securing access to health care. Both the Medicare program and the 1993 Clinton Health Security Act have dangers attributable to many causes. Chief among them is the penchant for hidden subsidies and the massive dislocations they cause—all the subject of the next two chapters.

CHAPTER 7

❖ ❖ ❖

Medicare: The Third Rail
of American Politics

THE OPTIMISM OF DAYS PAST

The debate over the rights of access to health care has taken place on at least three levels. The first attacks the problem as a matter of legal or moral theory. The second examines particular programs introduced to remedy observed defects in the basic system. The insurability of pre-existing conditions and institutional obligation to provide emergency care fall into this group. The third, and largest, topic is the comprehensive provision of health care to, if not all individuals, then to large groups of them. To most people, access to health care focuses exclusively on this question.

Medicare tops any list of large-scale health care programs. The system is enormous in both size and popularity, at least among its 37 million beneficiaries. Until recently, its political support as a program has proved quite invulnerable, and even the extensive and often acrimonious debates of 1995 and 1996 produced few if any important changes in either its set of entitlements or its revenue sources. It has been said more than once that Medicare is the third rail of American politics: "touch it, and you die." Yet martyrdom for some political figures may be the only viable alternative to the massive insolvency that looms on the horizon. The hospital insurance trust fund is estimated to run out of money by 2001 if not sooner, depending on the pessimism (or realism) of our working assumptions. The payments for physician services continue to escalate out of control. So although the Clintoncare invitation for universal coverage for all Americans could be, and was, declined without upsetting the status quo, Medicare raises much more stark choices for there is no place to hide. To be sure, its entitlements are politically vested, but they are also legally and economically precarious. Any legislative reform, driven by looming budget realities, will defeat the most entrenched expectations of its participants. The current program is not sustainable in the long term; yet none of the plausible fixes has proved to be politically salable. Today many third rails run in parallel. Before this saga runs its course, Congress may not be able to leap across them all.

It was not always thus. Medicare was first established in 1965 in a spirit of buoyant optimism typical of the carefree days of Lyndon Johnson's Great Society.[1] In the 1964 elections, Democrats had obtained 2 to 1 majorities in both houses of Congress, and Johnson linked forces with his liberal wing to defeat the depleted coalition of Republicans and conservative Democrats. His original proposal covered only hospitalization, but the response of the medical profession was to expand the bill by including payment for physician services to senior citizens. The collective judgment of the profession preferred the long-term injection of funds into its coffers to the hazy risk of long-term regulation, which came to roost some 15 years later. I can still recall my fiercely independent physician-father railing against Medicare on the ground that over time he who pays the piper calls the tune. But too few shared his apocalyptic vision. Hospitalization was combined with physician services, and Medicaid, the state-administered program of assistance for the indigent, was thrown in for good measure. Many proponents saw the initial expansion as only the first large step down the path to universal health care. If the elderly and poor came first, children would surely follow, and finally the entire population. If universal coverage was a good thing for some segments of the population, universal coverage for all would be so much better.

Even a cursory examination of Medicare's legislative history should leave the wistful reader with a powerful sense of the Nirvana that never came to pass. The Senate Report on Medicare, conscious of contemporary critics, stressed the actuarial soundness and solvency of Medicare's two key components—the Hospital Insurance (HI) of Part A and the Supplemental Medical Insurance (SMI) of Part B. In a section devoted to the Actual Cost Estimates for the Hospital Insurance System, the Senate Report repeatedly and fervently affirmed that "the committee very strongly believes that the tax schedule in the law should make the hospital insurance system self-supporting over the long range as nearly can be foreseen, as well as actuarially sound."[2] The Report then emphasized the "conservative estimates of cost" used to secure that result.[3] Testimony given at the hearings suggested that these statements were unduly optimistic, even when they were made, because the cost estimates of earlier failed Medicare proposals had already been shown to be substantially inadequate.[4] The projections found in the Report do not match well with the actual performance:[5]

YEAR	HI ESTIMATES*	HI EXPENDITURES*	DIFFERENCE
1966	1,037	999	-3.7%
1970	2,946	5,281	79.3%
1975	4,168	11,581	177.9%
1980	5,466	25,577	367.9%
1985	7,066	48,414	585.2%
1990	9,061	66,997	639.4%

* In millions of dollars

The 1965 Senate Report took a similar position for the SMI program. "The committee has recommended the establishment of a supplementary medical insurance program that can be voluntarily elected, on an individual basis by virtually all persons aged 65 and over in the United States. . . . This program is intended to be completely self-supporting from the contributions of covered individuals and from equal-matching contributions from the general fund of the Treasury,"[6] initially set at $6 per month per subscriber, divided equally between subscriber and the treasury. Once again the Report described the costs assumptions behind the program as "conservative." Indeed the Senate Report reiterated its confidence that "the $6 total per capita income of the system . . . will be fully adequate to meet the costs of administration and the benefit payments incurred, as well as to build up a relatively small contingency plan." The initial projections for this program were made for only a two-year period because the premiums charged for the service could be revised freely in subsequent years, making future predictions harder to make—a difficulty that persists to this very day. Although the projections were not made, the promise of the even division between beneficiary fees and general revenue contributions was not kept. The original 50/50 split between government and private contributions quickly altered so that by 1975 the private contribution was down to about 44 percent, and by 1980 it had dropped below 30 percent. Today it hovers just over 25 percent.

The legislative history contains one instructive tension that gives some hint of its future travail. The program was to be self-funding on the one hand, but eligibility for participation was based on current status, not past contributions. A similar ambiguity surrounded the start of social security, which gave its first generation of enrollees benefits that far exceeded the meager contributions they made to the plan, while casting the burdens on later generations.[7] Medicare took the same posture with its target population. Extending coverage "has been done, of course, with the knowledge that the current beneficiaries on the rolls have not made contributions specifically for the increased benefits or for the new benefits then being provided. Of course, this means that the benefits going to the already-retired group represent in a sense an 'unfunded' liability which has to be met out of future contributions."[8] From the outset, therefore, long-term plan stability required some extra contributions from general revenues or future plan recipients, or both. But no transitional shortfall can explain the precarious financial situation years later. For a program to misfire as badly as Medicare has done, some major design error has to be identified, not only in its original elaboration, but also in its subsequent transformation and administration.

THE SEEDS OF DESTRUCTION

And errors there are. The key mistaken assumption about Medicare, so common to all major legislative innovations, is directed to what might be termed the political half-life of the program. Statutes that are made by politics can be remade by politics in the absence of constitutional restraints. The cost and utilization estimates on Medicare all assumed that subsequent generations would not amend the basic program in ways that compromised its financial soundness. There was little awareness that the half-life of its entitlements was far greater than the half-life of the correlative structural limitations. Rather the legislators tacitly acted as though the two elements extended in parallel for the foreseeable future.

The pattern of justification articulated in the Senate Report echoed themes in the debates over the 1964 Civil Rights Act, which had just been passed a year before.[9] That statute was also promoted as a "mild and moderate" measure directed at two unexceptionable targets: Jim Crow in the South and explicit discriminatory behavior in both North and South. Every objection about the overreach of the program was met with an amendment designed to satisfy the doubters: professional testing was permissible; bona fide occupational qualifications were allowed; pensions could be actuarially based on sex; intention and motive, not effect, were the keys to liability; preferential treatment on the basis of race was not required or permitted; employers were not responsible for the differential skill levels of applicants; and, sexual harassment was not so much as a faint blip on the horizon.[10]

Over the next decade, the political culture and judicial decisions reduced the early compromises to distant memories. The Civil Rights Act became far more intrusive and powerful than even its supporters had hoped at the time of its passage. No longer could the nation be content with hitting the obvious targets; now all forms of pervasive and unconscious attitudes on race and sex had to be rooted out. Once launched, the Act legitimated a new civil rights establishment within government, within business, and within the bar. The passage of the Act altered the political balance and thus ushered in the age of further expansion. To protest the set of "horribles" at the birth of the legislation would have been castigated as fear-mongering or worse. To protest the changes in result thereafter was to reopen a debate that had already been closed: the basic principles of the law were firmly established, the only open questions went to its political implementation. The expansion of the statute from disparate treatment to disparate impact cases; the repudiation of the color-blind principle in the name of voluntary affirmative actions; the extended coverages for age, for pregnancy, and for disability all came within the mantle of the original movement. The moral of the story is to introduce any major program in stages: start with the program and accept any limitation necessary to secure passage and then bore away the limitations from within.

A similar political dynamic has overtaken Medicare. The original program was laced with caveats and reeked prudence from every pore.

But once in place, the program's scope could be expanded by regulations and amendments designed to fulfill its basic commitments. New classes of beneficiaries could be added to the rolls, most notably under the disability program added in 1973; new formulas for payment could be introduced, most notably to expand the taxpayer share for the reimbursement of physician services; new coverages could follow from administrative deliberation; new tax increases could be imposed—23 during the 30 years after the passage of the program; and new expectations could lift Medicare to a near-sacred Social Compact between the generations. Just as water flows downhill, so power and rhetoric move in one direction only. Grand programs expand inexorably—at least until they crash.

Medicare is doubly explosive because of the intrinsic boldness of its enterprise. The most elementary concern with economies of scale—with programs that grow less efficient as they become larger—should stand center stage. Medical care is not like power and light. It cannot be justified as a way to contain the excessive pricing of a natural monopolist. In fact, the system itself introduces government monopoly into the provision of medical care—a monopoly that does not erode with time or new technologies. The problems inherent with natural monopoly are, if anything, greater when the monopoly is of government origin. Why believe that any single provider can master the venture, especially when plagued by weak feedback systems? No isolated group at the center can match the sensitivity about costs and benefits that decentralized competitive markets can generate. Yet, oblivious to this peril, Medicare simply establishes a list of benefits and a set of corresponding prices. Because no list is self-defining, the process invites ceaseless lobbying efforts by vendors aching to place their goods and services on the approved list.[11] With reflection, Medicare establishes a single-payer monopoly for large parts of the health care market—a perfect microcosm of a command and control economy. These structural defects should have been obvious at Medicare's birth. The heady political economy of the 1960s, however, did not scrutinize new uses in state power; it basked in their reflected glory. This carefree equilibrium has come unglued over time. To mark the transition, it is unnecessary to rely on general speculation when we can closely examine Medicare's two basic programs: the Hospital Insurance package and the somewhat misnamed Supplementary Medical Insurance.[12]

PART A: HOSPITAL INSURANCE

THE ORIGINAL PLAN

The Hospital Insurance (HI) portion of the program is funded solely by a payroll tax levied on employers and employees (including the self-employed). These charges have increased steadily over time. The 1966 rates for the HI payroll tax was 0.35 percent each on employers and employees, capped on incomes up to $6,600 per year, for a maximum payment of $46.20 per year. No taxes were imposed on self-employed persons. By January 1, 1994, the rates reached 1.45 on both employers and employees, and 2.9 on self-employed persons, capped at incomes of $135,000 per person, for a maximum contribution of $3,915 per year on a broader base of workers. Inflation could account only for an increase of about $200 per year from the original base. As of January 1, 1994, the earnings cap was removed so that the 2.9 percent tax applies to all earned income. Thus, for high income earners, the Medicare hospitalization tax exceeds their basic social security payments. The heavy taxes imposed on workers today are not set aside in separate accounts to fund their future health care expenses. Rather they are turned over the United States Treasury in exchange for treasury securities that can be redeemed when funds are needed to pay HI bills. The Medicare payroll funds are thus commingled with general tax revenues and spent when received. The "assets" in the trust fund, therefore, are no more than promises from the United States that it will use *future* tax revenues to replace money already spent on *prior* Medicare obligations.[13] The program is less a trust fund and more a Ponzi scheme. Although its nominal balances peaked at $130 billion dollars in 1995, that nominal excess will be spent down rapidly over the next seven to ten years if current practices are continued.[14]

The government does not spend HI revenues directly. Rather, in the spirit of public/private partnerships, they fund Participation Agreements with various "providers of services," including hospitals, skilled nursing facilities, home health care services, and hospice programs.[15] The definition of home services is statutory: it includes part-time or intermittent nursing care (normally under 28 hours, but up to 35 hours per week with medical need); physical, occupational, and speech therapy; and medical social services, supplies, and equipment. The coverage does not include drugs, housekeeping, or transportation services.[16] The basic period of coverage for each "spell of illness" is 90 days,[17] with 60 "life-time reserve days," all or part of which can be attached to any one hospital stay.[18] A spell of illness covers the period of admission in a hospital or nursing care unit, with the key proviso that there must be at least a 60-day gap between the last day of one spell and the first day of the next. Finally, the number of spells for which a participant can receive hospitalization during a lifetime, or for that matter, during a year, is unlimited.

The basic fees for these services are dispensed by the program administrator, the Health Care Financing Administration (HCFA). The patient is responsible for an inpatient hospital deductible for each spell of illness, which is revised annually. That figure was $696 for 1994 and $716 for 1995. If the stay exceeds 60 days, an additional "coinsurance payment" equal to one-quarter of the original deductible is charged for each additional day of hospitalization. If the total period of stay exceeds 90 days, the patient can draw on the lifetime reserve period, but only by making a second set of coinsurance payments, equal to one-half of the original deductible for each additional day of hospitalization.[19] HCFA pays for the remainder of costs in accordance with its reimbursement formulas.

The government is a zealous agent for its patients, which prohibits patient payment of any additional fees for hospitalization covered by Medicare. A fairly extensive private market, however, supplies Medigap insurance for both the hospitalization and professional services not covered by Medicare. This hospitalization program covers the copayments required for both periods after the initial coverage period, and for 90 percent of hospitalization for a lifetime minimum of 365 additional days.

Medicare also imposes extensive obligations on participating hospitals. Hospitals must maintain peer review organizations (PROs) to review the quality and utilization of their facilities. They must agree to comply with the antidumping and emergency care provisions of EMTALA, discussed in Chapter 4.[20] They must also comply with a host of other obligations on sound billing, patient notification of rights, and the like. In addition, the hospital facilities must meet certain hospital care standards, or "Conditions of Participation," to remain in good standing with the program.[21] Failure to retain standing means the loss of all reimbursement from HCFA—itself a catastrophic consequence owing to the large proportion of Medicare patients in hospital beds.

All this is by way of preamble. The $64 billion social question was cost. How would this system of payment fare with cost-containment? The 1965 Committee Report was cautious but upbeat, projecting that responsible government action could meet the challenge. Thus the Report envisioned that HI would reach its steady state within a few years after its passage. It did so on the implicit assumption that the behavioral patterns of all players—physicians, hospitals, and patients, for starters—that held before Medicare would continue afterwards, even though the original Senate Report qualified its projections by saying "they should assume dynamic conditions as to both earnings levels and hospitalization costs."[22]

The Report's subsequent analysis reveals that only two considerations drove the estimates: social aggregates for both wages and hospitalization rates, which were thought to move in parallel over the life of the program. The allowable range of financial variation was around 50 percent—stunningly narrow, especially in hindsight. The most conservative model assumed that the rate of hospital utilization would move up more rapidly than wage rates for some short period of time and equalize thereafter, in steady state.[23] The moderate model assumed that the parallelism between wage rates and hospital utilization would be established at an earlier stage. Overall the feasible range was set at somewhere between 0.67 and 1.08 percent of the original $6,600 payroll, adjusted for inflation under various scenarios of wage earnings.[24] The upshot predicted (in constant dollars) a benefit payment of around $6 or $7 billion for 1982, instead of the $38 billion figure observed, which (even if adjusted for inflation) amounts to an underestimation by a factor of two. Any doomsday scenario was explicitly rejected. Thus the Report scoffed at the possibility that hospitalization costs could increase at 4 percent and hospital utilization rates would increase at 7 percent *for the indefinite future*—as they had done in the immediate past. After all, hospitalization expenditures could not "exceed 100 percent of the earnings of all workers in the country?"[25] "It is inconceivable that hospital prices would rise indefinitely at a rate faster than earnings because eventually individuals—even currently employed workers, let alone older persons—could not afford to go to a hospital under such cost circumstances."[26]

Unfortunately the Report's estimation of future costs was as wrong as it was confident. Errors of this size, however, do not just happen because actuaries cannot sharpen their pencils. The Report never addressed the political dimension, nor did it translate its projected aggregates—wages and hospitalization—into statements about incentives on *individual* actors whose self-interested behaviors could subvert the performance of the system at every juncture. Projections for the indefinite future do not begin to address how self-interested individuals and groups will milk the system for their short-term advantage—an advantage that could last for years, or at least until the rules change. Nor was it asked whether the Medicare system could yield changes in both the price and quantity of the services rendered. "The planners seemed to have overlooked the fact that if you shift the demand curve outward without moving the supply curve, prices will go up. The original 1965 cost projections allowed for a 10 percent increase in hospital admission rates among the elderly, but in fact hospital admission rates among the Medicare eligible rose immediately by 25 percent, the rate for surgical procedures by 40 percent, and the number of hospital days by 50 percent."[27] No surprise here.

Put at its most fundamental level, the Medicare program shows the imbalances that result from the now-familiar divergence between private and social costs. Individual users, acting out of self-interest, are more willing to consume resources provided by others than they are to consume resources they must provide for themselves. Medicare recipients (like all individuals) will not take into account the systemwide costs *to us* of their actions just because some tiny fraction of those costs redounds to them in the form of higher payroll or income taxes. The usual relationship holds: as the price to the consumer goes down, the demand goes up. The usual social conclusion follows: social resources are diverted from higher to lower value uses.

In this instance, the basic theory is supported by the evidence, which in many different settings indicates that additional investments in medical service provide little or no improvement in health care outcomes.[28] The Rand studies of private health insurance markets (where monitoring is better) indicate that individuals with more comprehensive health insurance make greater use of health resources, without any measurable improvement in their overall health.[29] Another study indicated that although patients treated in academic hospitals received far more care than those treated in community hospitals, the mortality rate of the two groups nine months after discharge were about the same, from which we can infer that the additional amounts of care provided little or no additional patient benefit.[30] Finally, another well-known study compared the health outcomes of Boston and New Haven residents. Although the former consumed twice as much medical care as the latter, the health outcomes in the two populations were, again, about the same.[31]

These and similar conclusions have been documented in a broad array of medical settings. The resource imbalances they represent do not disappear solely because health care is accorded among all goods some special or preferred status in law or social philosophy. Indeed, harping on the proposition that health care is an entitlement worthy of protection in opposition to the market creates a cultural climate that supports these excessive utilization levels. It is very difficult to accuse sick people of milking the system on Monday after bestowing on them some protected entitlement on Sunday. Sick people are not supposed to behave like market actors: to get that result, we could have stuck with a private market, which itself is far from perfect in constraining excessive care. Surely Medicare recipients are not supposed to consume less by virtue of their new-found status; so they must be allowed, if not encouraged, to consume more. No fragile sense of individual self-restraint will take root when illnesses are serious and the resources to cope are in short supply. The social expectations encourage high levels of plan utilization.

The basic financial structure of the original HI program only aggravated these tendencies. Before October 31, 1983, the reimbursement for hospital services operated under a system known as "retrospective cost-based reimbursement."[32] Hospital costs in individual cases were simply passed through to the government for payment, virtually dollar for dollar. The battles over allowable costs were largely confined to the question of whether certain indirect costs of hospital administration should be assigned to Medicare patients or to patients treated under some other program, such as an employer's plan. Allocating Medicare's "fair share" of the total expenditures gave rise to protracted and complex struggles, which inspired ingenious hospital cost allocation studies that loaded an ever larger share of costs to the reimbursable side.[33] But whatever the disputes about overhead and joint costs, bills for routine medical services were usually paid.

These titanic wrangles between hospitals and HCFA should not be allowed to detract from the main event: the impact of Medicare on patient behavior. The basic payment system worked at cross-purposes with any sensible system for rationing scarce resources. From the outset, the only payments that Medicare recipients made were largely independent of the amount of care they received. The initial deductible for hospitalization does not increase whether one day is spent in the hospital or 60. The additional cost to the patient for hospitalization from days 2 to 59 is therefore zero. Only when the hospital stay reaches 60 days does coinsurance kick in. As might be expected, the number of admissions that last into the coinsurance period is relatively few, and most people who take advantage of this period do so for a relatively short time.[34] The vast bulk of hospital days fell within the initial 60-day period.

Worse still, the basic incentives all worked to expand the utilization of hospital services. At the margin, hospital care was free to patients but reimbursable to hospitals. Hospitals had incentives, therefore, to cater to patient desires by providing the most comprehensive battery of (covered) tests and services that public funds could buy. The only line of government defense against overcharges required a showing that hospital bills were inflated to raid public coffers. But any floodgates that government officials could erect were insufficient to stem the tide of bills submitted for payment. The major cost control command when Medicare was enacted in 1965 is still in place today. Reimbursement is limited to "reasonable costs." The details were left to be worked out by regulations, guided solely by "the principles generally applied by national organizations or established prepayment organizations," which in turn allowed services to be rendered on a "per diem, per unit, per capita, or other basis."[35]

Unfortunately the private baseline of comparison was not fixed in stone, but itself was subject to market pressures that drove prices upward in *both* the public and the private sector. Now that one low-paying segment of the market no longer had to be served, outside charges to third parties could move smartly upward because any increase extracted from paying patients could in turn justify the higher reimbursements from Medicare. Within this framework, individual consumers have rough but insistent incentives to make the right judgments on what procedures to pay for and what to pass by. No external reviewer is likely to have much luck in deciding whether this or that procedure was "medically necessary" under the circumstances, when documentation of circumstances resides first and foremost in the hands of the patient and provider. Thus more extensive utilization of procedures went hand in hand with increased prices. Any external system of auditing was overwhelmed by the sheer volume of cases to process. For every case that was kicked back, a dozen could soon appear. It is easy for A to provide services to B when some impersonal C has to pick up the tab. The initial design of Medicare underestimated the risk of moral hazard and took insufficient steps to control it.

THE DRG

In one sense, however, the original Committee reports on Medicare were correct. This process could not go on indefinitely, and it did not. Medicare expenditures for hospitals went from $2.7 billion for fiscal 1967, the first year of the operation of the program, to $38 billion by 1983, far exceeding the "unsustainable" rate of increase that everyone had dismissed out of hand in 1965. Likewise, the percentage of HI expenditures moved up from 63.6 percent of total Medicare expenditures to 71 percent. The rate of inflation for hospital services averaged 6.6. percent between 1960 and 1950, dropped to 5.8 percent between 1960 and 1965, and then moved sharply upward to 13.9 percent from 1965 to 1970.[36] In 1983—as a product of the early Reagan years, and after some experimentation at the state level—Congress ended the cost-plus feeding frenzy of the earlier period.

At the heart of the new prospective payment system was a set of "diagnosis-related groups" (DRGs).[37] An administrative board establishes an elaborate grid to cover certain diseases and disease combinations. It then assigns for each class a distinctive rating to determine its appropriate length of stay and treatment pattern. The raw data in turn can be "converted" into a compensation schedule for each type of procedure. The system is called "prospective" because the payment for any individual case depends in the first instance only on its classification rating and not on the length of stay or successful outcome in the individual case. The system does not permit routine ex post increases in payment because of the unanticipated difficulties of treatment. Nor does it reduce hospital fees simply because treatment in a particular case was less costly than anticipated. To open the door to these routine recalculations would lead back down the path to cost-based retrospective payments, where hospitals could offer ingenious excuses for every hard case but remain strategically silent on easy cases.

To avoid the perils of excessive individuation, the DRG system pays by the pre-established averages per diagnostic category. The hospital is protected not by case-by-case adjudication, but only by the law of large numbers. It receives extra compensation for its hard cases by pocketing unearned compensation from the easy ones. It reimburses the government for the easy cases by taking care of the hard ones. Only at the extremes does a safety valve allow recomputation in extraordinary circumstances, beyond the control of the hospital, that could take into account changes in the patient or case load mix.[38] But with everything said, the DRG introduced a system of capitation payments, not by patient, but by procedure: so much per case period. Because the budget per procedure is fixed, the theory goes, the hospitals will now follow a strategy to maximize its profits subject to the external constraint—in theory, to supply efficient, low-cost treatment for patients.

An enterprise of this magnitude and complexity is buffeted from all directions from the moment of its birth. To start with the obvious, someone has to make the classification and to assign the appropriate cost figures. These DRG cost figures are administered prices, but they cannot be concocted out of whole cloth. Set them too low, and the system shuts down because the efficient provider of necessary services cannot recoup its costs over the long haul. Capping costs for all procedures at $100 results in the confiscation of hospital wealth, the end to the Medicare program, or both. Although current law provides no constitutional protection against these forms of takings claims, the political realities are such that Congress and HCFA cannot consciously push the rates too hard even in the short run.

This political side-constraint against wholesale bankruptcy may avoid the most glaring instances of government abuse, but it hardly serves to fine-tune the cost cuts in a system known to contain more fat than it needs. But how to set the rates when markets are silent? Current supply and demand considerations are hardly dispositive because the private demand of Medicare patients has been consciously severed from any demonstrated willingness to pay. So the only possible route is through a reconstruction of historical costs, subject of course to needed adjustments for inflation, which could take place at different rates in different locations and in different product markets.

Controlling inflation is only the first step in the process. All historical price schedules are tainted with the failures of its own prior judgments. The raw data must be massaged to remove the corrosive contaminants—capital costs, exempt costs, and certain nursing costs—

that seep into a reimbursement system targeted to medical services only. Likewise the architects of the DRGs thought it was imperative to recognize regional variations in the provision of hospital care—large urban, urban, and rural are the three main classes. The level of reimbursement also has to reflect differences in hospital type—for example, community versus teaching—because the latter supply more of the instructional resources needed to secure medical services in the next generation. Yet, in each instance, the choice of territory or wage level is contestable, as is the size of any teaching subsidy. Nor can matters come to a stable resting point. The recalibration for the DRGs cannot be done just once. Its rate structure must be continuously updated (annually under the law) to take into account the constant rate of change in treatment protocols and technology. As of 1993, there were around 492 DRG classifications.

The DRG system places a financial wedge between the patient and hospital that was not present under the older retrospective payment rules. The constant pressure on hospitals to contain costs could lead to withholding treatment that is by any definition medically necessary for patient care. But that objection, although true, cannot be regarded as decisive. *No* legal set of rules allows two people to act as if they were one in spirit; and certainly no set allows three "people"—hospital, patient, and HCFA—to display the enduring unity of purpose of a single person. To keep the administrative and incentive problem in perspective, no private insurer finds reimbursement an easy nut to crack, even in the absence of government regulation. Any coordination rule has room for slippage. Finding a single flaw in the incentive structure does not call for replacing it with a second system that regrettably may introduce a new and greater flaw of its own. The relevant inquiry is whether gaming the system poses more acute risks under some systems than under others. If the choice is simply between excessive overconsumption under the older retrospective payment system and conflicts of interest between patients and hospitals under a prospective payment system, the *global* choice for DRGs is easy. Prospective payment guards against the greater mischief and, for that reason, should be preferred.

The improvements that DRGs are designed to bring about, however, do not exhaust their probable set of consequences. DRGs do more than eliminate the traditional incentive for hospitals to run the meter. To maximize revenues, hospitals also receive strong incentives to strike out in novel directions. One frontier involves classifying procedures. When payment amounts did not depend on the choice of categories, diagnoses could be as candid as the bills were high. But once the classification determines the payment structure, it becomes the subject of intense pressures: "upcoding" is bracket creep for medical classifications. When in doubt, code a new admission into a higher DRG, or find that the initial diagnosis reveals two conditions instead of one, or demonstrate from the start that more expensive procedures are required for the same illness. The hospital has pretty good knowledge of its own cost schedules; and it also knows the price schedule authorized by DRGs. It also has a large first-mover advantage because it shapes the file from admission to discharge. If the reimbursement for coronary bypass with catherization is $150 when for coronary bypass without catherization generates $100, the built-in incentive to upcode the procedure exerts itself if, but only if the cost of the additional procedure is less than $50.

In principle the same problem can, and does, work in the opposite direction. If the cost of the additional procedure is greater than the incremental price allotment, why do it? The payment depends on averages, and a hospital can beat the system by economizing in appropriate cases, based in part on superior knowledge of its own business. The financial incentive to do too little will not of itself determine the outcome. A sense of professional responsibility, a fear of tort liability, or the prospect of accreditation difficulties might reduce the risk of skimping on medical care. But the inescapable truth is that any external system of supervision fights a losing battle in trying to counter the built-in advantage that hospitals derive from knowledge of their costs. The DRG system may have 493 categories, each category with thousands of cases, all different and all unruly. With the fixed compensation system in place, the temptation to cherry pick from the array of potential cases is great, and the safeguards against this adverse selection process are highly limited.

Not only does the DRG system introduce new problems, but it cannot counteract some defects inherent in the previous system. In particular, the system, far from addressing the rigid separation of geographical markets, tends to reinforce it. In a competitive framework, business tends to move to suppliers in low-cost regions. If gasoline sells for $.20 less per gallon in the suburbs than in the city, few city residents will drive to the suburbs just to find lower prices. The cost in time and money are likely to exceed any price savings. But, by the same token, it would be a grave mistake to assume that the price differential will have no effect on consumer behavior simply because most people will not consciously seek it out. City residents who live close to the suburbs, commuters to the suburbs, and weekend vacationers could all purchase gasoline in the suburbs. Thousands of similar hidden maneuvers will shift sales (and tax revenues) from the city to the suburbs in measurable amounts.

A competitive system of health care should show the same tendencies of migration across boundaries, owing to local and regional price differentials. Not all city residents would seek cheaper suburban care, but some could and would: the higher the price differential, the more rapid the move. The ratio of patients in the two systems should alter in ways that reduce the total burden: geographical competition should spur all hospitals to lower costs to preserve market share. Unfortunately the regional pricing of DRGs blocks that tendency because high-cost providers receive high reimbursement levels. The rules are directed more toward not rocking too many boats at one time than toward wringing inefficiencies out of the system. The government program blocks any effort to shift Medicare recipients to low-cost centers. Medicare recipients, in turn, are insulated from this inefficient cost structure and likewise have no pressure to search for cheaper providers. No competitive system accords this tariff-like protection to market incumbents. DRGs may begin life as cost-containment devices, but they quickly take on a second, less social function: the preservation of territorial divisions and through it the maintenance of nationwide cartel pricing.

An unprecedented exercise of political will could in principle address the regional variations in current price structures. But just what should it do? It is highly unlikely that any program of administered prices could replicate the regional variations that would emerge in market settings. No one has anything like the information needed to anticipate the constant movement in market shares or the size of the sustainable price differential. But even if we supposed that the impossible could be done, the reformed DRG price structure would still be missing the one critical element for effective cost-containment: *it imposes no direct constraint on patient demand.* The most that the perfect DRG system can provide is accurate costing of the cases after they come into the system. But it does not clamp down on the *number* or *types* of cases brought into the system in the first place. Let a 90-year diabetic be brought in for a heart valve operation, and the DRG system gives the procedure a very high score and thus awards the hospital substantial reimbursement for heroic efforts. To be sure, the hospital may not take some of these difficult cases where it does not expect to recover its costs. But the first-mover advantage gives it the power of initial selection, which the hospital will exercise in a way that aggravates the basic structural problem. So constructed, the DRG cost structure studiously ignores the benefit side of the equation. The Medicare payment does not depend on the anticipated outcome of the surgery, let alone any estimate of benefit if the surgery was successful. The treatment of the case within the bowels of the Medicare treatment is no different from a similar procedure on a patient 20 years younger with a far better prognosis. In the day-to-day operation of the system, it hardly matters that the payoff in patient health differs markedly between these two cases.

Think of the choices as seen from the patient side. Not one Medicare recipient in 20 knows the rudiments of hospital reimbursement. Not one in 200 should trouble themselves with the arcane issues that professionals find so hard to master. The principle of rational ignorance should control. The one fact that Medicare participants do know is that they pay very little for a great deal. General revenues pay for 75 percent of their hospitalization costs. The lesson, therefore, is unmistakable. Insulate the receipt of services from payment for services, and any rationalization of the reimbursement will only put the squeeze on hospitals. It will not constrain overall demand nor weed out those cases with low rates of return. Once again there is nothing special about health markets: subsidized services are consumed in excessive amounts.

All too often, however, the problem is not viewed as one of demand. Instead the culprit is regarded as new and costly technology that has to be provided to an expanding population base.[39] Of course, overall population is growing, and the population over 65 is growing more rapidly still. The introduction of new technologies continues unabated from magnetic resonance imaging to laser holography. But it is odd to see any reason for fear in either of these tendencies. In a well-functioning market, the change in age mixes *should* induce increased expenditures on hospital care in response to the long-term changes in underlying demand. Likewise, new medical technology in open markets presents no greater peril to the welfare of its citizens than the mainframe computers of a generation past: technology expands opportunities, and although these improvements should increase total utilization, they need not drive up unit costs with improvident purchases.

Yet once again there is a caveat. The optimistic scenario depends on individuals having to pay the full cost of their services. The cost-containment features of the ordinary rules of supply and demand could work with new medical innovations, just as they worked with computers. But once these expensive devices are introduced into a Medicare environment, all bets are off. The skewed incentives that drive utilization on other matters will, if anything, prove more influential. The ability to make sensible utilization decisions at the center will hardly improve so long as massive subsidies pervade the system. Within these constraints, introducing a new and expensive technology poses a continuous threat to overconsumption that justifies the gloomy prognosis on cost-containment. A DRG system may have prevented matters from becoming still worse, but it has done nothing to restrain the upward spiral in hospital utilization. When the right to health care is deemed priceless, it turns out to be very expensive.

PART B: SUPPLEMENTAL MEDICAL INSURANCE

BASIC DESIGN

The second portion of the Medicare program, Supplemental Medical Insurance (SMI), deals with compensation for physician services. Its structure differs from that for hospitalization, but the bottom line is the same. The system imposes no effective constraint on demand, and once again the reform efforts introduced under the mantle of the Resource–Based Relative-Value Scale (RBRVS) have proved unable to stem the tide. Because medical services differ in important particulars, however, it is best to recount this story separately.

Under the original design of Medicare, membership in Part B is "voluntary" to all persons who are enrolled in the hospitalization program of Part A, that is, to persons over 65 and to disabled Americans. The present financing calls for program recipients to pay around $46 per month. The original plan had required plan participants to pay 50 percent of the total costs, but in 1973 Congress tied future premium increases to the general rise in social security payments, even though medical costs were known to be escalating at a more rapid rate. Consequently, only 29 percent of the plan costs today are covered by premium dollars, whereas the remaining 71 percent of the bill comes from general tax revenues.

With ratios like these, the gain from joining the program are so pro-found that of the 32.1 million or so people over 65 who are enrolled in the hospitalization plan, some 31.4 million have signed up for physician services as well. For disabled Americans, the numbers are only slightly lower: of 4.1 million enrollees in hospitalization, 3.7 are enrolled in physician services.[40]

On the benefit side, individual plan participants are entitled to a vast array of services—in- and outpatient diagnostic and treatment ser-vices, physical and occupational therapy, speech pathology, home dialy-sis, clinical psychology services, vaccines, Xrays, and much more.[41] That system allows individuals to choose either fee-for-service medicine or enrollment in various kinds of managed care plans. Managed care plans have had a one-time effect on costs and utilization, but they have had lit-tle effect on the overall operation of the system.[42] As is the case with the HI plan, the SMI plan has grown mightily since its modest inception. For example, its expenditures in 1993 totaled $56 billion.

The cost side provides comprehensive coverage subject to two important limitations. First, individuals face a $100 annual deductible. That deductible had been set at $50 in the 1966 plan, but notwithstand-ing the acute financial strains, its increases have been kept well below the levels of inflation, for the usual political reasons. The second limitation is a copayment feature of 20 percent. Unlike the coinsurance feature for Part A, this component is directly proportional to the total levels of expenditures and thus varies generally with the age of the recipients. Thus, on average, older Medicare recipients have higher copayments than younger ones. In principle, this copayment requirement could place a genuine restraint on the willingness to consume physician services. By the same token, the copayment's influence on utilization of physician services can be reduced in two ways, one private and the other public.

MEDIGAP INSURANCE

The private method for reducing the effect of the copayment is through the purchase of so-called "Medigap" insurance, which means just what the name implies. A private insurance carrier offers, for a fixed premium, coverages that dovetail with the Medicare coverage.[43] The coverage in question applies to both Part A hospitalization and to Part B coverages for physician fees. In both cases, it reduces the amount of private cost to the receipt of medical services and thus increases the level of access to the system. Our first reaction might be to ask what objection could be raised against the purchase of additional insurance in a voluntary market. Normally none, but in this context the decision has a clear impact on the total amount of payments that must come from Medicare itself. Medicare beneficiaries purchase Medigap insurance on a lump sum basis. This insurance thus makes any individual decision to seek out physician services less costly at the margin than it would otherwise be and thus increases the physician utilization rate. The Medigap insurance, of course, faces a parallel risk of overutilization because it stands liable to pay the 20 percent copayment of the physician. Nonetheless it can charge a premium that allows it to make a profit.

To see the dangers of overconsumption, assume that the average $1,200 Medigap premium, the 1995 level,[44] translates into the ability to fund a $25 copayment for 40 physician visits, which equals 20 percent of the $125 total cost per visit. The Medigap plan makes money even if it induces an increase in number of patient visits from 30 to 40. The ten extra visits induce a $250 increase in payments, as the total moves from $750 to $1,000. But that private increase is paralleled by a $1,000 increase in Medicare payments because Medicare must pay $100 for each of the additional ten visits. That $1,000 in additional government payments is an incremental benefit to the patient not borne by the Medigap insurer. The empirical evidence bears out this result: "elderly individuals with Medigap insurance generate 67 percent more health care spending than those without, and they spend 15 percent more out-of-pocket."[45]

Because Medigap policies benefit both the private insurer and the Medicare participant, the issuance of these policies should *not* be a matter of indifference to Medicare's financial exposure and hence to Medicare itself. Accordingly, the key policy determination is whether Medicare should condition its grants by requiring individual recipients to pay the deductible out of their own pockets in order to counter the risk of overutilization. Just that possibility shows why it is incorrect to frame the issue as one of freedom of contract between the Medicare beneficiary and the Medigap company. Once the Medicare program requires individual payment of a deductible, a Medigap contract no longer counts as an exercise of freedom to contract, but as a potential breach of an existing contract. Any insurance carrier should be able to limit the purchase of second-tier insurance in order to limit its own exposure. A state-run Medicare program is no exception to this general rule.

Nor should that prohibition be unduly difficult to enforce. Efforts to evade the restriction by obtaining reimbursement of direct patient payments to Medicare need not be scrutinized on a case-by-case basis. They could be forestalled at a single stroke by banning the sale of Medigap policies, or at least by restricting their use. Ironically the current rules now cut in the opposite direction. They require a Medigap insurer to pay the full deductible and the full copayment in addition to the catastrophic coverage that must commence with the 151st day of hospitalization after Medicare benefits are exhausted.[46] The insistence that all supplementary insurance fill the gaps reflects the common perception that state-mandated minimum terms are necessary to prevent market exploitation. But the provision deflects the insurance away from its social function of handling low-probability events with high losses and converts it into a bill-paying service that encourages overexpenditure on small items that do not pose a threat to financial security.[47]

At the same time, the government requires Medigap copayment be complete; it does not allow hospitals to *waive* the deductible portion of the charges, claiming that such charges constitute fraud and abuse. That waiver has the identical economic effect as the Medigap insurance required in private contexts: it reduces the costs of the insured's entry into the system and thus increases the external costs borne by the insurer. Only the political realities account, therefore, for the inconsistencies within the system. Thus the boundary line between the cost-containment and access is shifted firmly toward the former, at the expense of the latter.

BALANCE BILLING

The second flanking maneuver on the deductible and copayments comes from the prohibition on "balance billing." Physicians who treat Medicare patients are not allowed to charge them any sums in excess of the 20 percent copayment for reasonable charges authorized under the statute. Although many physicians are content to accept the Medicare fee structure, physicians in high-demand specialties or physicians with high costs have been reluctant to do so.[48] As we might expect, the distribution of balance billing varies greatly. For 1987, about 40 percent of Medicare patients were treated without any balance billing at all; some 50 percent paid (yearly) between $1 and $200; and the remaining 10 percent paid figures in excess of $200, with 0.1 percent paying $2,000 or more.[49] The total sums equaled $2.3 billion compared to a total Medicare budget for physician services of around $25 billion. Balance billing thus increases the supply of physicians willing to serve the Medicare population, but it also reduces the ability of at least some patients to obtain it. As such, it became an obvious target for regulation.

The first line of attack came at the state level. The question was whether or not the states could require individual physicians who treat Medicare patients to waive their claims to balance billing. For example, Massachusetts directed its Board of Registration to "require as a condition of granting or renewing a physician's certificate of registration" that the physician not engage in balance billing of their Medicare patients.[50] Pennsylvania also banned balance billing. The challenges to the statute by various medical groups went down to a predictable judicial death.[51] In both cases, the courts held that the physicians could not complain that their property was taken because they voluntarily joined the program; nor could they show that Congress had precluded the states from regulating fees in its Medicare statutes.

The issue of balance billing also invoked a Congressional response. Medicare divides physicians into two classes: participating and nonparticipating physicians. The former are said to "accept assignment" from Medicare, which means that they will abide by the Medicare fee schedules and refrain from balance billing. In contrast, nonparticipating physicians do not accept "assignment" and thus reserve the right to impose additional fees.[52] Before 1984, a given physician could decide whether or not to accept assignment on a case-by-case basis. That election carried with it a price. The nonparticipating physician had to bill the patient directly for the full fee and thus risked delays and nonpayment when participating physicians could routinely recover 80 percent of their fees from Medicare.

That disincentive did not preclude the practice of balance billing, so more stringent sanctions were imposed on nonparticipating physicians. The Deficit Reduction Act of 1984 required nonparticipating physicians to decide *annually* whether to participate in the Medicare program on an all-or-nothing basis. No longer could physicians categorize their patients by their ability to pay or the ease of collection. Thus the price for receiving higher fees from some patients was to forfeit Medicare reimbursement in all cases. The relatively small volume of additional fees often did not justify the additional business risk, thereby increasing participation levels. Congress also imposed a price freeze on the fees that nonparticipating physicians could collect from Medicare patients.[53] The predicted response occurred. Although assignment rates have varied widely across states both before and after the changes, nationwide acceptance of assignment rates rose from 51 percent in 1983 to 67 percent in 1985 to 74 percent in 1987.[54]

Price freezes do not last forever. In 1986, Congress lifted the 1984 price freeze, only to replace it with a system of "maximum allowable actual charges" (MAACs) for medical services, which effectively capped physician fees at MAAC rates unless their average annual fees did not exceed statutory levels.[55] That system, in turn, yielded to yet another variation on the price control scheme that permits nonparticipating physicians to charge Medicare patients at most statutory maximum, which today is set at 115 percent of the allowed Medicare rates.[56] The constitutional challenge to that restriction was promptly dispatched on the ground that "participation in the Medicare program is voluntary" vis-à-vis the federal government. The court was not troubled that state law (as in New York) *compelled* physicians to render services to all patients "without discrimination as to the source of payment,"[57] that is, it required physicians to accept Medicare patients in their practice. Apparently the double dose of coercion is permissible because both pieces of the scheme are not authored by a single hand. Finally, balance billing has been banned for patients who receive treatment under both Medicare and Medicaid.[58] Once again, the political system has beaten back any effort to use prices to restrain patient access.

RBRVS

The debate over balance billing shows the greater political strength of Medicare beneficiaries relative to physician groups. Cost-containment has lost out to full access. But increases in volume on the system have provoked yet other responses to constrain costs, of which the most important is the Resource-Based Relative-Value Scale (RBRVS) pioneered by William Hsiao and his Harvard colleagues.[59] In form, the RBRVS seeks to introduce into physician payment scales the rationality of a pure competitive market. Hsiao describes the basic structure of the policy in terms that hide the worst of Harvard behind the best of Chicago:

> The RBRVS study uses a rational and systematic process to derive the relative prices that would have emerged from a rea-

sonably competitive market. Economic theory shows that competitive prices have socially desirable properties that promote efficiency and lead to optimum use of society's scarce resources. The RBRVS study developed methods and collected data to mimic the relative prices that would have emerged if we had a perfect competitive market for physician services.[60]

The procedures used to emulate this competitive outcome are, however, little more than a warmed-over version of cost-plus factor pricing. Thus Hsiao's research first made an elaborate classification of medical procedures and, for each procedure, assigned numerical values to three separate components: (1) physician work (2) practice expense (covering various overhead and administrative costs), and (3) malpractice.[61] The resulting numerical sums are adjusted first by a geographical factor and then by a conversion factor (CF) that translates points into dollars. The price setters can change the weights for individual procedures and for the CF. In practice, the weights given procedures are not revised routinely, but the CF is reexamined on an annual basis to reflect overall inflation rates, or more precisely the Medicare Economic Index (MEI), which is tied specifically to a narrower health-related basket of goods. In addition, the current scheme contains a built-in "volume control" intended to keep the total budget within some overall cap. As utilization increases, the CF is reduced to ease it back to its former levels.

In the early going, it was thought that RBRVS would increase primary care at the expense of secondary care. One confident prediction read:

> Payments will increase for internal medicine by 16 percent, for family practice by 37 percent, for otolaryngology by 7 percent, and for obstetrics and gynecology by 1 percent. Payments will decline for radiology by 21 percent, for thoracic surgery by 20 percent, for ophthalmology by 17 percent, for orthopedic surgery by 10 percent, for general surgery by percent, and for urology by 3 percent.[62]

But the smaller observed changes in practice reflect the powerful inertia of the status quo ante. Acquiring a working mastery of this complex system takes a professional lifetime, as experts from large medical centers battle within the inner sanctum of the HCFA. But understanding what is wrong with its basic design does not require similar expertise. It only demands some appreciation of the irreducible gaps between the RBRVS and the competitive prototype that it is supposed to mimic.

To start with the most obvious point, the mechanism for generating information differs radically between the two systems. The genius of a competitive market is that no single person has, or can pretend to have, the knowledge needed to determine the relative values of given inputs for different projects. Instead the system of market exchange uses a common medium—money—as the yardstick for determining relative values. Individuals and firms can determine how much they value the resource and then bid for it if value exceeds price. Owing to the impersonal nature of markets, competitors need not have any knowledge of the intended value that their rivals make of these goods. Bidders need only compare stated price with private value. No single actor in a competitive market "constructs" the prices that others have to pay.

This decentralized price mechanism thus economizes on the need for any person to make collective judgments about the relative value of particular goods and services. It also allows the benchmark to shift with the relative scarcity of inputs to eliminate both shortages and surpluses. The changes are not made discontinuously on centrally accumulated information; they are made continuously on privately acquired and privately valued information. The RBRVS has a built-in rigidity wholly alien to competitive markets.

Within this framework, any firm also has to reckon its costs. In so doing, it usually makes the same calculations that bureaucrats perform before setting the RBRVS. An insurance company writing health coverage in an unregulated competitive market takes into account, for example, age, sex, occupation, education, and prior medical history, and it assigns a weight to each factor before determining the total premium. The insurer then offers its product to consumers, who can decline or accept it. This second hurdle differentiates the competitive situation from the RBRVS. A competitive market generates powerful evidence that the cost of inputs is below the value of outputs. When the buyer purchases insurance, the premium covers the *entire* cost of the product, including the firm's cost of capital. It is possible to construct a relative value scale for quite literally thousands of potential products, but most of these products never reach the market because their inputs are too costly to allow their sale at a price that covers all relevant costs. The market throws up an effective *screen* to determine which cost calculations are sound and which are not. Finding a buyer is conclusive evidence that someone else values the output more than the seller values the inputs. Potential products that fail this one test remain on the cutting room floor.

The process for selecting goods for markets provides a radical disjunction between market and administered prices (which is what RBRVS supplies). To see why RBRVS offers technique without purpose, consider the cost of constructing a skyscraper with a single suite of offices located 500 feet above ground. Project costs include the cost of the site, the raw materials, capital, labor, general overhead, and the like. A building is then constructed for the computed price. It may seem easy, but this method avoids answering the critical threshold question: is the project worth the cost?

We can make the same point by exposing the confusion that resides in the common phrase, "the labor theory of value." In Lockean hands, the theory refers (imperfectly, to be sure) to the idea that individuals acquire the ownership of external things by "mixing" their labor with them.[63] The basic function of the Lockean theory is, however, limited to acquiring ownership of natural objects that are regarded as part of the original commons. After acquiring the land or things, individuals can improve them for use, sale, or both. Locke's theory does not fully explain why the unilateral action of single individual binds the rest of the world. It can be defended pragmatically as the best method for getting resources (or at least land and movables) into productive hands. No auction houses grace the state of nature, and, as Locke noted, requiring unanimous consent of all potential claimants only guarantees starvation in the face of plenty. So understood, the labor theory is justified as a convenient way to match persons with resources, and nothing more.

The labor theory of value also has its Marxian version that is implicitly reflected in RBRVS. Broadly conceived, that position holds that any object derives its value not from capital but from the infusion of labor. But it hardly follows that more labor entails more value, let alone value worth the cost of that additional labor. The hypothetical office tower is not worth $1 million just because $1 million in labor was expended in its construction. Someone has to value the output at the price to justify the sacrifice of input. Any so-called labor theory of value that attributes value to labor independent of demand has no descriptive or normative power.

This utter absence of a market filter renders RBRVS a worthless proxy for consumer value. The scale gives some clue as to the cost of the beast, but it offers us no independent confirmation of its worth. Sometimes that price reflects the benefits conferred, but sometimes not. For the buyer, the only precondition for using medical services is for private benefits to exceed private costs. Because the entire system is dedicated to reducing out-of-pocket costs for all medical treatments, overconsumption will be the order of the day *no matter* what pricing system is used between the government and the health care provider. No filter on demand, no working market.

One final sign shows that RBRVS has none of the properties of the competitive market that it is supposed to emulate. The market for tomatoes is competitive, but different grades of tomatoes command different prices. The market for lawyers is competitive, yet different lawyers charge different fees. The utter failure of RBRVS to reflect any fee dispersion means that Medicare administrators can capture none of the quality differentials usually (if imperfectly) priced by competitive markets. The monolithic quality of its rate scale does not reflect some startling discovery that all physicians perform the same procedures with equal skills. It is evident that the system of valuation is blind to the subtle interplay of forces that give competitive markets their dynamic quality.

THE POLITICAL STRUGGLE FOR LEGISLATIVE REFORM

The DRG and RBRVS constitute two sides of today's effort to run a system of administered pricing. Because neither program constrains demand in the futile effort to rationalize costs, the system chugs on as before. Yet as costs escalate, prices are not in place to moderate demand. Instead, the political efforts to reconfigure the system come in powerful bursts marked by brutal pushing and shoving, as government administrators sit in the middle of a political triangle, with health care providers of all stripes in one corner, Medicare beneficiaries in a second, and ordinary taxpayers in the third. As the level of tax increases becomes no longer sustainable, government operatives can move in only two directions—either fees to hospitals and physicians, or benefits to patients—or both must be reined in.

Both courses of action have obvious perils. Higher costs to Medicare participants result in lost access. Reimbursement reduction compromises the viability of needed facilities. So the struggle among benefits plans, reimbursements, and taxes continues far into the night, and it helped bring about the budget impasse in the fall of 1995—which, more than anything else, accounted for the Republican losses in the November 1996 elections. The President and the Congress could not agree on any fundamental restructuring of Medicare payments, or even on the size of the premium increases for Part B of Medicare. True to form, a Presidential veto blocked the major restructuring of Medicare, even as the President acknowledged the need "to slow the rate of growth in Medicare spending."[64] At one level, the President's concession seals the intractable nature of the spending cycle. A slower rate of growth (in real terms) for Medicare spending virtually guarantees that the program will occupy an ever larger share of national expenditures, without offering any justification for this huge investment.

Nowhere did the President address Medicare's root difficulty: the unsustainable size of its basic subsidy. During the 1995–1996 debates, the Democrats converted Medicare into an article of faith, the inexorable outcome of a social compact by the younger generation to take care of their elders—which should not be mistaken with the practice of children taking care of their own parents. The irony here should be palpable. The original 1965 Medicare deal set the government portion of professional services compensation at 50 percent of total cost. With the capping of recipient payments in 1973, that percentage drifted down over the next generation to close to 25 percent. The harsh Republican program, however, only sought to raise the levels back to 31 percent, a far cry from the original understanding, which even they did not dare to propose in the current political climate. The President's program acknowledged the long-term need for rate increases and called for a monthly premium rate that is only $8 less than that of the Republicans—to go into effect in the year 2002 when Clinton is out of office. But Clinton's short-term plan called for a modest rate reduction before the 1996 election. Political promises are wasting assets. Any promise to raise future rates is subject to nullification by the next administration that is equally preoccupied with its own reelection prospects. The President's position is not credible because all the hard choices come in the next millennium, where they are left for others to combat.

A second staple of the presidential rhetoric treated any criticism of the overconsumption of health services as a disguised protection of tax breaks to the rich. But that approach mistakenly assumes that these two separate reform programs should be linked at all. The case for tax reduction depends on the adverse impact of high rates of taxation on investment and labor. Those taxes should be reduced even if the question of Medicare were never on the table: the machinations of high-bracket individuals reduce their taxable income base so that the government obtains only a small increase in revenue for a very large loss in private income.[65] The main problem with Medicare is wholly independent of the tax structure. The pricing system of the program makes it impossible to constrain recipient utilization. That structural flaw has to be addressed wholly without regard to any issue of tax reform. Both systems are out of whack. Reform on both fronts will be blocked by either issue, let alone both together, as a question of redistribution from rich to poor. The key elements are the internal issues of resource allocation at stake in both regimes. The errors in Medicare are not offset by the errors in basic tax rates. The two problems only compound each other. To preserve the status quo is to make two errors, not none.

Yet the Republican rhetoric did little to blunt what seemed to be a clear political victory for the President, but their vetoed 1995 bill did at least struggle with the fundamental structural flaws of the Medicare system. To borrow from the language of the pension laws, the Medicare system at present functions as a *defined benefit* system. The logic is that the government first sets out the entitlements and then scrambles to fund them when the demands from the system pour in from every direction. As such, no budget constraint is built into the system at the front end. The risk of overcharges falls to the taxpayer. To combat this scheme, the Republicans proposed a MedicarePlus program[66] which comes much closer to a *defined contribution* system. Under this approach, the government assumes a fixed financial obligation to Medicare recipients, much akin to vouchers, that allows each recipient to purchase the Medicare set of benefits from a group of private providers that includes ordinary HMOs, various kinds of provider organizations, labor groups, and fee-for-services plans.[67] The great attraction of this system is that it allows private competition into the market for subsidized health services and thus promises some of the cost efficiencies that cannot be delivered by any system of DRGs or RBRVSs. The hope is that these inefficiencies could maintain the level of subsidized services while reducing the cash size of the subsidy.[68]

But the program was never meant to be because the Clinton veto statement denounced the bill on the ground that it "introduces untested, and highly questionable, Medicare 'choices' that could increase risks and costs for the most vulnerable beneficiaries."[69] The President's reluctance to experiment with market responses to the health care difficulty is predictable on simple ideological grounds. But even if limited weight is given to his arguments, the difficulties with the program are not easily overcome. The belated effort to convert Medicare from its present defined benefit structure to a new defined contribution structure must, perforce, bleed the implicit subsidies out of the system. As the program is now constructed, all participants may pay an equal amount into Medicare, but they do not withdraw, on an actuarial basis, equal benefits from it. The older the recipient and the sicker the recipient, the greater the implicit subsidy, both from the general taxpayer and, in some cases no doubt, from other Medicare recipients (that is, those who could be privately insured for less than their current Medicare contributions).

Under the current legal regime, however, no interested party has any strong incentive to quantify the size of these implicit subsidies because the ultimate payouts of benefits nowhere turn on that precise knowledge. All that anyone cares about is the level of general tax revenues that are brought into the program, and not their allocation among Medicare recipients. The situation here is not dissimilar to that which is found in other regulated industries. Before the Telecommunications Act of 1996,[70] for example, residential and rural phone service was heavily subsidized by commercial and urban accounts, but no one could give a precise measure of the subsidy involved. The implicit understanding of everyone was that the monopoly power conferred on the local exchange carriers could be used to provide subsidies to preferred recipients. The deregulation under the Act did not remove the obligation for universal service at subsidized rates, but its competitive provisions did remove the monopoly revenues that undergirded the older system. Now that implicit transfer payments can no longer support the system, Congress responded by decreeing that an "evolving" level of universal services had to be funded by "equitable and nondiscriminatory" charges imposed on all interstate telecommunications carriers.[71] But as befits a task of such complexity, the newly liberated subsidies could not be set out in the Act itself. Instead, the Act contains an explicit delegation to the Federal Communications Commission, which will be able to work out the required transfer payments, if at all, only after protracted hearings and disputes. Good luck.

The difficulties of introducing competition while preserving subsidies are not confined to telecommunications. Once again health, for all its special features, faces exactly the same difficulties. The Republicans' proposed defined contribution system, the MedicarePlus system, would have forced politicians to confront the size and distribution of these implicit subsidies. In effect, the idea is to give each individual Medicare member a voucher keyed to the present level of Medicare payments, perhaps reduced by 5 or 10 percent to reflect the size of the anticipated gains from private provision. But issuing every Medicare recipient a voucher of the same amount would give a healthy 65-year-old person an ample cushion with which to purchase first-class medical insurance, while leaving his 85-year-old counterpart substantially out of pocket. The vetoed House bill therefore keyed government payments to the "age, disability status, gender, institutional status, and such other factors as the Secretary determines to be appropriate, so as to ensure actuarial equivalence."[72]

One precursor of this system is the defined contribution program now offered to government employees today, the Federal Employee Health Benefit Plans (FEHBP). The Heritage Foundation has invoked this model to defend the defined contribution approach to Medicare by pointing out its greater flexibility and lower administrative costs by allowing individuals to purchase insurance from a wide array of approved providers, including ordinary insurers, managed care organizations, fee-for-service plans, and union plans.[73] Unlike Medicare, these programs are required to offer only a very narrow set of benefits, but otherwise they are free to vary and expand benefit packages as they see fit. The program has proved popular with government employees, so why not take it public?

Unfortunately, the critical differences lie hidden in small details. The FEHBP program is directed to a group of employees below retirement age whose members are healthy enough to work in the first place. The level of variation in anticipated health demands is likely to be small in that group. Hence the variation in premiums could be restricted as well. But the Medicare population is far older and has a far greater variation in health. In addition, the insurers will all have the option to accept or decline individual health risks. The adverse selection problem is real because those individuals with good health profiles will have lots of opportunities to insure; those with serious needs will not. The list of relevant variables set out in the Republican bill was not robust enough to counter the dangers. Even the best intentions leave some Medicare recipients with a government check below that needed to purchase insurance from the astute private carrier that retains the right to accept or reject customers at will. In a program of around 40 million recipients, a 1 percent misfit rate could yield 400,000 uncovered elderly and infirm individuals—in other words, a political crisis powerful enough to rock both parties.

The bill's guidelines did not solve the problem of rating, either. It is one thing to require that risk-adjusted calculations be made, and another to make them. Consider some of these complications. The vouchers in question are not being sold to persons at age 50 to cover their medical risks at age 65. They are sold to individuals who are already on the Medicare rolls. For those individuals who are currently being treated for serious medical conditions, the size of the known future liability is already large. If the only uncertainty in a particular case is whether an insured will require between $100,000 and $150,000, the voucher awarded for that person must be somewhere between those two amounts. The only insurable component of this cost is the last $50,000, and the lack of a broad database makes it virtually impossible to decide whether the applicable voucher should be set at $120,000 or $140,000. Nor do the calculations get any easier given the possibility that death will terminate the need for any future payments during the covered period. But whatever the answer, what is being marketed as a nominal defined contribution plan is really an estimated prepayment of anticipated expenses for future years. It is not likely that any government agency could make these calculations for each person on a yearly basis without overwhelming the system. The defined benefit program, notwithstanding its considerable failings, is spared these calculations. And it allows political institutions to conceal their compromises under the shadow of the law.

The problems with Medicare vouchers remain serious even for persons still in good health. The House bill contemplated risk adjustments for individual cases, but it did not make them or even prescribe how to make them. Nor did it take into account that the dominant sentiment in so many regulated insurance markets is to exclude, as improper forms of discrimination, the kinds of information that is indispensable for determining risk. Thus it is common in many jurisdictions to insist that automobile insurance companies ignore age, sex, marital status, or territory, notwithstanding that they are powerful risk predictors.[74] Could any voucher program have overcome the pressures of the antidiscrimination movement in insurance? One telltale sign that this bill would not have been equal to that task is that it refused, perhaps correctly, to confront the question of whether race, along with sex and age, could be used to ensure the "appropriate actuarial equivalence." The point is of no little concern given the race-sensitive data that is found in both hypertension and renal failure cases so central to the question of organ transplantation.[75] But unless some payment differentiation is made on those grounds, the insurance companies will select against black candidates because of their greater risks. Alas, even if that differentiation could be made, a full rating system might still prove unable to generate a set of accurate prices for insured. If that enterprise failed, the mispricing of individual risks could allow astute insurance companies to snap up the good risks and leave the government program saddled with the higher costs of the poor risks.

Even if we put the racial complication aside, the difficulties are far from over. It is one thing to say that sex is to be taken into account and quite another to indicate just how much it should be weighed and why. And sex is a dichotomous variable, easy to identify. Disability and institutional status is not so much a variable as a minefield. No one is quite sure what counts as a disability under the Americans with Disabilities Act, but the number of disabled individuals swells in response to the prospect of gains from exploiting the legal uncertainties. A similar field day could be expected here, as regulators try in effect to make judgments about the individual health status of every eligible person. Why such a fine cut? Because the private insurers will do so in their underwriting, forcing the government to keep pace in order to avert financial ruin. But once the rates are calibrated to known disabilities and disease conditions, we are no longer talking about pure health insurance. We are back to talking about a prepayment program with a small insurance component. Unlike the program for government employees, the regulations will have to calculate the insurance premiums for individuals who already have had strokes, or those who have Alzheimer's disease or kidney disorders. The government is not underwriting the insurance against future risk; it is paying compensation for risks that have already materialized. The more individuation that is introduced into the system, the more it appears that everyone will get the same amounts of care as they received under the older program.

The only way to obviate this impasse is to set premiums that refuse to individuate to this degree and that force some individuals to bear privately the losses that were covered under the old, defined benefit program. In the end, that tough line could succeed only if the fate of the least fortunate does not drive this negative political response to any reform of the entire system. Only if the government—meaning public opinion—is prepared to "just say no" to persons with heavy disabilities and little means to cope with them, can this problem be attacked,. However, that outcome cannot happen so long as universal coverage for persons over 65 years of age is treated as a nonnegotiable moral imperative. The defined contribution approach may push the margins back, but it suffers from the same objection (or has the same strength) of a market system. It is explicit about its choices and will say no to given individuals. And it is that reality that the current Medicare colossus cannot accept.

MEDICAL SAVINGS ACCOUNTS

Short of some dramatic initiative, therefore, the future political course has already been set. Political forces will stymie the comprehensive rationalization of the system. The impending difficulties will be met by a mix of higher taxes, inferior services, and longer lines, coupled with the purchase of private medical care by those who are able to offset the care from other sources. In an effort to spur that development, one popular step now is to introduce a Medical Savings Account, which would allow tax-deductible money to be placed into Individual Savings Accounts, from which money can be drawn without taxation if spent for medical needs, and with taxation if ultimately used for other purposes.[76] Under this system, individuals now in effect have first-dollar exposure to liability that will induce substantial behavioral changes at the outset. They will economize on medical expenses at the lower levels because the money they spend is their own, but they will not be so foolish as to refuse to spend money when the need is dire. The system could make a real difference at the bottom end by cutting out reimbursement for small payments and leaving Medicare to provide insurance against the risk of larger losses. It is a program that has the strong support of many Republicans, but which is deplored by many Democrats and for one reason—it undermines the implicit set of cross-subsidies that the current apparatus requires. The Democratic opposition to MSAs was so intense that Clinton compromised on that other most popular of initiatives, the portability of health insurance in the face of pre-existing medical conditions—just to limit its effect.[77]

Once again, the political debates over MSAs conceal the strengths and weaknesses of the system. The MSAs do have the unfortunate feature of expanding the current tax practice of subsidizing health care by allowing employers to deduct the premiums without forcing the recipients to take them into income. That practice began during World War II as a concerted effort to escape legal ceilings on wages. But keeping all medical premiums out of the tax system privileges one kind of personal expenditure relative to the others, without counteracting the great vice of all tax subsidy programs: overconsumption. The Medical Savings Account in effect restores parity between insurance programs that do not depend on employer contributions, but only at the cost of extending an unprincipled subsidy to a new domain. But political considerations again block the no-deduction alternative. Management and labor will move as one on an issue that provides benefits to both sides of the transaction, no matter what the adverse consequences to the system as a whole. The tax deductibility of health insurance is as politically untouchable as the deductibility of interest payments on home mortgage, and every bit as indefensible as a matter of first principle. Yet, in a world of second-best, the proposal may do more good than harm by inducing some restraint of spending for minor illnesses, one of the sore points of the current system.

IS THERE A FUTURE?

So what is to be done? As a matter of first principle, the answer is easy: never start down a road that promises to give subsidies; but once given, seek to limit them if possible. That second task is always tougher than the first because it is so difficult to undo the expectations and the entitlements that grew up in the interim. Thus on transitional questions, the present set of feeble alternatives may be the best that can be enacted. Raise deductibles and copayments. Reduce hospital coverage for the first week instead of for the first day. Allow greater choice in provider plans.

But hold on to no illusions. There is no political coalition that has the ability to stay the course for several years so that these transitional reforms have the breathing room to work some permanent benefit. The dominant likelihood is that deferring today's hard choices is to invite still harder choices in the long run. By June 1996, the trustees of Medicare could only report that the program would go bankrupt by 2001, not 2002. But results like that are the norm in an age where no one wants to be the bearer of bad news. The entire episode has only one silver lining— it could insulate us from similar programs whose ambitions exceed their success. So we should try to learn from our mistakes by avoiding still more ambitious programs for health care, by heeding the proposition that no state program can bridge the undeniable gap between wealth and utility—which brings us to Clintoncare, to which the next chapter is devoted.

CHAPTER 8

Clintoncare:
The Shipwreck

AN EGALITARIAN MOMENT

So much has been written about the rude demise of the Clinton Health Security Act of 1993 (HSA) that it might seem pointless to disinter legislation that has long been left for dead.[1] But some exhumation is warranted because the ideals behind the HSA still exert a powerful hold over public debate. James Fallows has written that a set of bad political judgments and scurrilous attacks sunk a program that was in reality no more complicated than the tort reform programs, routinely proposed by Republicans and far more desirable.[2] In her recent chronicle of the Clinton decline, Theda Skocpol portrays the Clinton health plan as the logical outgrowth to the original New Deal commitment to using government intervention to secure a better life for all Americans. To her, its failure rested not only on political machinations but also on "Reagan's Revenge," a theme she borrowed from historian Alan Brinkley's essay of that name.[3] A 20-year conservative attack slighted, in her view, the benefit of New Deal reforms by reducing the taxes needed to fund government programs and the bureaucrats needed to run them. This constant onslaught doomed Clinton's program that on its merits promised "simultaneously to make Americans more secure and the national economy more efficient."[4] It is odd perhaps to think that someone could intelligently make over one-seventh of the economy in less than two years. But no matter. To the supporters of the Clinton health care plan, the sins of the past decisively shaped the realities of the present.

Whatever the postmortems of the program supporters, optimism was in the air at the outset of the Clinton administration. The Clinton plan got off to a flying start by fusing egalitarian populism with public discontent with the overall state of the health care system. By 1993, the United States had achieved a rare double: the highest cost for health care in the world and the highest level of popular dissatisfaction with the system as a whole.[5] The most visible focal points of the present failure were the inexorable rise of medical costs to around 12 percent of GNP in 1990; yet simultaneously some 37 million Americans had no health insurance at all.[6] The following years showed continued growth in both total health expenditures as a percentage of GNP (so that it is close to 14 percent today) with still more Americans removed from the insurance rolls.

The lack of any constructive movement created an impetus for more extensive government intervention. At the height of the debate, Ronald Dworkin put the case for the Clinton plan and against free markets in forceful yet familiar terms. He protested the unequal distribution of wealth; he lamented the lack of information available to consumers in making medical decisions; and he deplored the practice of cherry picking—the selection of the best risks only—that would take place in an unregulated insurance market. Indeed, for good measure he insisted that a national health program would point the way for similar advances in housing, jobs, and education.[7]

Dworkin's analysis is typical of the attack mounted by the critics of the status quo,[8] but it offers a weak foundation for any comprehensive health care reform proposal. If wealth is unfairly distributed in the United States, we should correct that matter head on. But the task is surely more difficult than we would imagine.[9] From 1945 to 1973, overall annual increases in income averaging nearly 3 percent were shared uniformly across all quintiles of the population, seemingly without the hand of government intervention. From 1973 to the present, American efforts at redistribution intensified, but their consequences backfired. Overall levels of wages have stagnated, but the position of the rich, especially the very rich improved relative to the pack, whereas those at the bottom lagged behind and lost ground both in absolute and relative terms. The clear implication of this data is that major efforts at redistribution undermine growth while facilitating the political gamesmanship that transfers wealth to the well connected and adroit. Health care is subject to identical pressures, which would only be intensified by passage of the HSA or kindred legislation.

Next Dworkin is surely correct in noting that accurate information about the costs and benefits of various health programs is hard to come by. But at most we can identify only two antidotes to imperfect information: disclosure and simplification. Perhaps a doctrine of informed consent might alleviate some part of the difficulty, but only in connection with individual procedures. A national health program offers no sensible remedy for this ailment, for in and of itself it does not secure the disclosure of relevant information even as it constrains the ways in which medical care is obtained. At best, this information lament only justifies a limited set of focused remedies, not a vast system of central planning.

Finally, markets will price insurance according to perceived risk, but for the reasons developed here at length, this tendency should be applauded, not deplored. Accurate pricing gives people the incentive to reduce their risks in order to control their costs. Accurate pricing also cuts down on the amount of strategic behavior when various interest groups jockey to become recipients of government largesse. The dislocations with community rating programs frustrate any move to competitive health care and the efficiencies it brings across the board. But Dworkin, by focusing solely on the limitations of coverage after the fact, only sees the down side of market insurance, none of its benefits. Finally, like most egalitarians, he dismisses the effectiveness of charitable assistance and care.

Dworkin's arguments, repeated countless times by others, helped to fuel the initial burst of support for the Clinton health plan. But its weak intellectual foundations proved unable to fortify it against the political and intellectual pressures that followed once the details of its operation were laid bare. To see why the entire edifice crumbled, it is important to identify the political and business forces that the Health Security Act set in motion, bearing in mind that the political missteps of the Clinton team were not the only reason for the demise of Clinton's program.

THE SHORT UNHAPPY HISTORY OF CLINTON CARE

The first step in this inquiry is to summarize the once familiar milestones in the two-year fight over national health insurance. The development of a national health care policy was perhaps the centerpiece of the Clinton presidential campaign of 1992. Yet the program did not emerge full blown at the outset.[10] Rather, in the initial stages, the key feature of the Democratic platform was its opposition to the much more limited, mildly market-based reforms of the Bush administration. On the table at the time were several programs with some political cachet.[11] Managed care contemplated the replacement of traditional fee-for-service medicine with group care plans: the "play or pay" proposal would have required all employers that failed to insure their own work force to contribute some fixed percentage of payroll into the public plans that would; and the Canadian single-payer system had the government negotiate physician fee contracts within the confines of a global budget cap. Politicians and commentators trumpeted each of these approaches as a superior alternative to the mishmash of health care programs already in place.

Notwithstanding, that is, their obvious defects that have attracted their critics. Managed care programs herd individuals into programs that deny or limit their choice of physician and thus undercut the bonds of loyalty in the physician-patient relationship.[12] Pay or play plans invite strategic maneuvering by employers: only employers whose insurance costs are likely to exceed the Congressional payroll tax will choose the pay option. Employers with healthy work forces will choose to insure, so all the bad risk accounts are dumped into the public sector with insufficient funds to service them. The single payer system prevents this strategy, but it invites abuse by a government monopoly that can stifle innovation, squeeze individual physicians, and operate in a slow and arbitrary way. So much at least can be learned from the history of Medicare.

Unpalatable choices like these left Clinton, the fledgling President, a wide berth to surge beyond the conventional wisdom by offering his own ambitious plan. Its subsequent political history is well known.[13] The crafting of the HSA began shortly after the election when the President made, in retrospect, his first major strategic mistake by appointing his wife, Hillary Rodham Clinton, to chair the White House Task Force composed of key Secretaries (Treasury, Defense, Veterans Affairs, and Health and Human Services) and trusted White House advisors, including, of course, Ira Magaziner.[14] Simultaneous with the creation of the White House Task Force, the President's plan of action called for the formation of an interdepartmental working group responsible for coming up with recommendations for the plan. The working group was unwieldy from its inception, as it tried to meld into a single group some 300 federal employees drawn from the White House Staff, about 40 "special government employees" hired for the occasion, and a large, but unknown, number of special consultants who assisted the working group on an intermittent basis. The bridge between the Task Force and the working group was Ira Magaziner, one of Clinton's fellow Rhodes scholars, whose own consulting career had little or nothing to do with medical issues. He was a member of the cabinet-level Task Force and he presided over meetings of the working group. The initial publicity for this combined effort was highly favorable if only from the belief that constructive government actions could harness the market and thus soothe the personal anxieties that ripped at the hearts of large portions of the American public.

Its political execution was, to say the least, faulty. The initial timetable called for publication of a full plan within 100 days—by around May 1, 1993. Toward that end, staffers and experts, some 500 strong, hammered out daily position papers and policy alternatives that slowly wound their way up into Magaziner's inner circle. The composition of the working groups undercut the potential legitimacy of the system. The Administration decided to adopt a "left-in" instead of a "center-out" formulation. It sought to gain the advantages of a cohesive base even at the cost of some greater political legitimacy. Although most major insurance, business, and medical groups initially had decided to cast their lot for universal access, none of them was invited to the table to fashion policy. Nor were distinguished defenders of universal coverage, such as Alain Enthoven or Henry Aaron invited. In due course and in no uncertain terms, they made clear their dissatisfaction with the final product.[15] In addition, too much power was concentrated at the top. The common complaint voiced both publicly and privately was that the only judgments on which Magaziner relied came from his own head. He had little confidence in the ability of lawyers to make policy decisions or fashion institutional arrangements; he regarded trained economists as professional prophets of doom; and neither he nor Mrs. Clinton was willing to check their cost estimates with the experts at Treasury or in the various budget offices.

Nor did it help that task force deliberations were shrouded in secrecy, even if the operating procedure just managed to comply with the various federal mandates. One unsuccessful lawsuit failed to force open the deliberations of the working group,[16] but it had the desired impact of undercutting the public legitimacy of the deliberations. Mrs. Clinton's own participation was interrupted by the final illness and death of her father. For both personal and political reasons, progress in the plan design was more difficult to make than expected, and the working group formally disbanded in May 1993 with its work unfinished. Notwithstanding all the reversals, the Clinton plan at that date still enjoyed a fair chance of success.

Work on the program continued in the White House at a feverish pace over the summer of 1993. The Presidential work product appeared in two documents. The first, released on September 7, 1993, was the Preliminary Work Group Draft of President Clinton's Health Care Reform Proposal,[17] followed on October 27, 1993, with the 1342-page draft of the HSA, which no one could, or should, read today from beginning to end. (My eyes glazed over more than once, and I never made it through it all.) When first announced, the plan garnered substantial public support. A Presidential address on September 22, 1993, gave the plan a rousing sendoff with a stirring speech,[18] which promptly registered a 56 percent approval rate.[19] The large medical groups supported the program at least in principle, and the Republicans worked overtime to assure the eager public that they would engage in a responsible bipartisan effort to implement a program of universal coverage. Insiders trumpeted the proposal as the most important institutional reform since the New Deal itself.[20]

The honeymoon did not last. The public counterattack had started even before the details of the plan were made public. Critics had a field day in attacking the plan for its gothic complexity, its porous cost estimates, and its wishful thinking. Writing in the *Wall Street Journal,* Representative Dick Armey insisted "the Clinton health plan would create 59 new federal programs or bureaucracies, expand 20 others, impose 79 new federal mandates and make major changes in the tax code."[21] And he unveiled a complicated flow chart as the visual device to clinch his point. Writing in the *Wall Street Journal* on July 14, 1993, Martin Feldstein projected the effect of the HSA to imply that "a family with $40,000 of income would face a combined marginal tax rate of more than 60%: the new 10% health insurance tax, the current 15% employer/employee Social Security tax, the 28% income tax rate (raised to at least 31% to finance the projected health insurance shortfall), a typical state income tax rate of 6%, plus state and local sales taxes."[22] A year later, an opaque report from the American Academy of Actuaries hinted on plausible assumptions that the range of anticipated premiums ran "from 8 percent to 54 percent higher than the Administration's estimates."[23] With numbers like these floating about, small businesses—always more feisty than large corporations—lined up four-square against the program because of its high payroll taxes. Spurred on by the National Federation of Independent Businesses, it lobbied from one end of the country to the other.[24] The Health Insurance Association of America, which consisted largely of small insurance companies that stood to lose their markets under the Clinton plan, mounted an effective $15 million ad campaign featuring "Harry and Louise" that raised uncertainty about the HSA with the well-to-do middle-class constituency, further cutting the public support for its main premise.[25] Bill Kristol wrote his influential memos that treated the rebuff of the Clinton plan as a bellwether test of "welfare-state liberalism."[26] The Christian Coalition, a determined opponent of Bill Clinton, sparked local grassroots opposition to the plan.[27]

No single event marked the demise of the HSA. Rather, the program slowly ran out of steam. Erstwhile supporters deserted a sinking ship as popular unease rose, so that by March 1994 the country was at best evenly divided on the desirability of major reform,[28] a sharp switch from six months before. The Administration never issued a second authoritative version of the HSA that responded to the perceived ambiguities in the initial draft. Yet the waters were clouded by the publication of alternative plans, including one by Representative Jim Cooper of Tennessee (called Clinton-lite) that purported to be both less expensive and less intrusive, and another that called for a single-payer program, championed by Representative Jim McDermott of Washington and Senator Paul Wellstone of Minnesota.[29] Democrats in the House and Senate, however, never published a complete alternative text, although Majority Leader George Mitchell in the Senate and Richard Gephardt in the House were reported to have drafted one (or more) plans of their own. Delays in the legislative timetable pushed back key committee votes until the time to regroup ran out. Public sentiment during the August 1994 recess entreated Congress to go slowly on the overhauling of one-seventh of the economy. By September 1994, the fall elections overshadowed the health bill, which then died an inglorious death, tempered by some hints of future insurance reform—which led to the fight over portability of health insurance in the spring and summer of 1996.[30] The election of the Republican Congress in November 1994 blocked the resurrection of a comprehensive plan that once seemed unstoppable. Today few people think of a possible resurrection of a program for which there had once been such high hopes.

What explains the failure of the Clinton forces to capitalize on the centerpiece of their political program? To concentrate on the short-term mistakes of the dominant players misses the larger structural issues at hand. Nor does it work to simply catalogue the ideological and business interests of those who opposed the legislation, as if those who supported it were free of such base motives. The ultimate issues have to go to the merits of the plan itself. Gaffes and intrigues aside, the program could not succeed. The plan was the ultimate exemplar of a system of universal positive rights that paid insufficient attention to its correlative duties. The bottom line is a variation of Lincoln's famous remark: it is possible to subsidize some of the people all of the time. It is not possible to subsidize all of the people any of the time—which is what the Clinton health plan sought to do.

A CAPSULE SUMMARY OF A COMPLEX PLAN

The theme of "security" is one of the most powerful magnets of Western political thought. The classical writers stressed the "security of the person" and of "security of exchange" as one way of stating the importance of individual autonomy and private contract. But the phrase did not exhaust its power in a world of negative rights. The passage of Social Security in the 1930s showed how this same phrase could be used to bolster a regime of positive rights, largely by suppressing any reference to their correlative duties. It was just that stress on security that lay at the core of the aptly named Health Security Act, which echoed a familiar theme. Over and over again, the President insisted that job loss, pre-existing conditions, or individual misfortune should not place Americans at risk for the loss of health care coverage. His transmittal letter to Senator Mitchell and Representative Foley (both gone from Congress today) etched out the main theme: "The 'Health Security Act of 1993' holds the promise of a new era of security for every American—an era in which our nation finally guarantees its citizens comprehensive health care that can never be taken away." It then returned to the theme and noted the emerging social consensus: "For the first time, members of both parties have agreed that every American must be guaranteed health care."[31]

Having seized the high moral ground, the HSA broadcast its two collective core commitments: first, universal access to comprehensive health care for all citizens on equal terms, and second, cost-containment. The HSA sought to pursue both objectives simultaneously through a vast array of legal and administrative mechanisms in the best of all possible worlds.[32] Financing for the system depended on a mixture of payroll taxes, individual premiums, and, for its administrative apparatus, general revenues. The hope was to harness the innovation and dynamism of competitive markets in the service of positive rights of health care. To its supporters (but not its opponents), the program was centrist in its commitments and orientation.

The Clinton program quite literally thought it could have it all. In rapid succession, the Preliminary Report ticked off the advantages of the HSA: universal access, comprehensive benefits, choice of plans, equality of care, fair distribution of costs, personal responsibility, intergenerational justice, wise allocation of resources, effectiveness, quality, effective management, professional integrity and responsibility, fair procedures, and local responsibility.[33] Who could quarrel with these objectives—or ignore the catch? Other sections of the Working Group Report set out the administrative structure needed to deliver the goods. In its most minimalist form, that structure envisioned four distinct layers of government: a national health board; state boards under the supervision of the national board; regional alliances (sometimes called health insurance purchasing cooperatives, or HIPCs), and finally the health plans themselves.

The national health board was to be responsible for setting standards; for reviewing the plans submitted by the states for their own operations; and for implementing or preserving programs on its own initiative when the state plans were found not to be in compliance with the applicable standards.[34]

The states were to be charged with designing specific plans to meet the federal requirements; ensuring that the plans provided the required subsidies to low-income employees; certifying the proper participation of individual health plans; regulating their financial operations; and collecting data on the operations of the various consumer alliances that purchased health care for individual plan members within their region.[35]

The alliances were to consist of a group of employer-based organizations that joined to purchase their health care insurance from qualified primary providers at substantial discounts. These alliances could not "establish boundaries that concentrate racial or ethnic minority groups, socio-economic groups, or Medicaid beneficiaries."[36] Within these broad outlines, states had to define the specific territories for each of their local alliances. Metropolitan statistical areas could not be divided, and any alliance that covered a Consolidated Statistical Metropolitan Area within a state was "presumed" to be in compliance with the HSA. Side by side with these regional alliances were corporate and union alliances with more than 5,000 workers, which were allowed to stay out of the regional alliances so long as they met the same set of strictures.

Finally, the regional or corporate alliances contracted directly with several different health care providers offering a limited menu of plan types. Fee-for-service plans were on the list along with various forms of managed care alternatives. Each type of plan, however, was subject to a general requirement of community rating, whereby "[e]ach regional alliance health plan may not vary the premium imposed with respect to residents of an alliance area," except to take into account the different types of plans that could be offered overall.[37] It was never quite clear which companies would be allowed to submit bids to the regional alliances. Subject to these constraints, alliances had to ensure that every person within their region was enrolled in some plan. Toward that end, the HSA made it "the *obligation* of every eligible individual to enroll in a health plan."[38] If not selected voluntarily, stranded individuals were to be enrolled in some open group the first time they sought medical care. Universal access was not only a right; it was also a legal duty. But it was never quite clear what would happen to individuals who wanted to enroll in a plan that was not prepared to accept them.

This brief skeletal outline is incomplete, but it still contains enough clues to explain why the plan was stillborn on arrival, wholly apart from the political mistakes of the Clinton team. As drafted, the HSA sought to maximize three goals simultaneously: universal access, comprehensive benefits, and cost-containment, probably in that order. What the program failed to address was the fundamental tension between the first two of these objectives and the third. In the end, the negatives from universal care with comprehensive benefits swamped any putative gains from cost-containment.

The most elementary defect of the plan turned out to be its political undoing. Looked at dispassionately, the plan hurt more people than it would have helped. The Presidential rhetoric fostered the illusion that

all Americans are in the same boat. A closer look at the promised benefits reveals a highly skewed picture of the likely distribution of gains and
losses. The program of universal access would have necessarily elevated
more people into protected positions within the system. But which people are guaranteed—or obligated—to participate in the universal coverage regime?

ELIGIBILITY

The first cog in the political equation is to identify the plan's eligible participants. Philosophically speaking, universal access has not reached its
limits until it includes all individuals on the face of the globe, but no
domestic political process could ever generate so lavish a subsidy for outsiders. Universal coverage thus applied only to "every American citizen
and legal resident," and thereby *excluded* the millions of illegal aliens who
now receive hospital and charitable care.[39] Covering citizens made evident political sense because they can vote. Covering legal residents was
trickier, but because most pay taxes, it would have been hard to exclude
them from plan membership. The exclusion, however, of illegal aliens
was a far more anxious call. Illegal aliens typically receive education from
state and local governments. Refusing to enroll them under the HSA
would not have allowed private hospitals to exclude them from emergency care. If they could survive without guaranteed care, why couldn't
citizens and residents who, if anything, have greater wealth and knowledge? What moral principle justified excluding that portion of the population most vulnerable to the shocks of serious illness?

Cost considerations provide the answer but not a justification that
commands universal respect. The ACLU, for example, insisted that the
"Act's exclusion of aliens and incarcerated people is not only inequitable,
but also irrational in terms of financial and public health considerations."[40] Its bottom line was that this irrational classification exposed the
HSA to a serious constitutional challenge under the equal protection
clause. That attack that would probably lose in the courts under current
law, which does not yet make alienage a suspect classification,[41] but the
ACLU's message had some equitable appeal in the legislative setting. Yet
once that proposal was on the table, the demand for broader coverage
worked like a stealth bomber for the opponents of the HSA. Perhaps voting taxpayers could have been persuaded to swallow a fair-sized horse,

but no quasi-constitutional imperative could have persuaded them to swallow an elephant. Requiring the coverage of aliens was meant to force voters to an all-or-nothing choice. In light of the increased financial risks, the answer that came back was nothing, which at least preserved the status quo. But once the prospect of coverage for illegal aliens was put on the table, it could never have been entirely removed thereafter. No one could ignore the possibility of extending coverage after initial passage, either by legislation or litigation. The Medicare rolls expanded to covered disabilities, and Medicaid to cover pregnant women only in the second round. So this lingering uncertainty had to dim the prospects for enacting the HSA.

REDISTRIBUTION WITHIN THE CLASS OF ELIGIBLE PERSONS

Let us assume, however, that illegal aliens have been safely excluded, and we can investigate how universal access under the HSA alters the fortunes of citizens and legal aliens. On this score, the image of formal equality, invoked to prop up the bill morally, turns out to be an economic mirage. All Americans may have equal access to mandated coverage, but they do not secure equal benefits from that coverage. The formal equality concealed a massive disparate financial impact that spelled political disaster for the President. To see how the HSA plays out in operation, it is helpful to divide the public into a few well-defined classes.

One relevant class includes individuals who do *not* wish to purchase available health insurance because they believe they are better off without it. Young professional twenty-something workers in good health and without dependents fit that picture. Mrs. Clinton was quite happy to attack those individuals for their uncivil behavior. Her message: "We're going to tell individuals who think they can get by without [health insurance] coverage because they're 25 and believe they're immortal . . . when they end up in the emergency room and stick us with the bill, that we're not going to let it go on anymore."[42] But her threat was oddly incongruent with her chosen program. The projected image is one of young people excluded from emergency rooms because of their inability to pay. Sticking with that image in a market system could have well induced the targets of her wrath to purchase the cheap health insurance available to them. But Mrs. Clinton's mission was not to instill the libertarian creed, but to force the younger set to join health care plans populated by their elders. Yet as Lance Stell has pointed out, however well this political hard-ball played with (some of) the over 50 set, it "sowed the seeds of inter-generational warfare."[43]

Why? Because the economics were so clear. The "Friends" genera-tion *correctly* perceived itself as losers from a program that promises a high level of benefits to all. Whatever the political rhetoric, their private calculations compared their anticipated costs with their benefits. These calculations revealed that social insurance drained their resources pre-cisely because it contained a massive subsidy for others. Because the HSA blocked their exit from the program, of necessity it turned this genera-tion into a political force that was opposed to its adoption. The blunt les-son of public choice theory is that if you can't leave, you fight. Young people who stood to lose large sums from participation in a national health plan could have been expected to devote some fraction of their resources to forestall its adoption and to register their dissent at the polls. So, from the outset, the hard economic realities falsified collective moral illusions of the HSA's benefits to all Americans. There is no collective public identity. "The" American people are not benefited when some substantial segment of them—numbering in the millions—is hurt.

Universal coverage of course plays out quite differently for other segments of the uninsured population. Many of these individuals were older and had serious health problems, unstable job histories and bad personal habits. For them, universal coverage at a uniform average price offered a powerful inducement to embrace the system. Yet this pool was always small in size. After all, it never included the Medicare population over 65, individuals enrolled in the Medicare disability program, and perhaps individuals eligible for Medicaid. But the costs to the small number of hardcore uninsureds surely had to be greater than the premi-ums that they could contribute to the health plan. They were uninsured for a reason, and adding even a tiny number of hard-to-care-for individ-uals could force up the overall plan costs substantially.

Viewed in this light, universal insurance would have operated as a wealth transfer from low-risk uninsureds to the high-risk uninsureds, against the political grain. Yet that evaluation oversimplifies the analysis by treating the subsidies as unidirectional. Large subsidies to this group of high-risk cases would have come from subsidies paid by individuals who already had good health coverage under private or public plans. Yet poll after poll revealed that whatever misgivings they had about the state of health care generally, most Americans were happy with the health care that they received under their own private plans.[44] The size of this subsidy from the contented many is hard to pin down, but it could have been very large. After all, in private plans, a very small portion of the insured population pool typically generates huge portions of the overall plan expenses. Adding even 2 percent more high-risk individuals to the ranks (which translates to around 5 million people) could drive up costs by a far greater amount, now that equal access to comprehensive medical care for all was built in at the ground floor. Yet because this high-risk group was poorly organized and politically uninfluential, it could not be counted on to secure passage of the HSA.

Most critical to the political alliances on the access issue were individuals who already received extensive medical coverage under some private health plan or under Medicare. These groups are very large and, by the simplest models of voting behavior, are likely to form the control bloc in any political struggle over the adoption of the plan. Most of this group had divided sentiments on the subject of health care coverage: dissatisfaction with the overall operation of the system; satisfaction with their personal care. For such people, the Clinton proposals had only a negative effect. At the very least, the HSA injected a discordant note of uncertainty into their lives, for no one knew how long their own private health plans would be able to survive the systemwide transformation in recognizable shape.

This anxiety crystallized when Elizabeth McCaughey, writing in the *New Republic* in early 1994, drew the (technically accurate) parallel between the Health Security and Sartre's play "No Exit."[45] "If you're not worried about the Clinton health bill, keep reading; . . . If the bill passes, you will have to settle for one of the low-budget health plans selected by the government." Enough liberal democrats shivered at the prospect that the HSA as then drafted did not allow *them* to obtain any additional health care above and beyond the stipulated plan levels, or that it prevented *them* from purchasing medical care that anonymous bureaucrats, using unknowable standards, did not deem "medically necessary or appropriate." Her piece received instant attention, even beyond the select circle of *New Republic* readers, reaching a mass audience, for example, through *Readers' Digest.*[46]

The strength of McCaughey's attacks show that the article hit home. A close reading of the HSA leaves some doubt as to whether McCaughey's stark readings were correct in all the particulars. As McCaughey noted in a later article, the official government response to her position was one of denial: "There is nothing in this Act to prohibit any individual from going to any doctor and paying, with their own funds for any service."[47] But beware of the negative implication of that official denial: it was illegal, even under the administration position, to purchase additional *insurance* protection individually unless all members of the particular plan had access to it. On this score, one of the most illuminating provisions of the Clinton plan appeared to allow a variation of only 20 percent from the median to highest cost health plan.[48] The variation in the price of homes, vacations, and cars is far greater, but those markets have no government pressure to compress the distribution of expenditures across persons.

But these subtleties do not stop the critics. Theda Skocpol, for example, directs her unqualified wrath at McCaughey: "McCaughey included outright lies about the Health Security bill, for example, falsely stating that it would prevent patients and doctors from dealing with one another outside of officially approved insurance plans."[49] A harsh charge, but Skocpol's statement is wide of the mark as well. If it means to imply that individuals could opt out of the Clinton plan in order to purchase their own medical care in the private market, it is false. Plan membership was obligatory for everyone. And if it means to say that individuals can purchase additional medical insurance outside the plan, it is false again. Private persons could not band together voluntarily to choose their own insurer. The only element of individual choice that remained under the plan was to purchase extra care on a fee-for-service basis, in Switzerland, if necessary. But perhaps my reading of the plan is wrong. The ambiguities were never laid to rest. During the political struggles, the text of the HSA was never clarified to resolve these ambiguities in ways that would put the critics' claims to rest. Once again, a statute that had been touted as the fountain of security lay vulnerable to the charge of injecting new insecurity into the lives of some of its intended beneficiaries.

McCaughey's account struck a raw nerve because Clinton's solid upper-middle-class, liberal democratic voters were quite determined to secure universal access for others without limiting their own options for health care. Once they regarded their access to health plans as compromised, it was only a matter of time before the entire coalition became unglued. The Clinton plan oversold equality. Public support for universal health care only went so far as to guarantee a minimum safety net at the bottom. The core liberal democratic constituencies, including its public intellectuals and professional classes, had no inclination to accept limits on private health care that could be obtained at the top. Its conception of redistribution brought up the bottom to some acceptable level but left the top to spend its remaining wealth as it pleased. The Clinton plan crept toward a second and far more coercive approach when it sought to equalize lack of health care across the board. The ethicists often pushed for the more radical reform. The voters were prepared, just maybe, to accept some form of a minimum safety net for all. The safety net approach tolerates multiple tiers in health care that the egalitarian vision does not. And why should rich and middle-class people be told that they could spend their excess dollars on education, travel, or idleness, but not what they really care about—their own health and the health of their families?

The resistance to universal access was especially strong among the elderly who already had (and have) the best deal imaginable. Huge portions of their care are subsidized by payroll taxes (for Medicare hospitalization), by general revenues (for Medicare physician care), and by state and federal grants (nursing home care and similar care under Medicaid, which constitutes today the majority of that program's $80+ billion in expenditures). The AARP, however, did not gauge the political winds as astutely as it might. In November 1993 and February 1994, it refused to endorse the Clinton Health plan.[50] Only in the summer of 1994 did it come out behind the plan. At that time, it thought that its members would stand firm for the principle of comprehensive health care from which they had benefited under Medicare or would benefit come age 65. But the AARP's leadership underestimated the forces of self-interest. A torrent of angry members phoned headquarters at the end of that summer to protest the decision of the AARP elite to bolster the sagging Clinton plan, without first consulting the membership. The procedural point packed such punch because the rank and file wanted to preserve the status quo.[51] At crunch time, AARP members and Medicare recipients stood four-square behind universal access to medical care—for all persons over 65. They rightly understood that the greatest peril to their care came from offering the same entitlements to persons under 65. To meet that challenge, the HSA sought to rein in Medicare expenditures.[52] It is no accident that Medicare recipients became champions of the status quo, given their desire to preserve the two-tier system of medical care that is now in place.

The AARP's rank and file knew its self-interest. The present Medicare subsidy works in two dimensions. First, it subsidies health care; second, it subsidizes its program participants. The former gives the program its political respectability because health is a preferred good easily defended on fashionable neutral principles that denounce the insensitivity of markets for their failure to rank goods and services in accordance with their intrinsic worth. But the later—coverage for present recipients—gives the program its political muscle. Expanding access to include everyone expands the subsidy for health care, but by the same token it sharply reduces or eliminates any subsidy to present Medicare recipients. When all the accounts are balanced, the expanded subsidy for health care comes only at the expense of other goods and services that most people want. But subsidizing health care across the board *destroys* today's subsidy to present Medicare recipients. Only when the subsidies are reserved for a limited portion of the population will the transfer to health care work for their economic advantage. Expand the class of beneficiaries to include everyone, and, alas, everyone has to pay for the subsidy that they receive. The financial advantage of Medicare recipients under the present legal arrangements shrinks if it does not disappear altogether.

An oversimplified set of numbers tells the tale. Divide the world into two equal groups—present Medicare recipients and the rest of the population—and see how their fortunes fare before and after the Clinton plan is put into effect on some stylized assumptions that isolate the central issues of the debate. Here the present situation refers to the public funding of the Medicare program. The post-Clinton situation refers to the distribution of public expenditures and benefits under universal coverage. Relative numbers and not absolute magnitudes are used.

	PRESENT			**POST-CLINTON**		
	MEDICARE	OTHERS	TOTAL	MEDICARE	OTHERS	TOTAL
COST	50	150	200	200	300	500
BENEFIT	100	0	100	75	125	200

On these numbers, or anything close them, the situation is not politically tenable. Under the present situation, the outcome is socially inefficient because the total costs exceed the total benefits by 100. But it is also politically stable because the government expenditures generate a net benefit of 50 to the politically connected Medicare population. The external loss on the general population thus increases to 175. But come the transformation, the costs of the new program are borne by all portions of the population equally: each pays an additional 150, moving the total costs up to 500. The benefit profile, however, shifts radically. The decline in the level of Medicare from 100 to 75 represents the contemplated cuts in the Medicare program. The 150 increase in benefits to the non-Medicare population optimistically assumes that their additional benefits offset their additional costs, so that they are made somewhat worse off by the passage of the Act. As stated, it looks like a lose/lose proposition, which will not pass at all.

To be sure, these numbers are highly stylized, but additional realism does not alter the picture. So long as the net position of the Medicare population is compromised, Clintoncare could not get the support of the AARP rank and file. So, even if we assumed that the rest of the population, or some fraction of it, benefited from the introduction of the program, the political status quo could not be altered. If the program had brought with it administrative costs and allocative distortions, as clearly seems the case, the net position of both the Medicare and non-Medicare population would have deteriorated still further. No matter how the numbers are sliced, the political majority is not there.

As stated the numbers assume no level of altruism between the Medicare and non-Medicare populations. But the political waters are further muddied because the indirect benefits of medical care run across age and interest groups. To modify the numbers to take these indirect benefits into account only requires that we assume that current taxpayers do not receive zero benefits when their funds are used to pay for Medicare recipients. But when that qualification is added to the others, the basic insight still survives. A selective subsidy allows for one group to win, while the larger society losses. But an ostensible universal subsidy gives no one refuge from its social inefficiencies. Hence partial plans can prosper politically in ways in which universal plans cannot, which is one reason why politicians love programs with selective coverage, whereas supporters of limited government prefer more general rules. When the benefits and burdens of a program are proportionate across all members of a population, any program that generates social losses will generate individual losses for each individual, an outcome that unleashes powerful political forces against its adoption or retention. A world with selective benefits makes it easier for interest groups to game the system, which the supporters of the Clinton plan learned at their peril.

WHAT BENEFITS?

What is true about universal access is equally true about comprehensive benefits. The Working Group Report showed all the self-restraint of a small child in a candy store when defining benefit packages. On this score, more than anywhere else, the unwillingness to confront the green eyeshades in Treasury and the Congressional Budget Office proved fatal. The original wish list covered the waterfront: hospital services; emergency services; physician services; clinical preventive services; mental health and substance abuse services; family planning services; pregnancy-related services; hospice services; home health services; extended care services; ambulance services; outpatient laboratory and diagnostic services; outpatient prescription drugs and biologicals; outpatient rehabilitation services; durable medical equipment, prosthetic and orthotic devices; vision and hearing care; preventive dental services for children; and health education classes.[53]

The moral logic behind this impressive list once again decreed that all individuals benefited equally from more medical care, so no one should oppose it. Yet the practical politics spawned by the program induced every industry supplier to lobby furiously to keep their products and services on the master list, because exclusion from HSA spelled economic ruin. The final principle of inclusion thus covered all services with positive value to recipients, with scant regard for the ratio of value to cost, either for some class of services or in some individual case. No item gets removed by a test that asks whether the service or program can help someone at some time. Benefits to every medical program are greater than zero. But that is the right answer to the wrong question. The right question is whether the benefits exceed the costs, for which no information is generated in a socialized system.

This benefit package had universal appeal, but once again the designers of the plan fell prey to their own egalitarian rhetoric. The Clinton plan created social insurance, not market insurance. Social insurance contains implicit cross-subsidies that undermine the rhetoric of "our common destiny." The straight, private calculation made in the quiet of homes across America was whether the package is worth its cost, person by person. The final tally showed that the probable constellation of plan winners did not constitute a political majority, or anything close to it.

To start at the top, low-risk individuals viewed the expansion of mandatory benefits as a minus. They pay proportionately for a more extended service list from which they expect to draw only a limited set of benefits. The more comprehensive the set of benefits, the greater the number of individuals who wind up in the class of losers. Thus if low-risk individuals who would prefer to remain uninsured are conscripted into the pool, they want limited coverage to cut their losses. Including prescription drugs (not covered by Medicare) also waved a red flag to young and healthy individuals.[54] Supplying coverage for substance abuse and mental health—to target only two key items—counts as pure cost and no benefit for persons of sober habits who abstain from drugs and alcohol. Yet their payments would have been open-ended because the amorphous nature of the underlying disease conditions make it very difficult to restrict payment once coverage is allowed. To be sure, everyone understands the easy cases, but who could trust the psychiatric profession to give disinterested determinations for myriad lesser disorders, no matter how many fervid assurances they offer on TV talk shows?

No one should be misled, however, by the true observation that mental health or substance abuse coverage may be included today in some private health plans. There is no reason to doubt that in some industries the worker base is sufficiently young and educated that the costs of covering these conditions is not prohibitive. Individual firms could also be in a position to mount tight controls to restrain costs. But it is one virtue of a market that it does not require every firm to follow the strategy of the industry leader. If other firms hire workers from different pools or face different costs of supervising treatment protocols, they could easily decide to spurn the coverage that makes sense for its rival. The incentives are there to make the right choice no matter what other firms have done. The insistence that any program adopted by one company should be imposed on all is a recipe for mass overinsurance because it misses the critical role that variations in market behavior play. By focusing on the few firms that do supply some coverage, it ignores the lessons that should be learned from the many rational firms that avoid this coverage altogether, or limit it sharply.

To complicate matters still further, the benefit packages are no more stable than the eligibility rules. Once again, the ACLU position offers an accurate barometer of the political cleavages. Just try to pass a program without coverage for mental health and substance abuse. The ACLU denounced that approach as constitutionally suspect for its invidious elimination of benefits for society's most vulnerable. "[W]e oppose the Clinton plan's limits on outpatient rehabilitation services for persons with disabilities, and also limits on mental health and substance abuse services."[55] Once again, the political process lost some of its ability to moderate coverage as a concession to the problems of monitoring treatment or containing costs. Congress was told all or nothing, and nothing was the response.

ABORTION AND FAMILY PLANNING

The difficulties in setting benefit packages expanded beyond these grubby particulars to the explosive dispute of over coverage for family planning, including abortions. On this issue, the political coalition for universal coverage quickly became unglued because it became impossible to bridge the gap between devout Catholics and strong abortion rights advocates. The ACLU ranks a woman's right to a safe abortion at the top of the constitutional firmament. In a world where the state only guards negative liberties, this right is guaranteed by removing all criminal sanctions against giving or receiving an abortion, which now becomes just another medical service supplied by the market or a charity. Peaceful coexistence between supporters and opponents of the abortion right is (barely) possible in that world of negative rights. No woman can have an abortion for another, so that those who favor the practice may participate in it, whereas those who do not may stay off to one side. The situation is surely not ideal because the same separatist logic also defends infanticide within families (which no doubt is practiced covertly in extreme cases). But the pressure points for conflict are at least reduced when only criminal sanctions are at stake.

The struggle over right and wrong, however, burns far brighter in a regime of positive rights. Now that the state funds medical services, there is no place to hide. The supporters of funding can *rightly* insist that the state has a duty to fund abortions so long as it funds other prenatal services. Otherwise the state "distorts" the choices needy pregnant women must make between exercising their constitutional right to abortion and carrying their child to term. This position holds that the state may support both prenatal care and abortions or neither, but not the former to the exclusion of the latter. Yet public funding of abortions invites howls of protest from groups who *rightly* insist that it is immoral to tax them to fund homicide.

The Supreme Court has officially upheld the Hyde amendment that excludes abortion funding from pregnancy programs, but only by the narrowest of margins, 5 to 4.[56] Its decision has not quieted the turmoil over the underlying issue. The political pressures to include abortion funding, abortion counseling, and similar services in standard federal programs such as Medicaid did not disappear precisely because it is an *open* question whether to fund abortion under, for example, the Public Health Service Act.[57] Or under the HSA.[58] Catholic groups strongly favored universal access, but bitterly opposed abortion funding. The ACLU detected no constitutional imperative for the HSA, but insisted that the equal protection guarantees of the Constitution required it to provide coverage for abortions along with other pregnancy care.[59] Whatever the legal weaknesses of either position, the Democratic coalition on universal care came apart at the seams.

The conflict went deeper than abortion funding. The draft HSA required all employers to provide their workers with a standard benefit package. Must the Catholic Church pay for the abortions of its lay employees? Must Catholic physicians and Catholic hospitals perform abortions? The Clinton bill responded to this concern by providing: "A health professional or a health facility may not be required to provide an item or service in the comprehensive benefit package if the professional or facility objects to doing so on the basis of a religious belief or moral conviction."[60] That compromise provision did not satisfy the ACLU, which was willing to exempt individual physicians from performing abortions against their conscience but refused to accept the same dispensation to health facilities, including Catholic hospitals. "This provision not only goes beyond legitimate free exercise concerns, but also raises serious Establishment Clause problem by allowing any health care facility to impose its stated institutional beliefs on patients and individual health care providers."[61]

Needless to say, that declamation did not sit well with the overseers of large Catholic hospitals. But more to our point, it reveals the unyielding coercive subtext of a world of state-conferred positive rights. Quite simply, the twin demands of autonomy (religious or individual) and nondiscrimination can no longer be reconciled. In constitutional terms, the "free exercise" clause of the First Amendment is now in hopeless tension with the Establishment Clause of the same amendment, which embeds the basic tension in a single sentence, albeit with two clauses: "Congress shall make no law respecting an establishment of religion, or prohibiting the free exercise thereof."

Starting with the Establishment Clause, it is odd for the ACLU to insist that an institution "imposes" its views on others by refusing to supply them with demanded services. Where is the use or threat of force? The hospital does conscript patients into its beds against their will. But so long as a world of positive rights converts every provider into a common carrier, this core conception of freedom—the right to be left alone—is necessarily compromised, both for individuals and for institutions. The institution that wants to escape the universal obligation of service now asks for a preference that counts as an impermissible establishment of religion. The regime of positive rights, therefore, removes or compromises the protection previously afforded to negative liberties. The world of positive rights produces a constitutional overload: to allow religious organizations their ordinary liberties is to give them an illicit preference. To eliminate that preference is to snuff out their free exercise. Faced with this tension, the Supreme Court has thrown up its hands and has tended to reject both claims so that the protections of both religion clauses disappear into a void.[62] So it is back to the political struggle between the Church and the ACLU. The language of positive rights only conceals the deep tensions on abortions, AIDS, drugs, sex education, and a thousand other topics.

This constitutional impasse could not arise in a world of negative rights. No one hospital has a monopoly. Other facilities could and do offer abortions. Why then must the state force every institution to provide them? The refusal to deal inheres in all private institutions, so no religious institution receives any preference by exercising its ordinary common law right to exclude. Hence it is possible to respect freedom of association without creating the religious exemptions condemned by the Establishment Clause. The ACLU position is thus exactly backward on a critical question of civil liberties. Under the HSA, the free exercise claim triumphs unless the word "exercise" is read so narrowly as to include liturgy but exclude their provision of charitable services. The frictions that ripped the Clinton alliance on this one dispute helped bring about the overall demise of the HSA.

COST-CONTAINMENT?

The access and benefit provisions of the Clinton program produced both too much redistribution and too much conflict within the normal democratic alliance to command majority support. The Administration's only hope for assembling a winning coalition depended on the cost-containment portion of the HSA. Taken in isolation, cost-containment is a political winner because it benefits the median voter, who now receives the same level of medical services for less money than before. Any credible cost-containment program that did not expand access could have commanded wide support because everyone receives the prior level of benefits for less. Indeed, the systemwide savings would have improved access indirectly by lowering the costs of buying medical care.

The predictions become much murkier, however, when cost-containment strategies are packaged with expanded access, as in the Clinton plan. Even if its containment strategies had been fail-safe, different groups would have received different net benefit packages from the HSA. High-risk individuals previously outside the basic system could have rejoiced from the double benefit of better access at lower cost, but their ranks were never large enough to ensure the passage of the HSA. Those many citizens who would have lost from expanded access faced a more complex calculation: to net out the probable gains from cost-containment against their probable losses from mandated universal access.

The tension between cost-containment and universal access was apparent from the outset. The Democratic issue poll of May 1993 asked individuals to rank cost-containment against making health care secure for everybody. Among those with clear preferences, cost-containment came out ahead by 49 to 38 percent.[63] In the end the Clinton political campaign decided to stick with security—health care that is always there—because of its far greater resonance with the public at large. Hence the consultants decided that the dominant goal should be security.[64] But the issue is hardly that clear. Security may rank first in the minds of most people, contrary to the earlier polling data, but if that security is to be guaranteed by the political process, it remains subject to the whims of the political process. Your health care needs are not placed in the hands of a single political entity that can alter the benefits or protection. The health care is always there, so long as Congress does not take it away.

Stated in another way, health security and universal access don't turn out to be the same thing. Security for you means that your benefits cannot be taken away. It does not mean that other individuals have equal rights to the same benefit. Indeed, the broader the access, the less secure are the many individuals who already have coverage: the additional expenses could trim down the benefit packages or increase the waiting on queues. Talking about security versus cost does not quite capture all the nuances of the relevant tradeoffs. Talking about universal access against cost-containment gives a somewhat more accurate reading of the choice. In practice, that calculation turned out to be stunningly easy to make. Losses from broader access dominate gains from cost-containment—period. Weary and cynical citizens know all too well that governments can expand access with the stroke of the pen. Medicare and Medicaid have brought new individuals and new treatments within their capacious folds. Those political commitments were easily enforceable by individual recipients: to withdraw them triggers a raft of political, administrative, and legal maneuvers. Unfortunately, good penmanship does not implement cost-containment. Everything depends on the complex systems of unproved worth. The most casual exposure to Medicare and Medicaid revealed, even in 1993 and 1994, that unquenched consumer demand outwitted at every turn the cost-containment technologies of DRGs and the RBRVSs.

Political cost-containment thus has a record of failure, even for limited programs. Who could pull the rabbit out of the hat with universal coverage and expanded benefit packages? The prudent voter, therefore, does not bite at the apple. Cost-containment need not be proposed as part of a package that expands both access and coverage; it can always be put back on the table by itself. The President finally glimpsed the political dynamics when he backpedaled from his original all-inclusive coverage demand to compromises that covered, say, 95 or 90 percent of the population. But the overall instability of the HSA could not be cured by a half-hearted concession at the eleventh hour, especially one that irritated plan supporters without placating plan opponents. Once again, the HSA came up short.

ADMINISTRATIVE CHOICES

The Clinton plan also faced serious administrative problems in its determination to place all health care under one roof. Yet this could not be done without impairing the efficiency of health delivery services. Competition and free entry place powerful restraints on the growth of individual firms. Unwieldy firms lose out to slimmer competitors. A regime of positive rights, however, cannot rely on decentralized decisions to set firm size because all its revenue comes from taxation, which only the government can raise and spend. Because the federal government could not have provided health care itself, it had to rely on delegation: set standards at the center and then allow the states to organize delivery within their respective boundaries. Sensible delegation, however, raised a new set of thorny difficulties. How are the activities of the two layers to be coordinated?

One system of control uses national budget caps to limit the total amount of resources committed to the system. Thus the HSA contained elaborate provisions to implement a system of premium caps, which in turn limits the total contributions that plan participants have to pay into the system.[65] Likewise, the HSA contained explicit provisions limiting the ability of individuals enrolled in fee-for-service plans to buy additional services. Any such purchase was subject to "reasonable restrictions" that explicitly included both a utilization review and "prior approval for specified services."[66] Total expenditures from all sources would have been set from above. State officials would have been required to cut services or reduce payments to meet their budget targets.[67]

This disguised system of price controls was introduced to reduce the percentage of GDP spent on health care. But why? Restrictions on consumption make sense to limit the effect of embedded subsidies. Whenever A is told to spend B's money, his temptation is to spend too much. But this risk disappears when A must spend his own money because ordinary self-interest checks extravagant expenditures. In this market environment, premium caps senselessly prevent consumers from making the best use of their own money by shifting it to health care as they get older. By blurring the line between private and public expenditures, price caps brand the private purchase of medical services as a dubious or even criminal social act. Spending your own money becomes a form of theft because it is said to increase the cost of medical services to other individuals. Wholly overlooked are the two obvious responses. First, this shift in expenditure reduces costs elsewhere for other individuals. Second, the shift signals a movement of overall resources into areas of greater private demand. In contrast, price caps distort sensible responses in all private markets. Once again, the public regulation of health care services follows the ordinary rules of economic behavior.

The situation in reality was worse that this critique suggests. Although the National Health Board could limit expenditures, it could not administer them. The unsettled conflict was whether the state regulators should adopt (a) a managed care system under which several firms within a given territory compete for business on the basis of quality and affordability of services, or (b) a Canadian-like single-payer plan.[68] On so critical a structural choice, the experts could not agree, so the HSA left its defining choice to local option.[69]

Punting on that decision guaranteed a second-generation, state-level struggle over the choice of plan design. That struggle would determine everyone's health care costs. One neglected virtue of voluntary plans is that the charges for each person or family depend primarily on their individual or family risk profile. The firm that supplies the stated coverage at the lowest price (quality constant) wins. Let coverage be priced too low, and getting the contract produces a loss. Pricing it too high results in losing the deal. The rates of different firms tend to converge on the cost of coverage. Any change between plans will not cause a quantum leap up or down.

Not so with the choice between competing managed care units and a single-payer plan. First, if a single-payer system is less efficient than managed care operations, no one will escape the increased cost. In addition, because risk is socialized, the determinants of cost change. What each person or family pays depends very little on their own cost profile. Instead it depends on the risk profile of the group of which they are a part. As noted earlier, the Clinton plan restricted the power of the state to shape the districts in which various health alliances would offer contracts to members. But even my premium as a Chicago resident would have depended heavily on whether the state chose a single-payer plan or managed competition. In the first case, my rates would have depended on the risk profile of my district. In the second, they would have depended on statewide characteristics. Furthermore, rates under managed care would have depended on the boundaries of my territory. My premiums would have been lower under a plan that folded the suburbs into the City district, but far higher if the City had been treated as a separate unit. None of these territories is set in stone, so politics would have reached a fever pitch before the dust settled. The redistricting struggles for political elections give a glimpse of the battles that would have followed. In market health plans, a person's own risks, not the territories, determine rates. Not so with national health plans, where territories count for all, and individual risks are largely irrelevant. It is a tremendous shift.

The Clinton plan was in reality far more baroque. Its universal access proposal would have ultimately required a single massive provider in each territory. Stated otherwise, political pressures might have preserved separate territories, but not multiple competitive plans within these territories. The disintegration of competition starts from the cross-subsidies that the HSA built in at the ground floor. It wanted to facilitate competition only along certain designated dimensions, namely, price and quality of service. But it also prohibited the use of competitive forces in the classification or rating of risk. Simultaneously, it required open enrollment up to plan capacity and gave preferences for renewal to individuals within its group.[70]

The bottom line is that no insurer could have kept underwriting control over its insured population. It would have had to insure all the risks that came its way, while charging only those premiums established on systemwide averages, averages that need not have reflected the risk potential of its own insured population. The plan that excelled in providing, say, treatment for cancer, would have attracted too many cancer patients. The difficulties of adverse selection remain alive and well. Consequently utilization would have increased and premiums would not have kept pace. Successful medical and service innovation would have led to economic ruination unless the states compelled transfer payments from low-risk to high-risk firms. These endemic cross-payments would have required firms to compete in one arena, while paying each other's bills in a second. Could firm A examine firm B's books to see if its charges were excessive? Would an expanded audit function allow firm A to challenge firm B's choice of care? Regulation and state supervision could draw the firms ever closer until they are transformed into subsidiaries in a common venture under state control. Managed care and market competition are possible, but managed competition sounds more like an oxymoron and less like an industry structure. By degrees, the inescapable cross-subsidies blend many firms into one.

The allocation problems within state boundaries under the Clinton plan were matched by a parallel set of difficulties in coordinating the plans of different states. Within a market system, inharmonious state regulations pose constant challenges to the operation of any nationwide health plan. That problem, however, pales into insignificance when workers in national corporations must be scattered across the 50 different statewide systems. The HSA frustrated continuous coverage of workers who were transferred across state lines. Even nationwide corporations with over 5,000 employees would have had to comply with all the conditions imposed on other provider plans:[71] three plans for workers, including one fee-for-service plan;[72] community ratings;[73] anti-red-lining;,[74] special assistance for low-wage families;[75] and ministerial busy-work. For their part, multiemployer plans, such as those that cover many workers from different companies in the same industry, would have had "to reflect the unique and historical relationship between the employers and employees under such alliance."[76] That nebulous standard could invite endless review, inconsistent decisions, uncertainty, and delay. The political opposition to the HSA follows from a simple recitation of its content.

TAXATION

The Clinton plan would not have come cheap. Ideally its tax base should be designed to minimize the disruption of productive activities. But how? A four-fold increase in the tax on tobacco products was one obvious ploy.[77] Yet its revenue potential was strictly limited, for high taxes could drive sales and production out of business or underground. Then property, income, and sales taxes that were now collected for other ends would have to make up the lost revenues. The revenue base would have to find new worlds to conquer. In the end, it was like asking for the best location to detonate a hydrogen bomb in New York City—no one could say where. A stiff payroll tax ran into fierce resistance from small business alliances. A new income tax hike would have come on the heels of the previous Bush and Clinton taxes and would prove counterproductive. Martin Feldstein, for example, estimated that "while the Treasury gained less than $6 billion in additional personal income tax revenue, the distortions to taxpayers' behavior depressed their real incomes by $25 billion."[78] The effort to boost one new tax thus cuts out the revenue base for all other taxes. In the end, therefore, no one could find a dark place to hide the costs of the HSA. Pick your metaphor. Did the well run dry? Was the last nail placed in the Clintoncare coffin?

REFORMING THE PROFESSION

Tackling cost and access might have been sufficient work for one generation, but in its original version, the plan sought to do more: to reform the basic structure of the medical profession, especially with reference to training future physicians. Without question, medical services in the United States are out of whack. The Clinton forces decided that the best way to fix them was to shift resources from high-priced specialists into primary care, both to reduce costs and to improve the access of the poor to basic services. Unfortunately medical institutions are peculiarly resistant to major changes. Specialists do not want to sacrifice handsome incomes and years of training to resume the day-to-day work of general practitioners. Teaching, research, and residency programs are all geared to large concentrations of specialists whose distribution does not follow that of local populations. Research and advanced care tend to be situated in centers that serve regional, national, and even global populations. New York City and Boston are examples of major medical centers whose specialists serve broader markets.

Notwithstanding these cross-dependencies, the HSA aggressively contemplated reworking the internal structure of the profession in tandem with its other projects. Its provisions would have clamped extensive federal control over all residency and training programs through a National Council of Graduate Medical Education whose members would have been drawn from the ranks of physicians, health care providers, and ordinary citizens. That Council could have set the number of residency slots for each residency program.[79] The HSA required the Council to take into account not only regional needs and physician availability, but also "the extent to which the population of training participants in the program including training participants who are members of racial or ethnic minority groups."[80] It is a nice way of talking about federal quotas for medical education. The centralization (not to say probable destruction) of the entire system of medical education provoked howls of protest from the medical establishment who did not hesitate to inform their local Congressman and Senators (including New York's Senator Moynihan) of their distaste for the legislation. But once again, the matter was never resolved before the HSA went down to defeat.

CONCLUSION

In the end, the Clinton health plan richly deserved its fate. The plan that boldly promised something for everyone soon revealed its potential to do something to everyone. The inevitable cause of 1992 became the unbearable albatross of 1994. HSA's demise was a predictable—and welcome—casualty of democratic politics. Democratic institutions all too often allow powerful majorities to run roughshod over isolated minorities. Sometimes they allow well-organized minorities to rip off disorganized majorities. But democratic politics do not suffer majorities and minorities to join together in acts of political self-immolation. The special interests did line up against the plan, and for once they represented just about everyone.

No one should treat the problem of the health care in America as trivial, nor the plight of the uninsured as unworthy of a second thought. But with that said, the Clinton plan revealed the true weakness of its egalitarian impulse. It could have done little to improve the lot of the uninsured, but it would have done much more to reduce care and increase the cost of care for the rest of the population. A program like that does not benefit all Americans. In the end, we should work for legislation that helps some without hurting others, or better yet, that provides help across the board. Health care delivery is not just an aspiration; it is also a matter of performance.

PART TWO

❖ ❖ ❖

Self-Determination and Choice

Interlude

We have now completed our discussion of the manifold issues that surround the question of access. The simple point that remains is that the size of the resource base does more for the creation of good health than any political interventions designed to skew its use. That conclusion seems good in two separate settings. First, it is unwise to create rights of access to the health system to divert resources from other individual uses. The social goal is to maximize not only the years of life, but the years of good living before the onset of serious illness. Health expenditures therefore cannot be cordoned off to include only those spent on health care proper. They include, in part, all the expenditures that go to create good health and to reduce the need for access: food, clothing, shelter, and leisure for starters. Second, it is mistaken to try to improve health care by guaranteeing systemwide rights to access. At this juncture, the law of unintended consequences takes over and reduces the availability of the facilities and services to which access is, in name only, guaranteed. In the long run, at least, the use of social coercion for redistributivist purposes runs up against a resource constraint that it cannot avoid.

Part Two turns from access to deal with questions of self-determination and choice. In it, I examine a set of restrictions that the state imposes on choices that individuals want to make for themselves, and with their own resources. In many cases, the law today insists that individual judgment should not be honored on matters most vital to individual welfare, choices that have to do with life and death. The basic challenge is why these restrictions on freedom of action, freedom of choice, and freedom of contract. At a formal level, the questions of access are left behind. But in a practical sense, their influence remains. Thus the suggestion is often ventured that we would allow choice to individuals if only they had sufficient wealth to exercise it responsibly. We might, the argument continues, therefore change our attitudes toward organ transplantation, death and dying, and contracting out of liability if we have had some sort of universal health care system in place, thereby assuming the success of social programs whose soundness is very much in doubt. For the most part, I shall avoid stressing these interconnections and will return to one simple theme: By what right does the state prevent individuals from doing what they want with their own bodies, their own lives, and their own fortunes?

CHAPTER 9

❖ ❖ ❖

Alienability and Its Limitations: Of Surrogacy and Baby-Selling

PROPERTY AND EXCHANGE

The strengths and weaknesses of the general model outlined in the the opening chapters of this book should also be tested in the context of particular cases. The first of these object lessons concerns the problem of organ transplants. What is at stake in this exercise is a systematic comparison between two regimes—state control and voluntary private markets—that may be used to supply and distribute organs and other body parts and fluids. The current system is the antithesis of voluntary markets. It contains a flat prohibition against the sale of organs between private individuals and offers heavy encouragement of voluntary donation as the sole permissible means of procuring organs for transplantation. The charitable side of voluntary transactions is preserved, and encouraged, whereas the commercial side has been shut down entirely. Yet today, even charity only goes so far in organizing a market for organ donation. The donor may choose to make a gift of the organ, but normally has no control over who receives it, except in voluntary transactions within families.[1] Typically the organs are placed in a large pool that is administered by the United Network for Organ Sharing (UNOS), a quasi-public corporation that controls these matters.[2] The use of the word "sharing" in the title indicates the communitarian strain that pervades its operation. What is not explained is how organs can be "shared" as opposed to being merely allocated.

221

Given our present institutional structure, the ultimate disposition of the donated organ falls to a staff of anonymous bureaucrats who act on impersonal criteria.[3] The first is whether an appropriate histological match exists between the donated organs and the potential recipient—an issue that would remain of paramount concern even in a market system of allocation. Second, the nod between rival claimants may be determined by geographical location or by the length of time that the potential recipient spends in the queue. In principle, panels of citizens and experts could be empowered to award organs to worthy recipients, by making judgments of comparative virtue—today a task with few takers, but one discharged with great difficulty occasionally in the past. Instead, exclusive reliance is placed on two sorts of criteria. One stresse the technical measures of compatibility and future success; the other resorts to nonmarket systems of allocation, such as lotteries or queues, but never systems of markets and bidding.

To critique various elements of the current system of organ transfers, we must contrast it with the market system that the current law explicitly rejects. That task, in turn, requires some preliminary discussion of the general role that alienation plays in ordinary markets and other specialized contexts in order to set the stage for the more detailed discussion of organ transplantation, which then compares the desirability of the two rival allocation systems. Once that comparison is complete, I hope to persuade the reluctant and skeptical reader that the following counterintuitive conclusions are correct. First, no ad hoc principles should limit the sale or gift of organs from one person to another. Second, general principles call for a regime of alienability by sale, gift, or bequest, limited at most by certain safeguards to prevent fraud, neglect, or undue influence. It should not matter whether the transaction takes place from the dead to the living—so-called cadaveric transplantations—or between two live persons, whether or not related by blood or marriage; nor even whether the transplantation is lethal to the donor. Of course, there is a vast difference in the desirability of these transactions and in the likelihood of their occurrence. Yet their ranking can, and should, take place by voluntary means, free of state coercion and control. The common law rules that allowed commercial exchanges to operate side by side with charitable donations are both simpler than and superior to the current regulatory regime.

To see why, suppose for the moment that the basic bundle of ownership rights did include the right to sell or donate property. In this system, property would be far from worthless, but its value would be limited to its best use by its present holder. Each person would have to fend for himself in a world of scarcity and be self-sufficient in a way that would require him to build his own house and farm his own land. Specialization of labor would yield no gains because no one would be able to sell the product of his own labor and use the proceeds to purchase goods and services supplied by another. So long as value in use routinely exceeds the value in exchange, the prohibition on sale is of no consequence. But the vibrant operation of thousands of markets suggests that often the reverse is true, and that exchange is a source of benefit for all participants.

A system of exchange depends on a secure system of property rights. I may only sell what I own, and for obvious reasons, only I may sell it. Once transferred, that property may be used, consumed, or retransferred, either in whole or in part. By repetitive voluntary transactions, individual owners can create joint tenancies, leases, loans, mortgages, covenants, and easements in exquisite variation. And they can form business partnerships and voluntary organizations. These transactions are all driven by the prospect of gain from trade, whereby self-interested persons surrender one thing only if they receive something of greater value in exchange. Voluntary exchanges allow both sides to be better off than before, as measured by their own conceptions of the good. What is true of the buyer is true of the seller, what is true of the lender is true of the borrower. Each transaction is win/win for its participants, so the more rapid the pulse of trade, the greater the gains to all participants.

Gifts work by a similar analysis. Sometimes they have been criticized as "sterile transactions" because they do not create new forms of wealth.[4] Typically the prospect of mutual gains from trade takes on a reduced role, as other motivations dominate. Yet even here donors receive indirect benefits, often in intangible form, from making gifts to family and friends. In addition, the ability to make gifts today may have induced yesterday's efforts to create or amass wealth in the first place. The lack of direct economic benefit surely reduces the frequency of gift transactions relative to sales and other forms of exchange. But the relative infrequency of these transactions is hardly a reason to ban or constrict their scope.

The indirect benefits of voluntary donations make these transactions win/win as well.

In practice we do not see an indefinite number of voluntary transactions. The most powerful limitation on their operation is friction, commonly called transactions costs.[5] Buying, leasing, and mortgaging are not costless. Terms have to be negotiated; the parties have to be assured that they will receive clear title to the property acquired. All this costs money. If the gains from trade are smaller than the transactions costs, it is not worth anyone's while to proceed. Where the gains are larger than the transaction costs, the parties will go ahead with the transaction. These frictions never disappear, and at some point they bring the process of exchange to a natural halt. The higher the transactions costs, the greater the social barriers to useful exchange. One object of a mature legal system is to reduce the drag so that the transactions can go forward.

The presence of transaction costs does not justify denying enforcement of the voluntary transactions that are made. The presence of joint gains is sufficient to justify a *presumption* in favor of their enforcement. But that presumption might be overridden by showing that the transaction yields, on balance, a net social loss. In principle, that showing can only be made in two ways: defects in contract formation and adverse effects on third parties.

The first concern is *process based* and requires a showing that the anticipated joint gains to the trading parties are not present, which requires a demonstration that the transaction was not truly voluntary, but was induced by duress, fraud, or other undue influence that interfered with the ability of one side to make the correct subjective valuation.[6] If I put a gun to your head to make you sell your prize Rembrandt for a $1,000, you are not comparing the value of the Rembrandt to $1,000; you are comparing the value of the Rembrandt to the value of your life. Similarly, if I represent my fake Rembrandt as a real one, the $1 million price is far above what you would have paid if you possessed accurate information, even on the doubtful assumption that the sale would go forward. If you are too young or demented to understand an offer, you lack the capacity to evaluate the gains and losses of any particular exchange.

Finally, the most difficult legal category to deal with is that of simple mistake, not induced by the other party and perhaps unknown to him. The mistake also leads to a misevaluation of the property that is transferred or received in exchange. The prospects of joint benefit are likely to be dashed; yet the security of transactions will be undermined mightily if a steady procession of claims of mistake—manufactured, dubious, or real—is permitted to undo the investments of others. It is not surprising that the problem has never generated a uniform legal response, but has spawned legal doctrine that is both difficult and obscure.[7]

Matters become more difficult still when the issue is not whether these elements of duress, fraud, incompetence, or mistake are relevant, but whether they must be proved case by case. There is no categorical rule. In certain situations good sense leads judges (and ordinary people) to recognize the common danger signs. Any transactions between a trustee and a beneficiary is suspect because the former cannot deal at arm's length with the latter. Matters are only worse if you are old and infirm, perhaps near death, and in imperfect control of your faculties. These cases of undue influence, which loom so large in the health area, again yield no consistent solution at common law.[8] Sometimes the mere disparity in value between what is sold and its market price is enough to justify setting the transaction aside. Who can believe that the infirm widow wanted to sell the $100,000 farm for $100? Sometimes courts require proof of some pattern of undue influence, even in the absence of fraud or misstatement. Retaining *independent* counsel or advisors for the impaired person is typically a useful prophylactic against after-the-fact challenges to the deal. No market advocate believes that freedom of contract forbids making allowances for demonstrated differences in the capacity for rational discussion or calculation. Yet none accepts any generalized assumption of individual incompetence, sufficient to undermine not only the capacity to contract, but also the capacity to marry and vote. The stock cases of undue influence are difficult to decide. Fortunately the issue does not loom large in commercial transactions, where only the fit and hardy see fit to venture. The issue takes on a larger role in consumer transactions, but even here consumers are often protected by their ability to take standard prices from large retail operators. But on matters of health, the questions of competence and undue influence are of major concern. It is a pressing problem for any regime that deals with organ transplantation.

The second ground for refusing to enforce voluntary contracts rests on their adverse effects on third persons, so-called negative externalities. No exchange or gift takes place in a social void. The transfer of property from one person to another may have profound effects on the welfare of third persons who are unable to contract with the parties in question. In principle, these third-party effects could be either positive or negative, and in many cases, both types of effect are present simultaneously. If the net benefits to third parties are positive, the law has all the more reason to enforce a voluntary transaction. Happily that outcome is the most common for ordinary exchanges because the increase in wealth that the parties obtain from one transaction increases the trading opportunities of other parties down the line. But matters are more clouded when the external effects turn negative. Now the transaction is no longer a win/win situation across the board. In all cases, the central task is to maximize the gains from exchange, taking into account the welfare of outsiders. Two cases are thus relevant.

First, if those external losses on balance are *small* relative to the gains to the trading partners, the transaction should be enforced nonetheless. The alternative invites deep social paralysis. Any disappointed competitor could then demand compensation or block the transaction, which could then take place only by a committee of the whole giving its unanimous consent.[9] That approach leads to social folly in the long run. The uniform gains from alienation between A and B are replicated countless times. The persons who lose in the one transaction will gain in the long run from the overall soundness of the legal regime. Thus, for our purposes, only systematic losses to third parties should be taken into account.

Second, if the third-party losses are *large* relative to the gains to the transacting parties, a total ban is warranted. However, where these losses are of somewhat lesser size and controllable by other means, restrictions, short of prohibition, may be appropriate, or some compensation may be exacted from the trading parties before letting their transaction go forward. The ban or restriction is appropriate only where the following inequality is satisfied: third-party losses less any gains to the trading parties are greater than the administrative costs of their control. Thus if A cannot murder B, then A cannot hire C to do the job for him or purchase a bomb or an assault weapon from him. Yet, by the same token, a general ban on the sale of tools and metal would so disrupt the entire social fabric that lesser forms of restraint, more closely tied to the abuse, must be adopted if any restraints are to be used at all.

Similarly voluntary restraints on output or price between rival traders are usually prohibited because of the systematic social losses that they impose on third parties. The standard economic models show how the monopolist's gain is smaller than his customer's losses.[10] If relatively cheap judicial and administrative means of control are available, acquisitions and mergers could be banned or approved, subject to certain conditions (for example, partial divestiture of property) to protect these third-party interests. Yet even here, the dangers of regulatory overreaching (for example, as through a ban on predatory pricing, which destroys routine competition) are sufficiently great that considerable attention must be given to formulating the relevant rule.

Physical harms and financial effects are not the only forms of external harm invoked to block a voluntary transaction. Of ever greater importance today are various types of "soft" externalities, those third-party effects that focus on the subjective reaction and social response of outsiders to particular types of voluntary transactions.[11] Within the standard form of economic analysis, all changes in utility of third persons are relevant in principle: feelings of resentment, outrage, shame, and the like are no exceptions to the general rule. Every action by every individual could influence the well-being of others, so that the psychological and symbolic effects, if given free rein, could dominate discussions of external effects. In line with this renewed concern with soft externalities, the academic literature contains much learned talk about the danger of the "commodification" of certain goods and services (for example, prostitution), which causes women, and men, to think less of their own personal and sexual capabilities,[12] and which are often blended with more traditional empirical claims that pornography increases the level of physical violence against women.[13]

Speech is not the only area in which these soft externalities have been arrayed against individual liberty. The topic of organ transplantation also requires some consistent approach to decide whether these soft external losses justify restrictions on the freedom to alienate property, labor or, for that matter, part of one's self. It should take its cue from the constitutional tradition that protects freedom of speech, a tradition that rightly has been sharply resistant to taking these elements into account *ever*. My outrage at your silly political pronouncements is no reason to ban them; they only justify my response, which others could find sillier than your original statement. Obviously counterspeech does not work as well for pornography, but the dangers of excessive zeal are every bit as great.[14]

Taken over the full range of cases, however, our law rests on a well-conceived global faith that the positive external effects from speech, considered globally, offsets its negative effects. It is just too dangerous to try to single out that speech which is especially offensive and dangerous and subject it to a set of restrictions that no rival speech is subject to.[15] The isolation of some negative effects on individual listeners incorrectly biases the inquiry. Ideally we should take both positive and negative effects into account. Practically we cannot execute that comparison listener by listener. As a rough proxy, therefore, the right view is to treat the two effects as though they *cancel* each other out, even though we cannot be sure that this is the case. As with economic losses, the search has to be for some systematic negative bias from speech. Generally speaking, that point only comes after a statement defames a particular person, incites physical assault or harassment, or induces a breach of a promise or of confidentiality. Until those buttons are pushed, the speech should be, and usually is, left free of government regulation and coercion.

The risk of overrating these soft negative externalities carries over to transactions in human organs. My outrage at your sale of your organ is no reason to ban it any more than my pleasure at your organ sale is reason to compel it. Too many forms of conduct offend too many people for any legal system to respond to them all. Politically it is explosive to respond selectively to these frayed sensibilities. The appropriate rule for these psychic externalities is this: *ignore* them all, lest freedom of action, speech, and contract be drowned in a chorus of special pleas, which accentuate the negative and ignore the positive external effects of controversial speech, thoughts, or conduct.[16] Within legal discourse, it has been said, somewhat mystically, that these are all psychic bruises that count only as *damnum absque ininuria*, harms without legal injury. An accurate account treats them as real harms, coupled with real benefits. The precise balance of advantage in any case is too difficult to calculate, so the only safe course of action is to avoid the temptation to ban activities whose consequences are not fully understood. Soft externalities should not come in from the cold.

TOUGH CASES FOR ALIENABILITY:
BABY-SELLING AND SURROGACY

Before turning to organ transplants, it is useful to note briefly how this two-part framework applies to some highly controversial cases, most notably baby-selling and surrogate motherhood. The initial point is that there are enormous gains from trade between the parties. No one should gloss lightly over the genuine shortage of babies brought about by the absence of the price mechanism. State-supervised adoptions are often a monument to collective rigidity or worse, subjecting prospective parents to endless and intrusive inquiries about parental age, family accommodations, psychological profiles, personal habits, and sexual histories—all for humanitarian ends. To the extent that prospective parents can avoid the queues, anxieties, delays, and indignities of present official processes, so much the better. Whatever the objections to a system of baby-selling, that practice must be compared to the imperfect substitutes in place.

In dealing with surrogacy or adoption, the dispute boils down to the question of whether the transactional or external risks justify banning or severely restricting these practices. In both cases, the popular sentiment of indigant outrage says yes. In both cases, a calmer, less hasty response suggests that the correct answer is no. Start with the transactional risks. There is always some danger that women will be coerced into entering into deals by force or fraud. But little evidence is offered to explain why this danger is so pervasive that it cannot be countered on a case-by-case basis by the ordinary rules used to ferret out fraud, incompetence, or undue influence. Why assume that women of full age constitute a suspect class subject to manipulation and exploitation by the sophisticated and ruthless individuals with whom they are forced to deal? Like all protective regulations, a prohibition on baby-selling is a two-edged sword. It says to some people that women are to be kept outside commerce and are the better for it. It says to other people that women are so incapable of making reasonable judgments for themselves and for their children that they must remain wards of the state, even on the most personal and intimate decisions of their lives. The double effect of economic regulation of women is apparent in legal prohibitions on wages and hours applied solely to women, which were once favored[17] but are now much distrusted.[18] The issue does not disappear just because the welfare of a child is at stake. Assumptions of flawed competence are not easily confined to some chosen domain.

Today, although both the baby-selling and surrogacy markets do function, if only at the fringes, the anecdotal evidence strongly suggests that the women understand the high stakes in the transactions and proceed intelligently.[19] Women who are intent on giving up their children in the "gray market" usually take pains to learn something about the identity of the prospective parents and can ask for résumés and interviews to satisfy themselves that they are letting their child go into a desirable new home. The effects on the child are likely to be *positive,* given their bleak prospects if the transaction breaks down. Similarly, anxious couples bent on hiring surrogate mothers rarely go to someone who has never had children herself and usually screen the potential biological mother to weed out women whose psychological composition and family circumstances make them inappropriate for the task. Why ask for trouble? A regime of *enforceable* surrogacy contracts facilitates this process by inducing potential mothers to reflect carefully on whether they are ready to assume that role. The process, therefore, helps weed out women who are uncertain about their future psychological state of mind and thus reduces the possibility of regret that could prove so tormenting on all sides. A regime of fully enforceable contracts, therefore, increases both the security and frequency of these transactions.

That screening function cannot be discharged under a popular compromise advanced by Professor Martha Field. She proposes to treat the contracts as valid but unenforceable at the option of the biological mother, but not the biological father.[20] The single binding constraint on the mother is that she make a once-and-for-all choice at birth. Field expects that typically she will follow through on the original plans, as some 99 percent of the surrogate mothers have done.[21] If the contracting device is not allowed to weed the wavering mother from the field, greater reliance and greater expense must be placed on psychological testing, thereby deterring many willing surrogates uncomfortable with the newer rules. The upshot is that the rate of withdrawal would increase; and if it went even from 1 to 3 percent, it could have enormous impact on the formation of surrogacy contracts.

That wait-and-see option should not always be shunned. When a married couple wants to adopt a child outside of surrogacy, the birth mother may change her mind up to the last moment. She may keep the child and sever the relationship with the adoptive couple, with some bitterness and sorrow. With surrogacy, however, the breakdown of the contract does not spell the end of the relationship because the biological father is still the father. Instead of a clean break, an ugly custody fight looms on the horizon. Given the prospect, many couples will decide not to go ahead at all. The intermediate solution, therefore, will undermine the market, and for what? The gains from trade are palpable; the external effects are the creation of a new and wanted person. Why enforceable surrogate contracts should not be the source of rejoicing is perhaps one of the major mysteries of our time.

In surrogacy relationships, too much is also made of the point that the money paid is conclusive evidence of a breach of trust between the mother and her child.[22] But even in so-called gift transactions of the gray market, the adoptive parents may well defray the medical and legal expenses of the birth mother. Here, the mere fact that the state law imposes an upper bound on the amount of money involved, and on the purposes to which it can be used, is no insignificant detail. The simple fact that the expenditures in question are both bounded in extent and in purpose *may* effectively limit the ability of birth parents to make sales that disregard the welfare of their children. But, by the same token, why believe that parents of greater wealth will make on average worse parents than those with less, or that mothers will look only at cash bids for their offspring when they do not do so in other circumstances? The elaborate résumés that prospective couples prepare about themselves and their families, the screening, and the interviews suggest that in these adoptions both parties act as buyers, be it of the children or of the love and affection supplied to that child.

Nor should we worry in this context about the exploitation of the poor. If the buyer's examination of babies in this market is as serious as we would expect, the difficult question is how any poor woman could persuade cautious buyers that her baby is worthy of adoption. Her risk is exclusion, not exploitation. Thus an unregulated market would be selective in its own terms and would favor teenagers from good homes who became pregnant out of wedlock, women who had affairs before reconciling with their husbands, and mothers who had some major commitments with their children at home, but were morally opposed to abortion. It is not likely that prostitutes or drug addicts would fare well in this market because their conduct would compromise the healthiness of any baby they could supply.

The same conclusion applies to negative third-party effects. One obvious source of concern is for the child who is conceived and adopted. Here, Elizabeth Anderson, one of the leading opponents of surrogacy, has claimed that the transaction so commercializes the relationship that it undermines the parent-child bond. The "contract pregnancy commodifies both women's labor and children in ways that undermine the autonomy and dignity of women and the love parents owe to children."[23]

No one can deny categorically the possibility that some harm could come to the child after the transaction takes place, but three counterarguments meet the objection. First, the transactions are restricted to small infants. It is obviously inappropriate to impose them on children who have already formed attachments to their parents or guardians. Under those circumstances, greater caution has to be taken with respect to any permanent transfer. Yet this constraint also holds true for divorces, adoptions, and foster care placements, all of which face equally severe difficulties in placing older children. The difference is that market transactions will veer away from the problematic situations that these other arrangements have to confront head on. The market problem, therefore, takes care of itself even if baby-selling is allowed across the board. If some constraint is needed, a simple prohibition of sales transactions for children over the age of two or three should be easily enforceable.

Second, the risk of abuse is hardly zero or even negligible for the child who remains with its own mother. Poverty and family instability are highly correlated with the likelihood of abuse and serious injury, and these losses are compounded if the mother has either remarried or lives with a new boyfriend who is not the child's father. A full estimation of the externality effects must net out the harms averted with the harms created. The latter may be more visible, but the former are every bit as painful. So long as that balance is positive, the state should encourage these transactions. On this score there is, for whatever it is worth, an ever growing awareness of the dangers associated with a public policy that uses counseling and supervision to keep a child in a broken home no matter how grievous the past patterns of abuse. So long as the supervision does not run around the clock, the risks of serious injury remain. Exit is often safer, and it is more likely to happen if side payments to the mother are used.

Third, the parents who receive the child do not own it like some chattel, but they are subject to all the same obligations that the law imposes on natural parents for the safety and benefit of their children. The more accurate description of the situation is to conceive of all baby-selling arrangements as assignments of parental rights (just as in regulated adoptions) subject to the same duties of support, and to the same limitations on abuse and neglect, imposed on the birth parents.

Formally, at least, the situation is no different from the assignment of rights under contract, where the invariable rule is that the assignee of the original promise takes subject to all duties that had been imposed on the assignor.[24] Thus suppose that you agree to paint my house on condition that I first clean the interior walls. I then sell my house to X and transfer my right to have the house painted under contract. You may not still be obliged to do the identical job, but if you are, you can still insist that my buyer clean the interior walls just as I would have to do.

To repeat, the language of baby-selling, however colloquial, is inaccurate because it ignores the duties that devolve on the "buyers" of the child, who are subject to the same punishment for abuse and neglect as the biological parents. By the same token, moreover, they are less likely to commit it. Surrogacy or baby-buying is not some casual decision. Why would people scour the earth for suitable children only to turn around and hurt them? In fact, paying cash helps protect these infants from abuse. It signifies an investment that the new parents have made in the child, one that is lost or compromised by abuse. And the payment also marks them as persons with sufficient resources and interest to care for the child and to spend the emotional energy necessary to negotiate a difficult transaction. It is quite amazing how little empathy the opponents of these arrangements have with the life-wrenching situation of any of the adopting parties. Their objections are so abstract, stern, and uncompromising that ironically they miss the human struggle implicit in so perilous an undertaking.

With all this said, the attention given to harms to the child explains why some clear restrictions should be placed on any transaction that on its face ignores the network of parental obligations. It is inconceivable to think that a sale of a child into prostitution or slavery is in the interest of the child—unless abject and immediate starvation is the only alternative. A powerful predictor of abuse is the transfer of a baby to any person who does not assume the full parental role. Likewise, there should be an absolute prohibition against the use of any child as security for the repayment of debts, a transaction that reveals on its face the subordination of the child's welfare to commercial considerations. At a minimum, the transfers should be absolute and unconditional—there can be no return of children to the original parents if a serious disease or birth defect manifests itself after transfer, or if the parents obtain a divorce in the interim.[25] Some stability is surely required—although it is often lost in the countless cases of children who are shuttled about the foster care system, perhaps in part because of the want of a long-term baby market.[26] Indeed, the Department of Child and Family Care in Illinois is practically in political and moral receivership. Do we prefer systems like that to the range of private brokers and facilitators?

The world of soft externalities still remains. Once again, Elizabeth Anderson urges the standard position. "These degrading failures of respect and consideration on the part of the surrogate industry are of concern to the state, because they are embodied in relations of domination that deny surrogate mothers their autonomy."[27] The use of the term "domination" does not refer to any particular wrong directed toward any particular woman, but it posits a set of universal social relationships that presupposes exploitation, not mutual advantage, as the norm for exchanges between men and women. It acts as though women make all their decisions out of desperation, without consultation with their mothers, sisters, daughters, friends, and yes, husband. It treats coercion as a social given and a necessary truth instead of a regrettable occurrence. It also paints a frigid and hostile view of social relationships that is belied by the large number of the successful marriages and working families.

Lori Andrews's description of how women cope with these transactions has less philosophical angst but more robust common sense because she starts with specific anecdotes about successful surrogates.[28] Her account rings far more true than any broad-sided condemnation of surrogacy, and by implication baby-selling, as inconsistent with some idealized duties of women in modern society. Once again, like all protective regulations, these prohibitions are a two-edged sword. They say to some people that women are beyond commerce, and better for it. They say to other people that mothers (and fathers) are incapable of making reasonable judgments for themselves and for their children, and that they must remain wards of the state on the issues of greatest concern to their personal happiness.

Nor should we credit arguments that surrogacy or baby-selling transactions will "commodify" children. If it is evident to the opponents of these transactions that a child is not a sack of potatoes, it is equally evident to the participants. The word "commodity" carries with it the idea of trading in fungible commodities, which is certainly one sense of the term. But it is far from the only sense in which that term is used. When a parent speaks of his or her child as a precious commodity, the term is used with conscious irony. Ordinary commodities may be fungible, but the child is a precious commodity precisely because he or she is unique and irreplaceable. Why should the infusion of cash to a transaction dull the senses to this perspective?

The current legal position often plays off the fears of these transactions, but for all their ferocity, the substantive arguments are weak. Thus the Court in the *Baby M* case set them out in some detail.[29] First, it found baby-selling was "loathsome" because there is no assurance that the purchasers will be suitable parents. But the same problem arises in adoptions and foster care, so the decisive question is not whether baby-selling will sometimes fail—it will. Rather, it is whether the state or the birth mother is the better judge of that result. Of course, the empirical evidence remains hidden from view because the practices have never been allowed. Nor can one draw too many inferences from stories about how gray market adoptions misfire.[30] The key factor is never the fact of mistake, but its rate. Moreover, many of these transactions skirt the edge of the law precisely because of the legal prohibitions that hem them in on every side. As with all systems of regulation, only the hardy are prepared to enter when the price of mistake is disbarment and criminal sanctions. Behavior in gray markets offers only weak clues to the patterns of behavior after legalization.

The Court in *Baby M* also suggests that counseling, guidance, and access to a child's medical history are necessary for a successful adoption. But on this score, it never explains why the state is in the best position to provide these services, or why private market provisions of these services would not proliferate if the transactions were unquestionably legal. Today families routinely seek counseling in cases of death, disease, or divorce, as well as cases in which children have behavioral problems ranging from attention deficit disorders to dyslexia and beyond. The Court did not explain why the new parents would not *want* counseling services to ease the transaction and would not *want* information about the medical history of the child or its biological parents. Mysteriously it also ignores the obvious point that counseling services could be more cheaply supplied if the transactions were fully legal and not in the gray market.

From its dubious assumption about participant ignorance, the Court blithely concludes that the transaction cannot be voluntary even though all parties realize substantial gains. Yet what is the alternative? Do state adoption agencies have the resources or the inclination to provide these services when their overworked staffs labor under incredible budget constraints? Once again, individual transactions may go awry and require intervention. But fears of inadequate counseling offer only the slimmest of reeds for shutting down the baby-selling market. These transactions do not contemplate the killing of third persons, the fixing of prices, or even the insult and offense to strangers. These modest transactional difficulties have to be kept in perspective.

Finally, the decision says that the financial need of the birth mother could make her decision "less voluntary." Yet scarcity is a universal condition that drives all transactions and could be used to invalidate all transactions for food, clothing, and shelter if it could invalidate these transactions. The case is not, to repeat, one of hard-line duress or fraud; nor is it a case where necessity demands that a sale be made only to a single buyer if it is made at all. The transaction is illegal because it is made illegal. Whether the focus is on transactional difficulties or external effects, the arguments for banning these transactions fail across the board. The case for allowing surrogacy and baby-selling is, quite simply, that we cannot find sufficient reasons to displace the ordinary common law rules. The lesson is one of no little importance because it carries over to the problem of organ transplantation with, if anything, still greater urgency.

❖ ❖ ❖

CHAPTER 10

The Present: Shortages
Without Solution

A PERSISTENT SHORTAGE OF ORGANS

The discussion of the general principles governing the alienation of labor and property, and the specific discussions of baby-selling and surrogate mothers, together set the stage for dealing with the modern issues surrounding organ transplantation. No matter how powerful the general presumption in favor of alienation in modern society, equally powerful social pressures work to limit the free transferability of organs, certainly by sale and in many instances even by gift. The ultimate question is whether our present organ transplant policy is justified under the analytical framework just developed. Externality problems do not weigh heavily and transactional difficulties can be met with restrictions narrowly tailored to the risks of duress, fraud, nondisclosure, and incompetence. My basic position is that the current policy misfires because it rests on a misguided and perhaps immoral view of altruism, which is beset by two fatal weaknesses. First, the current altruistic policy overestimates the ability of detached generosity to meet the demand for organ transplants and thus tolerates inexcusable organ shortages. Second, its excessive confidence in donative transactions is improperly used to justify the ban on the social institutions—voluntary markets—that could help alleviate the current shortages. The constant appeal to high ethical and moral standards offers scant justification for the massive regulatory intrusion into this area, and we should all be far better off if altruism were confined to a more modest role: as a reason for private charity for those in need.

What is needed, in my view, is a total, frontal assault on the present legal regime that governs organ transplantation and on the philosophical outlook that sustains it. In order to place that critique in context, it is necessary to review the evolution of organ transplantation policy. The subject is of necessity a modern one, for no one has to fashion an organ transplantation policy before medicine develops techniques to perform organ transplants with relative safety and efficacy. Accordingly the issue did not receive considered attention from the earlier common law judges, who had plenty of other issues on their plates.[1]

More to the point perhaps, the technological obstacles that must be overcome before organ transplantation is a viable practice no doubt influenced the evolution of the biological and psychological traits of the human species. In the state of nature, a person could suffer many injuries—the escaped prey, the thwarted courtship, the bad turn in the weather. But the most deadly threat to any living creature is a physical invasion of the body. Although modern academic tort lawyers too often transform tort law into a bloodless exercise on the optimal prevention of accidents, the historical take on the subject was quite different. The key operative fact was physical invasion, and none was so dangerous as *corpore corpori*—by the body and to the body, by breaking bones and rupturing skin, as the Romans said. In the state of nature, these physical invasions always spelled trouble. Although there would be some strong biological urge to remove foreign objects from the body, whether splinters or bullets, no one has ever had a biological impulse to remove an internal organ, especially one that is in the pink of health. The biological aversion here is uniform and complete over recorded and unrecorded time. Thereafter, the psychological and emotional impulses on this, as on so many other issues, should be congruent with the underlying biological facts of survival. Just as strong territorial instincts undergird the institution of private property, and strong affective instincts nourish the family, so too deep instincts block the separation of any organ from self—a feature to which the blunt and elemental prose of Leon Kass makes a sustained and self-conscious appeal.[2]

Given our deepest presuppositions, any proposal to allow the free transferability of organs will probably fall on deaf ears, even before the onslaught of communitarian rhetoric drowns it out. The strong biological impulses are not rooted in the tenets of market economics, and the slow changes in evolutionary time are constantly at war with the radical transformations of medical technology. In light of these built-in obstacles, it takes a determined and detached rationalist to overcome the natural biological aversion, if it is to be overcome at all. In 1600, or even 1900, any court would have struck down a contract for the sale of a kidney. To all appearances, the seller had signed his own death warrant in a transaction of no benefit to anyone else—for it is far harder to receive a kidney than to surrender one. Likewise a court would have regarded any contract for the sale of a kidney for transplantation after death as ghoulish or worse. Recall that the social defense of freedom of contract rests on the assumption of mutual gain through trade. However, the contract for an organ sale for transplantation circa 1600 or 1900 does not reveal that potential, no matter how great the individual differences in subjective preferences and taste. Without that prospect of gain, judges would have decided the case as if there had been no consent, or no consideration, or no capacity; or they would have invoked doctrines of duress, or mistake, or contracts against public policy, or something—anything—to set the transaction aside. Yet now, when the technology has changed, should our attitude toward contract change as well? Why not, if the prospects of gain from trade between the parties are readily apparent to professional and citizen alike? We only ban transactions for the sale of organs because there is some reason to believe that these would, in fact, take place.

THE EVOLUTION OF MODERN TRANSPLANTATION POLICY: MEETING THE SHORTAGE

Turning then to the modern age, the scarcity of organs for life-saving transplants is the melancholy starting point for discussion for all sides of the transplantation debate.[3]

The tale of the numbers is quite inescapable, as shown in the table on the following page. We can easily observe the increases in the queues for organs. These increases, moreover, have become more rapid in all categories over time. Perhaps the most dramatic increases are in the queues for livers and lungs. These numbers carry with them a profound human message. In 1989, the total queue was only 40 percent of what it is today.

Lloyd Cohen, in his excellent and learned plea for a futures market in cadaveric organs, describes the consequences of the net imbalance in terms that have become only more urgent with the passage of time.

At the current level of medical knowledge and technique, approximately 15,000 Americans could benefit from a heart transplant, 22,500 from a kidney transplant, and 500 each from a liver or pancreas transplant.

How many cadavers suitable for organ harvesting are potentially available to meet the demand? The most desirable cadavers, though not the only ones suitable for transplantation, come from people who die of accidental causes. Each year approximately 60,000 die in automobile accidents alone. The Center for Disease Control estimates that 12,000 to 27,000 of these people die in a hospital. Thus at a minimum something on the order of 12,000 hearts and livers and 24,000 kidneys are potentially available for transplantation. This is six times the approximately 4,000 cadaver kidneys donated in 1983. Were those 12,000 hearts and livers and 24,000 kidneys available, they would be more than sufficient to satisfy the demand for tissue as defined by the current waiting lists and current definitions of clinical suitability. In addition, there would be more than enough to satisfy the demand of all categories of potential transplant patients, other than heart patients, even under the most liberal definition of clinical suitability.[4]

ORGAN	YEAR								
	1988	1989	1990	1991	1992	1993	1994	1995	1996
KIDNEY	13943	16294	17883	19352	22376	24973	27498	31045	34129
LIVER	616	827	1237	1676	2323	2997	4059	5691	7239
PANCREAS	163	320	473	600	126	183	222	285	319
KIDNEY/ PANCREAS	0	0	0	0	778	923	1067	1234	1462
HEART	1030	1320	1788	2267	2690	2834	2933	3468	3706
HEART/ LUNG	205	240	225	154	180	202	205	208	227
LUNG	69	94	308	670	942	1240	1625	1923	2274
TOTAL	16,026	19,095	21,914	24,719	29,415	33,352	37,609	43,854	49,485*

*United Network for Organ Sharing: U.S. Waiting List Statistics (November 6, 1996).

The more recent figures on the number of accidental deaths have not changed materially: about 12,000 to 15,000 suitable donors die each year. Of that number, only about 4,000 donate organs—a number that has not increased since 1983. About half the potential donors are not asked, and about 40 percent of those who are asked decline to give.[5] The potential supply of accidental organs is no longer sufficient to keep pace with the overall demand because the ability to use organs has increased vastly, whereas the number of motorcyclists (who die suddenly because of traumatic head injuries), if anything, has declined.[6] Nor has it kept pace with those who have abandoned the search as futile or have died before transplants could be performed.[7] The gain side of this picture does not require any real elaboration, whatever we think of the transaction from the side of the organ donor. Yet the supply is constrained for the most prosaic of reasons: no explicit cash price can be offered for the use of cadaveric organs, and transplants from live donors are found only occasionally for kidneys and occasionally liver segments. There are no sales.

Historically this development took place in stages. The Uniform Anatomical Gift Act (UAGA), now adopted in every state, took the first and welcome step by allowing donative transfers of organs at death, based on a prior expression of intention by the original donor. The requisite intention could be manifested by signing organ donor cards, effective immediately on death without probate. Thus section 1 provides: "Any individual of sound mind and eighteen years of age or more may give all or any part of his body . . . the gift to take place on death." Section 2 provides that in the absence of any gift by the decedent, a gift may be made by family members, stated in order of priority as spouses, adult children, parents, and adult brothers and sisters. Finally, section 3 restricts the class of donees to "hospitals, doctors, medical and dental schools, universities, tissue banks, and a specified individual in need of treatment." The UAGA did not address the question of donations from live donors; nor did it address the question of whether organs from cadavers could be made subject to sale, but left that matter for each state to resolve individually. The statute thus expanded the scope of transactional freedom by authorizing one important set of transactions whose legal status had previously been in doubt.

By the time of the National Organ Transplantation Act of 1984,[8] the locus of power on the matter switched to the federal government and with it came a resort to state prohibition: a ban on the purchase of organs, just when the new generation of immunosuppressive drugs (for example, cyclosporine) increased the success rate—and hence the usefulness—of organ transplantation. The statute makes it a felony punishable by fines up to $50,000 and prison terms of five years "for any person to knowingly acquire, receive, or otherwise transfer any human organ for valuable consideration for use in human transplantation if the transfer affects interstate commerce"[9]—as it always does. Human organs are broadly defined to include "the human (including fetal) kidney, liver, heart, lung, pancreas, bone marrow, cornea, eye bone, and skin."[10] The statute then defines valuable consideration to include all payments in cash or kind subject only to a narrow exclusion that covers "reasonable payments associated with the removal, transplantation, implantation, processing, preservation, quality control, and storage of a human organ or the expenses of travel, housing, and lost wages incurred by the donor of a human organ in connection with the donation of the organ."[11] The strategy of the act is to allow cash payments or other goods and services to offset out-of-pocket losses that are otherwise incurred, but to bar the transferor of the organ from making any profit above and beyond those amounts. The explanation for the ban on profits in the Senate report is brevity incarnate: "It is the sense of the Committee that individual organizations should not profit by the sale of human organs for transplantation." The Committee adopted a different view for blood and blood derivatives because these "can be replenished and donation does not compromise the health of the donor. . . . The Committee believes that human body parts should not be viewed as commodities."[12]

The ban on the private sale of human organs was not imposed in a void. The 1984 National Organ Transplantation Act put in its place a rival system for the centralized control of organs that sought to respond to the position of both the individual donor and the vast class of potential recipients. Because the statute had precluded the sale of organs, the only possibility left was the gift of organs at death. (Gifts during life are hardly a viable option except within families.)[13] How then to induce gifts when purchase was ruled out as an option? At root, the current legal regime takes the same attitude toward organ donation that public television takes toward voluntary contributions. The dominant strategy is to promote awareness and to reduce the private costs that individuals have to bear in making the contribution. Toward that end, public-spirited organizations can alert people to the possibility of donation, can encourage people to sign the donor cards authorized under the UAGA, and can develop public advertisement campaigns to increase contributions. But the evidence suggests that only a tiny fraction of the population has taken advantage of this option.[14] Few people wish to contemplate their own mortality when healthy, and few next of kin can think rationally about the question of organ donation when they are stunned by the sudden and accidental death of an adolescent or young adult who was in perfect health. Even when these cards are signed, transplant teams normally will not operate without the approval of family thereafter.

BEATING THE SHORTAGE?

REQUIRED REQUEST

The issue of organ shortage is by any measure the dominant constraint on the system and has if anything grown more acute with the increased level of success found in organ transplantation.[15] What then can be done? To bolster the low level of voluntary contributions, Arthur Caplan proposed in 1984 (the same year as the National Statute) that *solicitation* become an obligation and not an option.[16] The duty attaches to the attending physician of the deceased and requires them when practicable to inquire of the next of kin whether they would consider an organ donation.[17] The solicitations for organs are tempered by an informed consent obligation, so that the physician must tell the next of kin of their right to decline participation in the program.[18]

Several states have taken this approach.[19] Some small pilot studies found a substantial level of increased participation in these programs,[20] but the initial doubts of the durability of these programs for the total population seem to have been borne out, given the flat level of organ donations over the past five or so years.[21] Thus, eight years later, Caplan himself summarized the results of his own research on the effectiveness of required requests in the Upper Midwest in these words: "We have found that a lot of requests are being made and a lot of families are saying no."[22] Most physicians who have struggled in vain to save a life are often not up to the heavy emotional battle of persuading the family to authorize organ transplantation.[23] Likewise, some anecdotal evidence suggests that some physicians may have been overzealous or tactless in their requests and thus created a backlash that in turn reduces the supply of organs.[24] Indeed, the process may easily get out of hand. Some physicians could be tempted to keep respirators going until the requests are made, even knowing that the patient's organs are unsuitable for harvesting.[25] In those cases, therefore, where the program does increase the supply of organs, that increase comes at a cost in terms of the hopeless lives prolonged and the unnecessary family and personal tensions.

Still the shortage remains. No one should ban making requests, and a good deal has been done, and doubtless could be done, to ensure that those who make the request strike a sympathetic and responsive chord in potential donors and their families.[26] But it is too late in the day for any false hopes that improved execution will expand the possibilities on this frontier.

PRESUMED CONSENT

Because voluntary gifts will not succeed in ending the shortages, and purchase is not allowed, why not just take the organs? In health matters, the claim is (usually) not so bald, for the proposal is in reality to introduce a regime of "presumed consent," so that the donation goes forward unless there is actual knowledge that the donor objected while alive or that the decedent would have objected as well. These statutes have usually been restricted to cornea transplants, but they invoke presumed consent to cover skin and bone as well. Efforts in California, Maryland, and Pennsylvania have been made to expand the reach of these statutes for all, but thus far none has been adopted; and even after adoption, their constitutional prognosis would be far from clear.[27] Several European countries have reported increases in organ donations after adopting presumed consent statutes.[28] Ironically the presumed consent regime shows far less respect for personal autonomy, here of the decedent, than either the gift or the sale alternative. Nor does this system of selection target the doctrine of presumed consent to those individuals who are most likely to consent in fact. The program, therefore, runs into the powerful objection that it could conscript organs from religious individuals in violation of their deepest beliefs and those of their next of kin. Do we really want to say that after death, a person's wishes count for naught if someone else has a greater need for his body? A system of voluntary gifts *or* voluntary sales avoids this problem because in both cases, those who strongly object to any form of transplantation need not enter the market at all.

Nonetheless, in the one reported case, the presumed consent statute was upheld against the challenge that it worked as a taking of the deceased's property without his consent and for a nonpublic purpose. *State v. Powell*[29] sustained a Florida statute that authorized the harvesting of corneas for transplantation on order of a medical examiner, unless (a) it interfered with an autopsy, or (b) there was some *known* objection by the decedent or the next of kin.[30] The statute is distinctive because it authorizes the harvesting of the cornea without first finding and notifying the next of kin, or obtaining their approval. In sustaining the statute, the court first noted that the common law recognized that the next of kin had no property interest in the commercial or material use of the decedent's body, but conferred on the next of kin only the limited property right needed to conduct a burial.[31] Thus a relative cannot recover the body or use it for security for funeral expenses; nor can the body be the subject of a gift in contemplation of death, or the object of larceny or theft.[32] The limited protection afforded to the next of kin at common law was found to be insufficient to create any property interest strong enough to stand up to state legislation. Here was one instance in which a common law right was accorded a constitutional status sufficient to trump a contrary legislative determination.[33]

Powell contains one important conceptual ambiguity. One route to its outcome assumes that neither the decedent nor the next of kin has any property interest in the body that can withstand legislative power. A hint of that view is found in the Court's statement: "Under the facts and circumstances of these cases, we find no taking of private property by state action for a nonpublic purpose in violation of article X, section 6, of the Florida Constitution."[34] Taken literally, the last part of this sentence could be interpreted to authorize far more than the use of a decedent's corneas without consent. It could be read to override any and all religious traditions and to permit state authorization of the use of *any* organ not only on a presumed consent theory, but even when a physician knows of actual opposition to the use of any body part from the decedent or his next of kin. Holding the body as a res nullius means that, in the private context, no person can resist the claims of the first possessor (which is why the right of burial in the next of kin had to be specially preserved by the common law), and in the public context, no one could resist the claims of the state. In light of the enormous concern paid to individual choice and autonomy everywhere else in the area of organ transplantation, it would be odd, perhaps indefensible, to give such short shrift to the common law rights of the decedent or the next of kin. The better interpretation recognizes that the prohibition against commercial uses of the body was only designed to ensure that the next of kin acted as a trustee for the body, not as an outright owner. A dead body is not an object for private gain or for state plunder.

A second interpretation of the *Powell* decision is far less troublesome. It may well be that the decedent or the next of kin is not an owner, but the common law rights, while not ordinary property, still count as a form of personal liberty or limited property that must always be weighed in the balance when determining the scope of the legislative power. Alternatively stated, we could argue that a taking of individual property indeed occurred, but that it was justified under the exigencies of the case. Such is the import of the words "[u]nder the facts and circumstances of these cases" in the sentence quoted earlier. Adopting this second approach means that the state statute amounts to a prima facie violation of an individual interest, be it in liberty or property, which obligates the state to justify its action. In this connection, the specific arguments that can be arrayed in favor of the cornea program allow a court to uphold this particular statute without necessarily giving its imprimatur to any and all legislative initiatives dealing with dead bodies.

The list is impressive. Corneas are small and easily removed from the body with a minimum of physical intrusion, so much so that the ordinary observer could not detect their absence; that typically no religious beliefs are directed toward the removal of corneas; that large percentages of corneas could be used to restore eyesight, even when harvested from persons of advanced age; that waiting to obtain the individual consent before harvesting the cornea results in the degradation of most corneas so that they are no longer usable; that the population, both the very old and the very young, who need these corneas to prevent blindness has increased; and that advances in surgical techniques have vastly improved the chances that any cornea implant will take. All of these points were set out with great clarity in *Powell*,[35] and any grand statements about liberty and property interests, or the lack thereof, are best read as inviting a class-by-class balancing test, and not a massive authorization of state mandated organ transplantation.

Stripped of all the rhetoric, *Powell* is at root a case where the size of the gains are enormous relative to the size of any losses. Where on its face the program could at some time benefit virtually any person, these gains are evenly distributed as well, so that the statute is not a form of class legislation with distinct winners and losers. So long as we have good, independent reason to believe that the court has correctly assessed the relative magnitude of gains and losses, why on utilitarian grounds would we oppose this particular statutory initiative? The counterargument is an absolute respect for individual autonomy in its strong Kantian version, not only as a means of social welfare, but also as an end in itself, no matter how destructive of social welfare. Here the price tag in human terms for that respect is very high indeed; the good utilitarian would countenance this limitation on the interference with individual self-control on the familiar grounds set out earlier. The case is one of *necessity* (both public and private) where the transactional barrier (the delay in finding next of kin) is fatal to the prospects of voluntary transfer. The broad distribution of benefits and burdens means that all persons are compensated in kind by their eligibility to receive the corneas. If all this were not sufficient unto the day, the overall statute could easily be saved by requiring that some small contribution be paid to the next of kin or perhaps donated to their favorite charity.

Taking this line still leaves us open to the argument of the slippery slope of government domination of all markets, but that objection can be met for corneas, even if not in other cases. A welcome discontinuity leaps out between the removal of a cornea and the massive intrusion necessary to remove a solid organ from the body; and the two types of procedures are likely to bring forth a major difference in the level of family resistance. This program has been around for sometime now and has not sparked any sustained public opposition: there is surely no reason to upset a workable state of affairs. Some slopes are just not that slippery.

The far harder question is whether we should push presumed consent beyond corneas for major organs because of the inability to increase the number of voluntary donations by education and other means. But even here, the web of social pressures imposes sharp limits on what can be done. The presumed consent statute will have little or no effect in the majority of cases where members of the family are present and able to voice their objections to the transfer. Indeed, it could have precisely the opposite effect and lead people, ever resentful of state authority, to withhold their consent. In any event, it is unlikely to do anything about the substantial number of cases in which requests for donations are refused by the family. And if organs are harvested from an individual whose family has religious or other objections, the entire organ donation program could fall into discredit. There is every reason to support a system of voluntary donations, even if we are skeptical, as I am, that it will work. The presumed consent movement is not likely to succeed any more in the future than it has done in the past. The use of a takings-like power has an important but limited place. It is necessary to deal with the challenge of markets head on.

CHAPTER 11

❖ ❖ ❖

Transplantation: The Supply Side

MARKETS AND ORGAN TRANSPLANTS

The failure of the existing solutions in this area drives us back to the insistent question of what should be done to improve the supply of organs for transplantation. The argument has been made several times that we should consider introducing of a market in organ transplantation in order to improve the supply, but far less frequently that market mechanisms should be used to allocate the organs collected among recipients.[1] In light of what has already been said, it is important to make the case that no combination of gift and takings approaches, however structured, can adequately remedy organ shortage. Only clear and unambiguous adoption of the market mechanism on both the supply and the demand side offers an adequate social response to the overall problem. Let us take up the two sides of the market in separate chapters.

SUPPLY SIDE: THE FUTURES MARKET

By every account, the supply side shortages are created in part by the inability to use price mechanisms to increase the number of persons who are willing to take the time, trouble, and risk to become organ donors. One proposal to alleviate this shortage contemplates the conscious creation of a future or options market for organ donations. The contracts in question will be entered into by persons in the prime of their life, even though the organs will be harvested, if at all, only when that individual dies. The agreement allows the individual to obtain either some ready cash at the time that the contract is entered into or to make some additional cash bequest at the time of death. Even if this market is constrained to post-mortem donations, there could be complete freedom on the prices paid, the time at which it is paid, the duration of the contract, and the conditions, if any, that are attached to the payment in question.

The variations that have been proposed are legion. Schwindt and Vining proposed that the government be the sole purchaser of these organs. A flat fee would be paid at the time of contract, and the government retains the right for collection throughout life.[2] Henry Hansmann countered with the observation that the contracts could be for shorter periods of duration, say, on an annual basis, without any government monopoly at all. Instead, any health insurance company could authorize a rebate in its premiums in exchange for the right to harvest the organs if death occurs during the policy period, thereby allowing competitive forces to set the premium size.[3] Lloyd Cohen's preferred future system is one in which individuals sign up today, using perhaps the same marketing intermediates, but they receive compensation only through their estates, when and if useful organs are harvested.[4] The proposals, moreover, are all compatible with any system of organ distribution after they have been acquired: lottery, technical regulation, queuing, or market.

Proposals of this sort raise questions at several distinct levels. Which system of payments is likely to introduce the greatest increase in the number of organs supplied? Here it is critical never to underestimate the importance that shifts in terms have on the incentives of the parties to contract, and that there may well be a difference between the various schemes that could speak to their relative efficacy, chiefly in minimizing the associated transaction costs. Certainly if the constraints against sale are relaxed on the transferor's side of the market, *all* these variants should be allowed. The objective is for the market to select the format likely to produce the largest benefit net the heavy transactions costs necessary to include persons within the system and to ensure the harvest of organs when and if that opportunity arises. Jesse Dukeminier warned of these costs as early as 1970 when he noted that the practical problems surrounding the creation of a futures market could easily prove insurmountable.[5] Indeed, he is right to observe that the paperwork and logistics pose the greatest threat to the operation of this proposed future market in organs. The likelihood that any suitable donor will die within any given time period, say, five years, in a manner that allows the retrieval of organs is very slight indeed. If we put the chance of death for some-one at age 25 at 1 in 500 and assume that salvageable organs will be recovered without complication in fewer than half the cases, it is likely within the course of a given year that only 1 in a thousand contracts will result in usable organs. If we assume that the value of all harvestable organs per person is in the $25,000 range, the total gains from the trans-action will be exhausted if the administrative costs per person exceed $25. Unfortunately a contractual strategy that pays a uniform figure to all insureds may well miss important variations in the appropriate level of payments to different groups of its insureds: some insureds may be too sick to donate organs, and others with suitable organs may have a very low risk of accidental death. These difficulties are only compound-ed when we factor in marketing costs, regulatory risks, contractual dis-putes, physician noncooperation, and potential liability for organs with latent but deadly communicable diseases.

One way to increase the present value of the contract is to extend the duration of its effective period beyond the five years just mentioned. But now counterbalancing difficulties will emerge. The age at which har-vesting takes place will rise, which in turn should lead to a decline in usable yield. In addition, people may move away from their original homes, perhaps even out of the country, so that the logistics of keeping tabs on who is inside or outside the system will increase as well. Although the number of contracts with a positive yield may increase, the transac-tions cost per contract will increase as well. The two effects will tend to cancel each other out.

The blunt prognosis is that each variation of the basic futures transaction will find it difficult to respond to the "problem" of low yield over a long period of time. If the size of these transaction costs exceeds the potential gains from trade, the market will shut down even if allow-able under law, and we will be back to the constant pressure for dona-tions either by card or from the next of kin at death. With organ cards, no financial institution has to bear tomorrow's transaction costs or worry about enforcing its exclusive claim to the organs in question. With the next of kin, the issue of delay between promise and performance is measured in hours not years. The absence of a price has advantages that the cash market for future donations is not likely to overcome.

Some evidence of these advantages is found in Lloyd Cohen's recent account of the Spanish practice that encourages cadaveric transfers from the next of kin by paying funeral expenses up to some stipulated amount.⁶ The program does not broadcast its exchange component: the request for the organ is not accompanied by a promise to pick up funeral expenses, which is only announced later. But the practice itself is sufficiently regular that any official in a hospital setting can make known the anticipated quid pro quo. The entire process does serve a useful function in softening the hard commercial edges that might otherwise be offensive. The money is used for purposes that are closely connected with the life, and death, of the decedent. It may be that the money is paid directly to the third party. Yet the organ procurement organization, whose position is quite different, appears to be paid on a commission basis. The upturn in organ donations that accompanied the introduction of the new practice cannot be easily attributed to some new-found source of altruism. It looks as though the financial incentives, suitably packaged, made a difference largely because the uncertainties of the future market were avoided.

The creation of a futures market in organs carries with it yet another complication with strong religious and cultural overtones. Does the decedent have the last say in practice, or does any objection by a spouse or a next of kin block the entire transaction after the fact? The practice of giving under the Uniform Anatomical Gift Act (UAGA) has been aptly described as one of "multiple vetoes," that is, a situation in which the decedent, the physicians, or the next of kin can block the transaction, no matter what others will do.⁷ These deep-seated social expectations will not disappear just because the futures promise is made in exchange for cash. To be sure, the UAGA provides that where the decedent has spoken, the family is bound, and the same legal rule could in principle apply to any purchase.⁸ But the social practice is surely otherwise, both for gift and sale, so that the objection by even a single remote family member will stop the voluntary donation.⁹ In death as in birth, the principle of self-ownership is itself at low ebb. The decedent ceases to be an independent person and becomes part of a familial group, someone who is not autonomous, someone whose wishes may be made to bend to those of the group—or so many people feel. This sense of continuity across the generations is common enough on matters of property law, where the current owner of land will not sell it to strangers even though he has clear legal title. The social claims of the next generation act as a powerful, but informal constraint on a legal regime that fosters freedom of alienation. Recast into the language of law and economics, no decedent has a full set of social property rights in his own person. Because these rights are limited at death by the claims of others, no system of advance contracts can provide good title to a buyer; and so too any promise of a future gift. Outsiders will sense this difficulty and accordingly will be reluctant to enter into any contract that requires legal enforcement in the face of strong popular resentment to any intrusion of commerce into family affairs. What reason is there to believe that this future market will emerge if blessed by legislation that does not disfavor it in some back-handed way? My prediction is clear: this market will not work even if it were made legal. I also wish that this market were opened up so that the resourcefulness and imagination of others could prove me wrong.

LIVE DONATIONS

Is there then any option to the system of coerced donations that is so commonly observed? Here I think that much more explicit attention must be paid to the possibility of allowing sales by living persons.[10] Clearly this will not be a viable market for heart or pancreas transplants, but it could work elsewhere. Indeed it could work whenever live dona-tions work within families. Fortunately the live-sale option is feasible where shortages are greatest. The transfer of one kidney is certainly a viable option; so too the sale of bone marrow. It is also possible to remove, and hence sell, some portion of the liver. So long as a healthy donor retains a substantial portion of the liver, its overall regeneration is possible.[11] To be sure, not all persons might be suitable transferees; since obtaining some minimum mass is critical, small children or adult females are more likely to be successful recipients than adult males. Yet even if the live transplant markets only catered to a portion of the needy population, it would help all others by reducing the queue for cadaveric transplants. The shortage of organs for transplantation could be attacked on many fronts at once.

The advantages of live transplants are substantial, and these should be set out before dealing with the inevitable impassioned objections. First, the value of the organ transplanted relative to the costs of transac-tions is likely to be large. In principle, it should be possible to get quite precise tissue matches,[12] because the organ is not harvested and shipped to its proper recipient in a crisis-like atmosphere. The organ can be stored, as it were, in the donor until the ideal recipient and time have been found. Once removed, the organ in question is far more likely to be useful to the recipient: organs taken from living donors generally have greater vitality. In addition, the transplant can be planned in advance so that both parties are in the same hospital, or, if necessary, the same operating room, to allow the quick transfer of an organ, just as is done with live donative transplants. With a high level of gains and greater time period, a wide range of safeguards can be introduced to ensure that transfers are not made on persons whose health cannot stand them or who are not psychologically fit to make the decision in question. Because time is no longer of the essence, potential transferors and their families can deliberate well before the moment of crisis and avoid making decisions of this sort when grief is at a high pitch. Because the transferor is still alive, the multiple veto problem, which is present at death, no longer poses a serious obstacle to voluntary transactions. Because the transferor is not ill, he need not have a lingering fear that physicians want to hasten his death in order to pounce on his organs.

A market of this sort should become well organized because it is highly unlikely that suitable medical matches can arise from random contacts between donors and recipients. The probabilities of a medical match are far too low. A bone marrow match between a random donor and recipient is around 1 in 60,000, which hardly justifies the cost of individual transactions.[13] It takes a thick market with lots of information on record to develop a database large enough to match buyers and sellers. Within that framework, prices could likely become well established and standard protocols explicitly developed to respond to the inevitable raft of contracting problems. Brokers and advisors can be used to match patients with recipients and to inform them of the relevant risks. Standardized disclosure and informed consent forms could be prepared as well. After the taint of illegality is removed, any number of other services could be incorporated into the underlying transaction. Mechanisms could be developed to secure payment both before and after the operation is performed; warranties for further care can be given in the event of post-operative complications; liability for medical malpractice can be preserved; life insurance can be purchased on the life of the organ donor for the benefit of his or her family.

The strong attacks on this exercise of contractual freedom are no more valid here than in other areas.[14] Thus it is often feared that transactions of this sort will exploit the poor because they will have greater financial incentive to take the risk in question. One answer is to restrict participation in the program to those whose net worth or annual income is above a certain minimum figure. But we should reject this selective authorization as a form of invidious discrimination against the poor because it assumes that they are unable to make responsible choices on matters of such gravity.[15] The better answer dismisses the charge of exploitation on the ground that it is no more sound here than it is in any other context, be it for minimum wage or surrogacy contracts. The basic logic of markets is that people will only surrender what they value if they receive in exchange something of greater value. The poor can advance through trade just as the rich and can rise in wealth and social standing by hard work and good fortune. There is no reason to think that this relationship of mutual gain will not hold with organ transplants where the stakes are far larger than in many other markets. Any concern with fraud or duress is overstated in light of the range of alternatives that should become routinely available on both sides of the transaction. In any event, the helpless poor are not likely to be targeted for organ transplants (any more than as surrogate mothers). Because their ill-health reduces the medical value of their organs, any exploitation of the helpless will not be of advantage to the would-be exploiter.

Indeed, the point here can be reversed, for the presence of compensation might ease the evident transactional difficulties. Early on one patient noted that "he feels diffident and rather ashamed to ask someone to give a kidney, and for peace of mind he would much rather be able to buy a kidney from a potential donor."[16] Conversely the absence of the compensation alternative is far more likely to increase the level of psychological coercion applied to family members. Thus the question of undue influence and tense interpersonal arrangements can easily arise in family settings, where live organ donations are now permitted and they indeed constitute around 30 percent of the kidney transplants.[17] Sometimes heavy social pressures is used to overcome a natural reluctance to donate precisely because the financial inducements are not available. In one well-known case, *In Re Guardianship of Pescinski,* the potential recipient,[18] Mrs. Elaine Jeske, age 39 with six minor children, had lost both her kidneys and was in dire need of a kidney transplant. Her brother Ralph, age 43, with nine of his ten children still at home, refused to get involved "because there would be nobody to take over his farm and he felt he had a duty to his family to refuse."[19] The demand that he make a gift put him in a terrible all-or-nothing situation—either way. He just might have been willing to undergo the transplant if his other siblings had been in a position to offset his risk of financial loss. Within a family setting, however, it is unlikely that the transaction would take the form of a front-end lump-sum payment.

Now suppose the relatives had been allowed to pay for the cost of additional help that might be needed on the farm, or to provide some disability or life insurance protection as well, or even to pick up the payments on the home mortgage or farm equipment for some period of months. Now the compensation serves to transform what would have been a win/lose situation into a win/win situation, or at least one in which Ralph's private losses might have been far smaller, so that he would have been willing, with confined generosity, to give the kidney. To be sure, a new round of bargaining difficulties is presented as Ralph could hold out for more than is offered. But now some combination of legal and social sanctions could well bring matters under control. As it was, Mrs. Jeske's sister, Mrs. Lausier, went to court in an effort to order tests on Mrs. Jeske's brother Richard, an institutionalized, catatonic schizophrenic, to see if *he* would be a suitable transferor. Richard's guardian ad litem strongly opposed the application on the ground that an organ removal was not for the benefit of the ward and his contention prevailed in the case: sacrificing the autonomy of the mentally incompetent is not a winning argument. Is seeking and paying a commercial donor any worse than this situation?

A second objection often goes hand and hand with the first: the creation of a payment market for organs will cannibalize voluntary donations. The argument was first made with respect to blood by Richard Titmuss, who claimed that paying for blood would not only induce inferior blood to be presented, but would also reduce the level of voluntary gifts.[20] According to Titmuss, keeping blood noncommercial would lead to the best of both worlds: better blood at lower financial cost. Responding to Titmuss's claim requires us to disentangle the issue of blood quality from that of altruistic donation. On the first issue, Titmuss feared that the prospect of payment would induce persons to donate bad blood for private gain. His point is correct, but only if no system of personal liability is in place to force the donor to make good the losses caused, and science cannot develop an independent method to monitor the quality of blood.

Taking the points in order, Titmuss's first assumption is surely correct and remains largely so today. Although someone who knowingly donates AIDS-contaminated blood is liable in tort, successful cases of this sort are hard to find. On the second issue, medical science has made much progress in the 20 years since Titmuss wrote, chiefly by developing reliable tests for both hepatitis and AIDS. These tests reduce the need for social proxies. Today, therefore, the focal point for blood is on the regulation of blood banks and other professional conduits, and here we can easily dispute the appropriate mix of industry self-governance, tort controls, and public regulation.[21] As the ability to test blood increases, all of these precise techniques will dominate altruism as a device for quality control. Because typing of organ tissue requires a detailed medical workup in any event, monitoring is always part of this process. Today the choice of gift versus sale contributes less to quality control for organs than it once did for Titmuss.

Titmuss's second point, however, continues to exert enormous influence because, no matter what the setting, the likelihood of entering into a gratuitous transaction is reduced if someone else is prepared to pay a hefty fee for the same organ. If, therefore, the creation of the paying market reduces the size of the nonpaying market, perhaps markets do inject a counterproductive element into the social efforts to increase supply. Indeed one of the most frequently voiced objections to the entire system of commercial markets for health care is just this, that it undermines the sense of altruism that communities must have to survive as communities, and not just as loose assemblages of autonomous and disconnected individuals. Titmuss marshals an impressive array of testimonial evidence in support of this proposition, and the success of altruistic donations for blood in both England and the United States has been one of the key empirical arguments for relying on voluntary mechanisms for organ donations as well. Thomas Murray's influential defense of the ban on commercialization, for example, follows his lengthy endorsement of Titmuss's work on blood. Murray writes:

> Relationships governed by markets keep moral and social dimensions to a bare minimum. Gifts, by their open-endedness defy such minimization. Impersonal gifts such as blood or body parts or charity may not regulate relationships between specific individuals, but they serve other functions

by regulating larger relationships, and honoring important human values, precisely those threatened by massive and impersonal bureaucracies. . . .

Gifts to strangers affirm the solidarity of the community over and above the depersonalizing, alienating forces of mass society and market relations. They signal that self-interest is not the only significant human motivation. And they express the moral belief that it is good to minister to fundamental human needs, needs for food, health care, and shelter, but also needs for beauty and knowledge. These universal needs irrevocably tie us together in a community of needs, with a shared desire to satisfy them, and see them satisfied in others.

Finally, these gifts remind us that wealth is merely a means to an end, and that not all valuable things can be purchased, among them love, friendship, fellow-feeling and trust.[22]

His arguments misfire at several levels. Starting with the most specific point, Murray is insensitive to the major impact that matters of apparent detail have on the level of voluntary donations. No obvious extrapolation connects the level of voluntary donations of blood to the level of donation for solid organs. Note these points of difference. Blood, as has been often said, is a renewable resource, so the donor's level of sacrifice required is low. Blood is taken at a preappointed time from persons who are in good health and, in some cases at least, is donated for the benefit of a specific person. Implicit noncash systems of compensation are adopted even in donation cases, such as the right to receive blood at no charge or on favorable terms in the event that the donor or his family should require it on some future occasion. But there is no reason for an exclusive noncash economy. A commercial market does exist side by side with the voluntary market, without having driven it out of business.

More fundamentally, Murray misunderstands both how markets operate and the relationship between market and altruistic behavior. No ongoing market could operate if the performance of each contract depended solely on its legal enforcement. Many contracts are not one-shot arrangements, but are part of loose, ongoing arrangements that depend on trust, reputation, and the prospect of future gainful interactions. We do not "buy" trust by making a payment to a trading partner; but we do buy trust by honoring short-run burdensome commitments in order to induce long-term confidence from trading partners. Nor are the intangibles irrelevant. In business, maintaining employee morale and customer trust is key to long-term success, so much so that the higher an individual moves within the organization, the more critical the attention to these organizational intangibles. No one in business could recognize Murray's caricature of business practice as anything other than the road to commercial suicide. Flexibility, responsiveness, loyalty, and worker and customer satisfaction are common, perhaps indispensable, inputs into successful firms. By contrast, large impersonal bureaucracies emerge when UNOS seeks to develop its own "equitable criteria" for organ transplantation.

Most important, perhaps, is Murray's mischaracterization of the social role of altruism and thus his overestimization of its fragility. First, market behavior (rightly understood) can prosper side by side with altruistic behavior. Charitable schools, churches and hospitals all have paid employees who chose their careers (and the salary reductions that may go with those careers) with the knowledge that market institutions can support charities, even more than charitable institutions can support markets. So long as the arrangements are clear to the participants, there is no reason to suppose that charities will perish from the face of the earth because they cannot compete with ordinary exchange relationships. The massive rise of charitable giving at the height of laissez-faire and before the advent of the income tax shows that the asserted contradiction between the two modes of discourse, charitable and market, is the figment of modern political philosophy and not the stuff of ordinary human affairs.[23] Most people exhibit a far greater ability to tolerate moral ambiguity about their multiple social roles and purposes than the communitarian vision of the world is prepared to acknowledge. Businessmen and women know full well how to work at the office during the day and on charitable affairs at night. They are sophisticated enough to recognize that ethics is situation dependent: family, friends, work, and politics need not all work in accordance with the same rules. No one disputes the Beatles' proposition that "money can't buy you love," but the proposition does not require any form of *ban* on the payment of cash in certain human relations. It is possible to have affectionate relationships with people who have worked as maids and gardeners, and trust is often engendered by paying wages promptly and making loans or advances to employees with sudden financial crises. It is also commonplace for many people to make gifts or bequests to persons who have been in their personal employ for many years.

Introducing cash or other market mechanisms for organ transplant does not eliminate the need for altruism; it is better understood as refocusing its direction at its appropriate targets. The physician who operates on a sick child may well be paid by a charitable fund that is collected by the hospital in which he works or by the friends and family of the patient. That physician may agree to some reduction in fee to take into account the financial condition of the patient and her family. But even more to the point, the key question is not whether altruism is appropriate, but who should be the altruist. Before the prospect of organ transplantation arose, everyone thought that the bereaved family was in need of special concern and support: friends made dinner, covered at the office, or contributed to a fund to cover extra expenses. Yet most modern tracts on ethical conduct assume a level of individual self-interest in ordinary social interactions that is far in excess of the observed social practices of unregulated persons.

The inability to see how charitable and commercial institutions interact has powerful consequences in dealing with organ transplantation. Unfortunately the modern ethical approach to organ transplantation works a strange inversion. Those who should be recipients of charity are asked in the name of altruism to sacrifice a second time, often for some nameless person. Why here? If the commercial market for organ transplantation were developed, the burden of altruism would fall on those who support medical and hospital services generally, or the family and friends of some specific recipient, and not the family whose loved one has been taken away. When the focus has been shifted, altruism can function more sensibly, just as it does for the many services already funded by charity. The only sacrifices that need be requested are financial sacrifices, which can be asked broadly of individuals in accordance with their wealth and personal involvement. There need be no element of personal crisis and time pressure on them to make the decision, as is always the case when the full burden of apparent altruism is placed on the putative donor or his family. A society that treasures altruism need not place a unique and nontransferable burden on those who are least able to bear it. It can combine market with charitable mechanisms to locate altruism where it will do the maximum good. It can add a charitable deduction to function as a kind of matching grant for individual charitable gifts. The community of needs can be satisfied by the community at large. If the decedent or his family wants to contribute in whole or in part, so much the better, but altruistic institutions and individuals can function without banning the commercial sale of organs.

Yet with all this said, will this live-transplant market work if allowed? It is difficult to make any confident predictions because the market has not been tried, but the concerns are surely worth addressing. One plausible fear is that we could not hope to see any supply of organs that is responsive to price. But why? Supply is elastic in virtually every other context, and it should be elastic here too. Remember that the entire population need not get involved in order for it to be viable. Even if the United States were the relevant market, a positive response rate of one-tenth of 1 percent would leave 250,000 people in the market, far in excess of today's shortages. The skeptic should *not* question whether he should do it, but whether some small fraction of the population might and whether that fraction might be increased by some change in price. For these purposes, it is irrelevant that 99 percent of the population would not alter its behavior if the price of kidneys were to double. The same is true about variations in the price of a Rolls Royce. But if the relevant pool of donors moves from 0.1 percent to 0.12 percent, that translates, as a first approximation, into a 20 percent increase in organ supply. And no one's background intuitions are so well developed as to rule out that possibility in advance.

Next, it is critical to respond to the disquieting precedents from overseas experiments. Reports about the sale of Indian kidneys to sheiks from the United Arab Emirates rightly note that the rejection rate after transplantation is so high as to make the entire procedure at best useless and at worst deadly. It is just that kind of procedure that a legal market in this country could avoid because the institutions involved could provide some form of warranty as to suitability and typing of relevant organs. As is always the case, no easy extrapolation can be drawn from the well-documented failures overseas. The prospects are that an above-board market in this country could do far better than the gray markets overseas. It hardly will do to ban voluntary transactions by predicting that no one would participate even if the markets were legalized. Try it out and see who is right.

CHAPTER 12

Organ Transplantation: The Demand Side

Any complete analysis of organ transplantation also requires an analysis of the demand side. Even if organs could be procured by some market mechanism, once acquired, they need not necessarily be sold to the highest bidder. In addition to sale, the state could distribute organs lotteries, technical matches, and waiting time, alone or in combination. Indeed, the current system of organ distribution involves some combination of these factors. Some description of the basic system is needed to make the overall discussion intelligible.[1] Before the passage of the National Organ Transplantation Act of 1984, no comprehensive database matched organs with their potential recipients. The Act filled this gap by creating in the federal government the Organ Procurement and Transplantation Network (OPTN), whose general charge is to oversee nationwide organ procurement and distribution. OPTN has not assumed direct management of this venture, but has delegated large portions of its authority to a private organization, the United Network for Organ Sharing (UNOS), whose exhaustive rules regulate the collection and distribution of transplant organs.

UNOS could have operated simply as a clearinghouse to facilitate organ matches by letting potential organ recipients and their physicians know what organs are available and, in a market regime, at what price. Yet the second part of UNOS's mission shows how easy it is to veer from facilitation to coercion. The basic statutory plan also authorizes government grants to "qualified organ procurement organizations" (OPOs). These nonprofit bodies receive reimbursement under Medicare for kidney procurement and are also responsible for developing procedures for acquiring nonrenal organs for use in transplants not covered by Medicare. As a condition for receiving their grants, these groups had to join UNOS and follow its medical standards and criteria for organ procurement, preservation, and transportation. In its original design, UNOS was only one avenue for procuring organ donations. Physicians and health care institutions were free to go elsewhere for their organs if they thought it wise to do so.

The original network obligation was to "assist." "The Organ Procurement and Transplantation Network shall (D) assist organ procurement organizations in the nationwide distribution of organs equitably among transplant patients."[2] The term "equitably" could have be read to encourage broader distribution to increase the likelihood of good matches. Yet the 1986 Budget Reconciliation Act gave OPTN (acting through UNOS) more coercive powers. As James Blumstein writes: "instead of serving as a publicly funded resource for improving the efficiency of the procurement and distribution system, UNOS took on the role of a nongovernmental or quasi-governmental regulatory body." He continues:

> UNOS bylaws require that all transplant programs of a transplant center come into 'full compliance with all UNOS membership criteria.' If UNOS approval of a transplant program is not secured, a transplant center must 'not perform any further transplant of the applicable organ until after it has established full compliance to the satisfaction of . . . UNOS.' Thus, a hospital with an organ transplantation program that does not satisfy UNOS's membership criteria is for all practical purposes not able to continue its transplantation program at all. It is not just a question of a hospital foregoing access to the UNOS network, or even foregoing access to Medicare or Medicaid payment for transplantation (in circumstances in which such support would be available.) The stakes are much steeper. Unless a hospital drops its non-UNOS-qualifying transplantation programs entirely, the hospital would be obliged to 'forego Medicare and Medicaid payment for *all* services, not just transplant services.'[3]

The unfolding of UNOS thus marks the familiar transformation of a government agent into a government monopolist, here through the operation of a quasi-private corporation that piggybacks its authority on that of HHS.[4] Now the central question is to what use UNOS will put its enormous political power. Surely not toward promoting open competition between various providers of transplant services. Almost like clockwork, the UNOS regulations impose stringent guild restrictions through minimum requirements for transplant surgeons, supporting staff and equipment, and facilities. In addition, they protect existing transplantation programs by making the start-up costs for new programs greater than the cost of expanding older ones. An "established transplant program" in one organ is able to start a program in a second organ with a two-year grace period before it has to comply with UNOS standards, but a new program must meet these standards immediately.[5] Sometimes it is difficult for a new program to begin at all because one of the governing standards addresses the survivability of individuals who previously participated in the program. The legislation creates a state-controlled cartel, not an information coordination system.[6]

The UNOS criteria also reflect the same bias toward a command and control economy. The philosophical underpinnings are set out in the report prepared by the Task Force on Organ Transplantation, whose work was done pursuant to the 1984 Transplantation Act. The Task Force Report begins with a strong affirmation of the dominant role of altruism: "The Task Force clearly adopted the position that organs are donated in a spirit of altruism and volunteerism and constitute a national resource to be used for the public good."[7] Consistent with that view, "the Task Force concluded that implementation of equitable access prohibits any element of commercialization on the distribution of organs."[8] But the rejection of commercialization was not accompanied by an alternative solution worthy of its name: "Given the scarcity of organs and the costs of transplants, we believe that the most ethical means of organ distribution is to rely on medical criteria."[9] Excluded from the mix are such issues as "age, lifestyle, access to a social support network, and previous transplants."[10] Why age and lifestyle are not medical was not explained. The one additional criterion that survives the Task Force view and is incorporated into the law is a constrained version of the rule, first in time is higher in right. "If two or more patients are equally good candidates for a particular organ according to medical criteria of need and probability of success, the principle of justice suggests that length of time on the waiting list is the fairest way to make the final selection."[11]

The implicit maxim of this system is that "each person should count for one and only for one." That principle shuns any effort to differentiate between the moral worth of individuals, but it assigns to each person the same unitary significance in the grand scheme of things. That principle is used as well in political elections, where each voter gets to cast a single ballot in an election regardless of the size of his stake in the outcome. Systems like this guard against obvious forms of favoritism and bias, but at the same time they exclude consideration of genuine differences that might influence an allocation scheme—a necessary concession in any nonmarket system of allocation. Once inside the Task Force world, only one criterion can determine the allocation of organs: the maximum survivability of organ recipients. How that can be done without taking into account such factors as age, lifestyle, and social support network is once again left to the imagination. But even within this truncated framework, much work has to be done. UNOS's self-assigned task is to design a medically sound system of allocation that treats all patients fairly and that maximizes the levels of organ donation while minimizing the risk of organ wastage.[12]

The current rules (with one important exception) follow closely the original task force recommendations. Thus UNOS created an elaborate point system to determine, for example, who gets a kidney first.[13] Key to the operation of this system are the principles of antigen matching. An antigen is, roughly speaking, a protein located on the surface of a foreign tissue capable of stimulating the host to attack the tissue on which it is located. A transplanted kidney or other tissue with antigens not found in the host is perceived as a foreign substance that white blood cells promptly attack. The better the match, the less likely the attack. As all persons, save identical twins, are genetically different, no perfect match is ever possible. The antigens at each of three key sites, or loci (with two antigens at each loci, one from each parent) are highly relevant to the probability of transplant rejection. Before July 1, 1994, only a perfect 6-antigen match (and no specific family member donee) placed the kidney into the national pool. Kidneys with less than a 6-antigen match were rated by a point system that determined the relative suitability of recipients. As of today all matches are done on a national basis.[14]

Before the 1995 UNOS revisions, the highest possible score for an imperfect match was 15 points. Up to ten points were determined on the basis of matches, and four points were awarded to those "presensitized" individuals who matched well with a particular donor, but who fared poorly against the overall pool and who may have rejected a previous organ match.

Of particular relevance was the so-called "O rule."[15] Type O blood is the universal donor, which can be given not only to O recipients but also to A, B, and AB recipients as well. Persons with Type A blood can receive O or A blood, but not B blood. Similarly, persons with Type B blood can receive O or B, but not A blood. Persons with type AB blood are universal recipients who can receive blood from any donor. Given this scheme, persons with O blood are universal donors, but can only receive blood from other O donors. In light of the restrictive sources available to them, the current regulations grant a preference for O organs to potential recipients with type O. The upshot is that an O recipient with a somewhat inferior match could take preference over an A, B, or AB recipient with a somewhat better antigen match. More precisely, type O organs will go to O recipients, except in those cases where there is no antigen mismatch with non-O-type candidates. In principle, the O candidate with a zero match could prevail over an A or B candidate with a 5-antigen match, but because O blood is the most common type, it is far more likely that the successful O recipient will have a good antigen match with the organ.[16] Finally, one point was allocated to that patient who has been on the list for the longest time. When added together, these compatibility measures determined who prevailed under the system.

The basic UNOS system thus spurns the use of any market mechanism, but UNOS does not explain why any alternative devices—technical criteria, queues, and lotteries—are superior to a market system. The weakness of these allocative mechanisms, relative to markets, has been considered countless times in other settings, and for most goods and services market methods of allocation have emerged superior to their alternatives. Queues impose costs on the buyers of goods without giving offsetting benefits to the sellers of those goods. They necessarily dissipate real resources to alter distributions without any clear explanation as to why or how. The gas station lines that grew during the price-control days of the 1970s belong to the dim past, but no one gets rich waiting in lines. Prices shorten the queues and thus eliminate the downtime. Organs may be more important than gasoline, but the same principles apply, and the levels of waste in waiting are, if anything, far higher.

Lotteries, for their part, avoid waiting and delay, but they afford inferior assignments of goods and services. Those who value the goods more highly than others have no better chances than anyone else. If the goods allocated by lottery can be traded, the inefficiencies of lotteries are measured by the costs of the second transactions, or the foregone gain from trades that could not be consummated because of high transaction costs, whichever is less. However, in a world that makes trade impossible—and organ transplantation today is surely that world—the losses of lotteries are measured by the difference in value in the hands of the winners and the losers. Surely the world can find some place for lotteries. They are commonly used, although not without objection, as devices to raise revenues in lieu of taxes, or to decide who wins the door prize at a school raffle. In those contexts, they function solely as a pure transfer system, with no independent negative consequences on resource allocation. Here the stakes are far higher. No one wants to assign surgeons to individual cases by lottery. No one thinks it high praise to say that liability for medical malpractice resembles the outcomes of a lottery. Why attach any moral virtue to a lottery for organs?

For their part, technical decisions—give the organ to the party with the best organ match—are surely involved in any sensible regime of allocation. No market participant would bid on an incompatible organ or even one that in all likelihood would be rejected. But the public use of some rational criterion still falls short because it necessarily overlooks two important points. First, we have no reason to expect a one-to-one correspondence between biological matches and private demand. Someone with an imperfect match could well have a stronger demand for the organ than does someone with a perfect match, even if the first transplant is less likely to take than the second. In essence, the ultimate gain from the transaction is, roughly speaking, measured by the likelihood of success multiplied by the gains from success. Hence the higher likelihood of success for one recipient could be overshadowed by the gains from transplantation to the second because of life expectancy, income, family situation, or quality of life factors. Where both parties have ample wealth, it is not clear who would bid higher; and even if the only concern were some abstract measure of utility, higher utility does not correlate perfectly with superior antigen matches.

The explanation is not hard to find. The very considerations that UNOS ruled out of bounds are just those that private recipients would take into account in setting their preferences. Recall the basic list of excluded characteristics under UNOS: "age, lifestyle, access to a social support network, and previous transplants." Start at the top. Why should age be irrelevant? It is not irrelevant for voting, marriage, retirement, or, indeed, in the fitness of organs for donation to others, where again younger is better. Ceteris paribus, the younger the recipient, the more likely the transplant will take, so the probability of success is higher. An organ for a 40-year-old person might extend life expectancy for 20 years, perhaps more. The same transplant in a person of 75 is likely to last for only one-fourth as long. Why ignore a fourfold difference in life expectancy because of a 2 percent difference in the chances that the transplant will take? The point has major consequences.

When individuals make their own decisions on whether to invest in their human capital, they surely take into account the period over which that investment will pay dividends, and their reduced ability to learn new skills, or maintain older ones.[17] One reason why 50-year-olds are less willing to retool than 30-year-olds is that they (or should I say, "we"?) have 20 fewer years in which to recoup the costs of their investment. Another reason is that with age they are less likely to have the adaptability and agility they possessed when younger. To the law's great discredit, the age discrimination statutes treat age as irrelevant when everyone knows that it is not. The British system in practice (or so we are told) categorically denies transplants to individuals over the age of 60. It is surely not difficult for UNOS to add or subtract points for age to offset any diminished chances of success. Yet our technical system responds more to abstract political imperatives of what should be done, at the expense of overall human happiness and success.

The refusal administratively to take into account lifestyle is perhaps more defensible because of the difficulties in externally evaluating what people have done and how they are likely to behave in the future. We would have to scramble to defend a system that favored hikers over couch potatoes, or the reverse. Yet even insurance companies make their underwriting decisions and price their coverages to take into account these intangibles. I can recall years ago that an insurance salesman insisted on visiting my home before issuing a policy, doubtless because he thought that additional knowledge he acquired about my habits and home could reduce his company's risk. To be sure, public bodies are too rule-bound to wade through the intangibles. However, individuals can do so, at least on their own account, without having to, or being able to, hoodwink anyone else. People whose lifestyles reduce the probabilities of a long-term successful transplant will tend to bid less for an organ or will be less likely to persuade charities to assist them. The predictive effects of lifestyle can be incorporated informally into the system without asking public bodies to pass on these delicate factors that, however soft and slippery, should never wholly disappear from view.

The same analysis also extends to access to a social support network. Individuals who can rely on an informal network are more likely to follow the appropriate dietary and exercise regimens needed to make a transplant work and are less likely to have the mood swings and depressions that could compromise their success. Administrators may not be able to make these judgments, but ordinary individuals can, both for themselves and for their families. Once again, the UNOS rules treat as socially irrelevant the critical factors that they are not able to evaluate intelligently. In contrast, any bidding or charitable system would readily take them into account.

But what of previous transplants, which now have failed? Here the basic problem is how to interpret the data. One obvious question is how long the previous transplant worked. A heart transplant that is rejected after one week is hardly a good reason to try another if the organ is available. But one that has lasted a decade or more points in the opposite direction. Transplants are likely to wear out, and the very fact that a recipient has shown the personal resilience and fortitude to cope with one transplant may well make him a better candidate for a second. Disregarding the prior record thus cuts UNOS off from useful information, which on a closer examination could cut in either direction, depending on the case. Once again, the decision makes sense for a public body that cannot delve into the refinements. But the individual knowledge dismissed by UNOS would surely be taken into account in any private system of allocation, charitable or commercial.

UNOS does, however, have some independent requirements that do survive, notwithstanding its general disdain for the "soft stuff." Its guidelines, for example, exclude current alcoholics as candidates for liver transplantations, but should some penalty be imposed on persons whose need for a liver transplant is causally connected with past alcohol use?

The case for this position need not rest on the assertion that the prognosis of success for the reformed alcoholic is poor, but could rest on the ground that in a world of excessive demand, past alcoholism is an effective moralism—a form of nonprice rationing that cuts out a large enough portion of the population to be meaningful.[18]

This approach is vulnerable on a number of grounds, however. People with other disabilities are not normally excluded from participation in programs, so alcoholics should not be banished from the community, any more than people who drive without seatbelts should be excluded from emergency room care. Sometimes, it is said, that their choice to drink was not voluntary but subject to genetic and social influences that we only dimly understand, or that efforts should be made to encourage their rehabilitation (as opposed to discouraging the initial flirtation with drink). In other areas, reformed alcoholics at least are treated as having disabilities, for which protection is provided under the antidiscrimination laws, most notably, the Americans with Disabilities Act. Or, finally, that the predictive power of prior alcoholism is weak, given that a liver transplantation is, as has been said, a powerful way to sober up a once-wayward drinker. In general, it is not possible to come to closure on this issue in a public setting because it is easy to conceive of at least some alcoholics (reformed or not) who might stand in the queue ahead of other individuals whose personal flaws are attributable to mistakes in lifestyles that are studiously ignored under UNOS. But a bidding system could treat this as one factor among many to take into account without having to make external justifications for public bodies. There would be no need to give one set of preconceptions or the other pride of place in the stripped-down social calculus.

Still another exclusion is far more insidious. The Americans with Disabilities Act is not only about disabilities. It is about Americans, permanent aliens included. Just as Medicare and Medicaid limit eligibility to citizens and permanent nationals, so too the current UNOS guidelines provide that normally no more than 10 percent of the transplants at any one transplantation center should be performed on nonimmigrant aliens.[19] Here again we encounter the dark side of altruism—a systematic and formal exclusion of outsiders for reasons that are wholly unrelated to their moral case for recipient status, at least in a world in which ability to pay and personal characteristics are all deemed irrelevant. The best explanation for this limitation is political: altruism for the group is a powerful exclusion of outsiders who don't vote and don't pay taxes.[20] But that justification is hardly moral unless the community of man gives national boundaries special weight and import. One great advantage of markets is that they do not respect territory and thus can transcend the localism of political life with its built-in territorial limitations. Only governments can restrict the sales of artwork overseas. Markets facilitate their movement. So here, too, the communitarianism of the UNOS position shows how easy it is to turn a system of exclusionary rules into a protectionist regime with a high moral tone.

RACIAL DISCRIMINATION IN ORGAN TRANSPLANTS

The heavy dependence on these technical criteria on its face should have one advantage. It should insulate UNOS from criticisms that its decisions are subject to unfair political influence or pressure. Yet, owing to how transplant organs are allocated, that has not proved to be the case because the racial questions that have divided so much of American life have also invaded the closed world of organ transplantation. The root of the problem lies in certain inescapable technical and demographic facts. The first of these is that antigen matches correlate along racial lines. All things considered, it is likely that a black recipient will do better with an organ from a black donor than from a white donor. The opposite is true as well: white organs will have lower rejection rates in white recipients. In addition, it turns out that whites and blacks have differential success rates with dialysis and transplantation. Controlling for other variables, blacks on average have a successful rate of transplantation that is somewhere between 10 and 20 percent below the same level for whites.[21] Yet, by the same token, blacks appear to be better able to tolerate dialysis than whites. Looked at as a technical matter, it appears that white recipients should have greater prospects of survival and should by the impersonal criteria adopted by UNOS receive a disproportionate share of organ donations.

That conclusion is accentuated by other well-known patterns of organ donation. One conspicuous feature of the present program of voluntary organ donations has been the relatively low level of participation by blacks.[22] The source of the difficulty rises on two fronts. First, there is a major reluctance on the part of many blacks to become voluntary donors into the system. The language of altruism often affords cold comfort to individuals and groups who think and act as outsiders to the system and who believe that any organ they contribute will benefit a white person—a form of redistribution across races they do not prefer. High levels of distrust and misinformation and the suspicion of public officials no doubt generally compound the problem. The lower the level of civil connection, the lower the levels of participation.

To compound the problem, a disproportionately large number of blacks relative to the whites populate the waiting lines for kidney transplants, largely because of the higher frequency of blacks suffering from end-state renal disorders (ESRD). For example, in 1988 there were 4,865 cadaveric transplants in a population of 67,778 white dialysis patients, but only 1,486 transplants in a population of 36,591 black dialysis patients.[23] Although blacks constitute about one-eighth the total population, they make up over one-third of the kidney population. On average, about 7 percent of the white patients and about 5 percent of the black population received transplantations each year, a difference of about 40 percent. The waiting time for black transplant recipients was nearly twice as long as it was for whites. (13.0 months to 7.6 months).[24]

The disparate white/black ratios have their origins in the technical modes of selection: the insistence on an antigen match that was designed to minimize the chances of kidney rejection. The overall policy of the administrative decision was (at least before the 1995 rule revisions) to treat all lives as equal, regardless of individual circumstances, and to maximize the total number of lives saved, without regard to race and (as is so typical in these matters) without regard to ability to pay or to cost. The disparate impact arose solely because of the correlation between race and antigen typing that makes white/white or black/black matches more likely than white/black ones. Once the result is known and documented, however, the practice, if continued, becomes vulnerable to the charge that it constitutes an intentional form of discrimination.

The next question, therefore, is whether the justification put forward—treat each life as though it were equal to all others—can withstand a showing of disparate impact. In part, the answer to this question depends on the rate of decay from improper matches. If a bad match led to fatal results, no one would be in favor of ignoring the technical data to achieve some collateral ethical advantage. But if the differences relate merely to probabilities of success, the sentiments on this question can easily change, so that the smaller the loss of effectiveness, the more potent the arguments for modifying the existing system. It turns out that survival rates are far higher for a perfect 6-antigen match than for a partial match. But even within the class of perfect antigen matches, white survival rates are around 8 to 11 percent higher than black survival rates, both before and after the introduction of cyclosporine.[25] With the improvement of immunosuppressive drugs, the importance of matching in determining survival is diminished, especially for less than 6-antigen matches.[26] Although it is an open question as to whether the differences that remain are large enough to matter—technical studies are divided on the question.[27] Immunosuppressive drugs have powerful side effects for which the less use the better.

This state of affairs has led to proposals that the system of allocation be altered to account for these differences, but ironically these proposals move in two directions. First, one school of transplantation experts continues to adhere to the proposition that the maximum number of lives should be saved and thus seeks to develop ever more refined matching mechanisms.[28] Others take precisely the opposite tack, that is, to downplay the importance of matching owing to the increased effectiveness of the immunosuppressive drugs.[29]

Any reduction in the salience of technical criteria could in principle lead to the rise of lotteries and queues as methods of allocation, at least in a nonmarket world. Wayne Arnason and Ayres, Dooley and Gaston have a very different set of policy objectives. It is to take the occasion to give blacks some systematic preference in the queuing mechanism. The preferences proposed have taken one of two forms. Ayres, Dooley & Gaston seek to operate within the structure of the UNOS point system, but to award additional points (up to 4) for "rare antigen matches" to offset the likelihood that they will have "less than a ten percent chance of qualifying for one of the antigen matching preferences" under the standard system.[30] The proposal has, however, an explicit racial objective, which is to make certain that disproportionate numbers of transplants will go to blacks, "without resorting to race conscious points."[31] The effort then is to forge a system of formal neutrality whose assured outcome tilts the balance toward black recipients.

For Arnason, black donors could be allowed, in an extension of the principle of the UAGA, to make directed donations of their kidneys, that is, to specify that these kidneys should go exclusively or preferably to black recipients. Currently the UAGA requires that a specific donee be named for the designation to trump a higher rating on the UNOS matching system. Arnason's proposal is to extend that option to *class* gifts, at least those by blacks and for blacks. What justifications can be offered for these two schemes? Let us consider first the modifications to the original UNOS matching system and then the directed donation rule.

UNOS MATCHES

The initial question about the Ayres, Dooley & Gaston proposal is how it ties into large social debates about the relevance of race in society. Any appeal to "diversity" does not seem relevant to the issue at hand because we are not talking about the composition of a classroom or a workplace. UNOS rhetoric to one side, the benefits of organ transplants are quintessentially personal, not collective. In addition, no ingenious explanation can justify the preference as rectification for a past wrong. Ayres notes that the neutral antigen testing counts as the "but for" cause of the current racial imbalance. However, there are other causes as well, including the high level of black kidney illness and the low level of black participation in the donation programs. Neither of these causes is attributable to past abuses or to present discrimination, much less Jim Crow. It is dangerous to look around for remote causes to present events, while overlooking the far more potent causes of the current imbalance. It is the combination of high levels of black kidney disorders and low black participation that places the unwanted stress on UNOS's technical matching system.

The simple fact that a larger percentage of blacks do have ESRD suggests that, looking at the kidney program as a whole, there already is a major redistribution of wealth through both special kidney programs and general Medicare and Medicaid programs *from* white *to* black, under the same type of unmotivated neutral criteria that are at work in the kidney selection area. Blacks, as a group, receive more benefit from the kidney program than they contribute. Yet no one should claim that this program constitutes a form of racial discrimination, let alone affirmative action, in light of how its eligibility requirements and practices were formulated. Nor should anyone, within the framework of current programs, claim that whites should obtain better access to any dialysis program because, pro rata, they have contributed a greater fraction to its cost of operation.

Ayres, Dooley & Gaston recognize "this difficult issue of framing,"[32] but do nothing with it. In their view, one set of implicit biases cries out for relief, whereas implicit biases in the opposite direction stay just as they are and never count even as offsets for other biases that cut in the opposite direction. Their limp ground for this tunnel vision is that transplantation of cadaveric kidneys is a "discrete" public concern, notwithstanding its intimate connection with substitute forms of medical treatment for the same condition.

It is difficult, of course, to revisit the entire debate over race relations in the context of one particular program. But two quick remarks do seem appropriate. First, with each passing year, it becomes harder to justify any form of racial preferences as rectification for official wrongs that were committed 30 or 40 or more years ago. The intervention of subsequent policies, which have cut in the opposite direction, makes these actions too remote to count as credible explanations for our current problems. Immediate causes explain more recent events. Second, even if these past wrongs did cry out for rectification, it is hard to see why it should be channeled through this program. Other forms of rectification do not require a sacrifice of human life to achieve their ends. So why concentrate the present forms of rectification in areas where they are likely to do the most harm. Even a larger state subsidy for ESRD (and it is quite large already) would give disproportionate benefit to blacks without compromising the internal integrity of the overall program.

From that it seems to follow that awarding rare antigen points for the reasons stated cannot be justified. In its 1995 rules revisions, UNOS did not incorporate this requirement or give any explicit racial preference. But it did act in ways that were directly responsive to the criticisms of Ayres and others by reducing the number of points given for a perfect antigen match, from 10 to 7, and adding points for waiting time (1 point is added for each year on the waiting list).[33] The net effect of these alternations is, as was intended, to increase the likelihood that black recipients will receive kidneys. The criterion on which they fare less well, matching, is reduced in importance, whereas the criterion on which they fare better, waiting, receives greater importance.

This modification of UNOS rules could be justified as an effort to overcome institutional rigidity and to meet the charge that UNOS guidelines cannot move fast enough to respond to changes in technology. Ayres, Dooley & Gaston, for example, went to great pains to show the influence of medical developments on the overall allocation scheme. A market system, however, does not have to wait for any institutional shift in response to new information about the survival rates of recipients with partial matches. Any potential bidder for a kidney (even those who receive charitable support) takes into account changes in the prospects of success as soon as they occur. Blacks can bid up their offers to take into account the improved rates of success without having to first persuade a national convention of the merits of their position. By the same token, they might be less likely to bid in light of their lower level of success with grafts and their better toleration of dialysis. Taking into account those differentials is studiously avoided under current policy, notwithstanding the explicit but wavering concern with maximum survivability. However, those differentials would be factored into the decisions made in any market system, where it would tend to increase overall survival rates. Using a bid system would allow foreigners to participate in the market on the same terms as American citizens and permanent aliens—and to infuse their funds into the present system. The weighting of points just drops out of the picture altogether in a bidding system, which not only includes all potential players, but which also takes into account the "soft stuff" that UNOS technocrats are forced to exclude. Under this framework, the only question to be asked is whether the blacks deserve some explicit cash subsidy that is denied to whites—a hard-sell indeed.

Nor can the UNOS adjustments be defended as the outgrowth of neutral scientific calculation. They were not. It is an old saw in the law of racial discrimination that formal neutrality can disguise discrimination. What credence should be given to Jim Crow's neutral rule limiting the eligibility to vote to individuals whose grandfathers had voted before the Civil War? At the passage of the 1964 Civil Rights Act, supporters and opponents alike were aware that ostensible neutral criteria could be used as a pretext for discrimination on the grounds of race or some other forbidden character. Neutrality has the virtue of preventing many forms of public impropriety by keeping explicit racial preferences from being enacted into law. But, it is only a necessary and not a sufficient condition for stopping government abuse. The residual discretion that remains under some neutral principles still leaves open avenues for official abuse.

The major attraction of a neutral rule, then, is inextricably tied to the advancement of overall social welfare by preventing *relevant* criteria (for example, waiting time) from being pressed into the service of partisan interests. A teacher who said that he favors a neutral grading system (count spelling errors) because it gives whites the highest grade is trying to beat the system, not to work within it—and would everywhere be made to pay the price. The same reproach should be directed toward any neutral criterion adopted to advance black interests at the expense of white interests by flipping the criterion (ignore all spelling errors) to obtain the opposite result. Neutral rules work best when they are formulated and executed with neutral intentions. The right question to ask is which rule would you adopt if your population were all white or all black—the very kind of psychological counterfactual situation that the criterion of neutrality was designed to escape in the first place!

These basic arguments carry over to the troubled thickets of organ transplantation. The system of technical allocation noted earlier reduces total levels of human satisfaction and for those reasons alone should be changed. But once within that framework the only acceptable task is to maximize the *aggregate* level of satisfaction of all individuals. In its own evaluations, UNOS ignores differences in longevity and the quality of life, and in the context of this controversy, it is useful to follow its lead. Within its chosen framework it should not be acceptable morally, no matter how attractive politically, to prefer a distribution that consciously opts to save 50 black and 100 white lives by means of kidney transplants when an alternative technical system could save 40 black and 120 white lives. It is not possible to devise any explicit moral criterion that prefers 10 black to 20 white lives, any more than the reverse. Why then tolerate its implicit adoption?

Ayres, Dooley & Gaston support their revised system of points by appealing to rules that favor O-type recipients for O-type kidneys.[34] Presumably that same argument could be used to defend a neutral criterion that is enacted to advance partisan interests. The nub of the argument is that the O preference favors one class of recipients over another, even though it reduces the total number of lives saved. At first blush, one tension between unequal access and overall number of lives saved has been resolved in favor of the former. Once UNOS makes that compromise, it should be free to make similar adjustments in other areas.

To this position, a number of responses are relevant. First, and most obviously, the preferences for O recipients is not a racial preference and thus does not trigger the same range of political or emotional responses. The entire structure of American constitutional law does not treat all distinctions alike, but reserves special attention to public distinctions made on grounds of race. Even when departures are made from that rule, as in the case of affirmative action, the level of argument on both sides is intense. It blinks at reality to assume that any nonracial distinction should, or would, capture the public attention of a racial classification. Could we imagine any outcry against the O-type rule if it had no racial impact whatsoever?

But even if we let this point pass, under the current UNOS rules, the O-type preference may well make sense on classical efficiency terms.[35] In an ordinary market system, we would expect to see O-type recipients bid more fiercely for O-type kidneys because they have nowhere else to go. Honoring this preference inside a state allocation system duplicates this market preference in a regulatory framework. As noted by Lloyd Cohen and Melissa Michelsen, it does so for good overall logic.[36] To assess the efficiency of a kidney allocation system, it is a mistake to look at each matching in isolation from all others. Suppose that, on the initial match, the O-type recipient has a 50 percent chance of success and the A- or B-type recipient has a 55 percent chance. Prima facie the preference for the A- or B-type makes sense. But the judgment is far less secure when dynamic considerations are brought into play by asking what happens to the long-term operation of the system. In particular, any person passed over in the initial match is still in the pool. An A- or B-type recipient might be able to receive 65 percent of the new kidneys made available. The O-type recipient might be eligible to receive less than 50 percent. By making the more difficult match first, the allocation rule leaves the more suitable recipient in the pool and thus increases the probability that both matches will be successfully made. Hence the O-type rule might well be justified by its overall efficiency, for the same reasons that O-type individuals would bid more vigorously for O-type kidneys in an open auction. In the long run, it saves more lives.

These calculations are not set in stone and might prove incorrect in the fullness of time. But if so, one dubious rule serves as an ill-precedent for the second. If those calculations are incorrect, the O-type rule should be removed forthwith from the UNOS system. Either way, the rule affords no support for UNOS's recent decision to twist its ostensible neutral rules to build in implicit racial preferences on organ matching. If no explicit racial judgment is permissible, a covert racial judgment is scarcely better. The subterranean influence of race on UNOS allocations removes the last shred of principled defense for public control over organ distribution. The high moral aspirations of the present system cannot withstand the pounding by political influences, just as the standard models of interest-group politics glumly predict.

DIRECTED DONATIONS

The Arnason proposal, which would allow blacks to specify a preferential for black recipients, raises a very different set of considerations. His willingness to sanction directed donations rests largely on the belief that the new incentives will stimulate a higher level of black donations. He may well be right because it is highly unlikely that potential organ donors have the disinterested generosity attributable to them in the UNOS literature. But if Arnason is correct, a raft of other queries follow on the heels of the original proposal. Money, for example, is likely to improve the incentives to donate still more. Yet purchasing organs remains strictly forbidden, beyond the pale of respectable discourse.

More importantly, even in our shadowy world of coercive altruism, it is fair to ask whether *all* persons should be allowed to make race-specific class donations. Does—should—Arnason's logic allow white group (or subgroup) preferences (for example, Italian or Jewish) to be taken into account in the donation process? At one level, bending the current rules in this way does not help remedy the underprovision of organs for blacks and should therefore not be encouraged. Globally, however, Arnason's incentive arguments cut exactly the opposite way. The first order difficulty is not any perceived imbalance in the pool; it is the shortage of organs to go around. *All* persons should be able to designate the class of eligible recipients in order to increase the available supply of organs in the pool. Oddly enough, the recent switch from local to national pooling is likely to exacerbate the difficulty on both sides of the pool. For all people, the clear preference of personal designation will be local, precisely because, as Adam Smith recognized long ago, all people are less interested in benefiting those who are at a distance from them than those who are close at hand.[37] Surely organ donations from blacks located in black communities are likely to *decrease* under any program of national distribution if there is any reluctance to provide assistance to whites, especially those located at a distance. But lest we gravitate instantly toward local allocation, the counterbalancing factor cannot be ignored. The broader national pool does promise a better technical match for organs by allowing the consideration of a larger number of potential donees. Once again, within the framework of the current law, it is hard to make any abstract determination as to the relative strength of these two offsetting effects.

Any program for directed donations receives a very different analysis within the framework of a market system. The question of national versus local quickly drops out because all persons are allowed to enter the system, on either commercial or charitable donations. Nor would it be necessary to have to make peace with Arnason's effort to carve an exception to the current practice of anonymous recipients. In a market, the seller can set whatever terms and conditions he or she wants to impose on the transfer of an organ. If blacks only want to transfer to blacks, or women to women, or lacrosse players to lacrosse players, so be it. The harder question is descriptive: will blacks choose to adopt this strategy if it means forgoing income that they could otherwise obtain from an organ sale to a white? Or would they choose to sell and donate some portion of the proceeds to their favor charity? These are points on which we are all entitled to make predictions, but the choice is of behaviors not ours, but theirs. The entire system of guidelines could be rendered a thing of the past; the moral tension between color-blindness and affirmative action would cease to be an issue of public import. The vast sums of money that are now spent on deciding whom to exclude from the program and why could now be spent on purchasing organs for persons in need, based on the usual charitable principles set out earlier.

CONCLUSION

In sum, the question of organ transplantation offers a vivid demonstration of the coercive failures of a system that cannot deliver the altruism it promises. In its concern to help everyone, it adopts a set of restrictions and limitations that are far more destructive than the practices likely to emerge in a system of markets. The parochialism of the system becomes manifest as the demands of interest-group politics work themselves into the fabric of the administrative order. Yet with the enormous outpouring of moralizing and a parallel expenditure of resources, the initial shortages have only become more insistent. It is an unhappy mixture of the sacred and the profane. The political consensus, however, is impervious to the manifest evidence of its own failures and cannot correct the troublesome imbalances that become ever more apparent with each passing year. Here the blame has to be laid not on technical issues, but at the doorstep of the moral philosophy of false comradeship that underpins the entire legal regime. With results such as these, how can anyone deny, at least for organ transplants, the perils, if not the immorality of, official altruism?

CHAPTER 13

❖ ❖ ❖

Active Euthanasia

It is an inevitable truth that all people will die. But it is far from inevitable when they will die or how they will die. The questions that I shall examine here concern the set of legal rules and social conventions that deal with the thorny and contentious issues that surround death and dying. The issue is hardly one that is confined to our own times. Debate over how people should die and what their physicians may do to help them die raged without interruption from ancient Greece and Rome to the present time.[1] The questions that are raised today are the same questions that have been raised throughout the history of medicine. To what extent should individuals have the *right* to control over decisions of life and death, most particularly by way of active euthanasia? Any analysis of this topic begins with two simple questions: Is the basic autonomy principle adequate to handle the problem of euthanasia? If so, what response to euthanasia does that principle require?

In grappling with this issue, one key distinction dictates the structure of the present law. On one side of the line, the right to refuse treatment, the right to discontinue treatment, and the right to withdraw treatment are all held to fall within the exclusive control of the patient. In some cases, these rights are disregarded by physicians who, it appears, are frequently not aware of patients' wishes to avoid cardiopulmonary resuscitation, or, if they are, simply ignore them. All too often, physicians keep patients in intensive care units, in considerable pain, for periods of 10 days or more immediately before death.[2] Coping with these systematic departures from accepted norms presents enormous logistic challenges.

283

If changes in physician culture do not come about voluntarily, perhaps some pointed lawsuits for breach of contract could bring the point sharply home. But for normative purposes, no one disagrees that these frequent lapses are just that: lapses. They do not constitute a considered retreat from the principle of patient autonomy, sanctioned and approved by the law.

Rather, the question presented here is what should be done in end-of-life cases. For all we know, a fair bit of covert, active euthanasia takes place side by side with the regrettable heroics to prolong life. But cases of active euthanasia will remain buried underground even when they accord fully with the wishes and intentions of dying patients and their families. No physician, not even Jack Kevorkian, will invite the loss of license and criminal prosecution that can follow from the simple proposition that active euthanasia is illegal everywhere in the United States.

To some eyes, at least, the juxtaposition of these two starkly different legal regimes raises serious doubts that are not easily put to rest. I am one of those people. I have no desire to challenge the first half of this equation, which allows patients to refuse treatment for whatever reason they see fit. But I do want to enter the debate to insist that the principle of patient autonomy that undergirds the right to refuse treatment also supports the right to active euthanasia, not withstanding our nationwide ban on the practice. Our universal legal prohibition on euthanasia functions as an unsound limitation—or too subtle refinement—of the principle of individual autonomy. The same unfortunate attitude that bans active euthanasia also requires a backstop prohibition on assisted suicide. Consistent with our general framework, we must ask whether this full set of restrictions on personal choice in life and death situations is justified as a means to overcome some problem of collective action, to control some dangerous externality to third persons, or to prevent some regular and systematic form of patient abuse. I believe that none of these asserted grounds for intervention is compelling enough to rein in the freedom of choice that presumptively all persons should enjoy over their own bodies and lives.

This part of the book addresses these controversial issues. This chapter concerns the scope of the autonomy principle in active euthanasia cases. Chapter 14 addresses the complications raised by the issue of physician-assisted suicide. Chapter 15 deals with concerns of patient abuse, with special reference to the experience from the Dutch system, the only nation that permits, if only as a matter of prosecutorial discretion, the practice of euthanasia. Chapter 16 explores the relevant constitutional issues in anticipation of a definitive Supreme Court ruling on the question. Chapter 17 extends the analysis to deal with cases of choices made by and for incompetents.

THE AUTONOMY FLIP-FLOP

One of the most evident paradoxes that riddles the entire area of health care is the inconsistent and partial application of the autonomy principle across a wide class of personal and institutional decisions. As was evident in our discussion of organ transplantation, the autonomy principle has been rightly invoked to block, in all but rare cases (chiefly corneal transplantations), the prospect of forced donations of organs from either living or deceased individuals. At the same time, the autonomy principle has been given short shrift as a possible foundation for allowing individuals, during life or after death, to sell their organs to other persons. Instead, the rival principle of community altruism has dominated the field, which tolerates near-coercive regimes such as required request and presumed consent and imposes the manifestly coercive prohibition on voluntary sale. Notwithstanding our present policies, I believe that a rule that treated voluntary gifts and voluntary sales with equal dignity, while subjecting both to the same safeguards against duress and misrepresentation, would function far better than the present command and control system over organ transplantation.

At first blush, the disputes over euthanasia seem far removed from those that swirl over organ transplantation. Euthanasia is usually the province of the old and of those who have severe chronic conditions. That class of individuals is not the normal class of organ donors, which tends to include young persons who die of traumatic injuries, but occasionally a poignant case pokes through to establish an intimate connection between the two. Several years ago, the *New York Times* carried the story of a fully competent 48-year-old woman who suffered from a terminal case of multiple sclerosis that had already induced quadriplegia.[3] The woman had already made clear her wish to die. Her last wish was to become an organ donor after death. At her instructions, her physicians weaned her from the respirator, and she died after several hours of labored breathing. During the time it took her to die, her internal organs were so damaged by the want of oxygen as to be rendered unusable after her death. Alas, the limitations against euthanasia impeded her ability to make one last voluntary gift. But for what end? Is it really better that this woman suffered pointlessly for several hours while her organs deteriorated? Is there any doubt that she would have accepted active euthanasia, by strangulation if necessary, in order to preserve her organs for donation? Yet the prohibition on active euthanasia made it impossible for anyone to propose, let alone execute, a course of action to which she would, I suspect, have readily acceded.

This sad tale not only chronicles a human tragedy, but it also underscores a philosophical point. The root difficulty in forming coherent policy on matters of death and dying is identical to that found in connection with organ transplantation. Our basic orientation displays too much equivocation and waffling on the role of patient choice and patient autonomy on matters of death and dying. The basic position reveals a sharp, almost jarring, duality on the entire matter. It is taken as gospel on all sides today that the individual patient who is competent is fully entitled to choose whether to accept or to decline treatment,[4] or indeed, the maintenance of essential but routine life support systems for nutrition and hydration.[5] The right to refuse treatment applies not only in those cases in which a person suffers from a terminal illness, but it also extends to people capable of living for many years so long as they have external support. Thus in *McKay v. Bergstedt*,[6] the Court (with the explicit support of the state) upheld the right of a 31-year-old quadriplegic to be removed from a respirator so that he could die a natural death, and thus avoid the calamity of outliving his devoted father and being consigned into the care of strangers.[7] In dealing with these matters, the right to refuse treatment or support has gained strength over time until it now counts as one of the few "absolutes" on the medical-legal horizon. In principle, an array of state interests can be lined up against it: preserving the sanctity of life; preventing suicide; protecting innocent third persons; preserving the integrity of the medical profession; and encouraging benevolent actions.[8]

In ordinary cases, none of these interests seems to bite. Paradoxically, being vested with a right to refuse treatment has as its chief value the right to decide what kind of treatment to accept. If we can accept or decline surgery at will, we can pick from a large menu of choices in between and decide which type of surgery to have and when. Here the absolute right of choice works in the same fashion as the absolute right to refuse to deal in the marketplace. No one ever made a fortune by refusing to enter into all transactions. The absolute nature of the right is critical for allowing individuals to shape the transactions that they do enter, without having to receive prior state approval.

It is one thing, however, to make rights absolute when the rivers of life run smoothly. It is quite another to accord the right that same absolute status under extreme conditions—which is why the common law rules of necessity play so critical a role in the design of the overall system. The problems of death and dying raise just these questions of ultimate choice. In the medical area, an ever stronger social consensus has turned these compelling state interests for regulation into jelly in the face of a persistent refusal of treatment by people who wish to die because they have no prospect of regaining a bearable existence. The individual situation may be one of dire straits, but it is also one in which nature nullifies the prospect of rescue. Within this context, the domain of individual choice becomes larger and more secure. In extremis, a person's right to refuse treatment, both in moral and in legal terms, is *never* conditional on his ability to make the right choice, that is, a choice that others, with full knowledge of the situation, would uniformly regard as rational for him. Instead, the issue is rightly regarded as one that contains an irreducible element of subjective choice: the proposed treatment may require an individual to endure future pain, to place additional burdens on family members, and to bear additional expense that eats up money slated for the provision of loved ones.[9]

These cases, perhaps more than any others, require a delicate calculus of benefits and burdens. However, the task of measurement and comparison is so elusive that no one person should ever presume to speak for someone else who is able to speak for himself. The legal system rigorously takes a back seat on the matters of choice and allocation and leaves the imponderables to be weighed by the person who, as a general rule, is best able to deal with them: the individual patient. Here this judgment is made secure in the knowledge that it will be wrong in some cases. It is easy to tell war stories of individuals who do not know what is in their own interests, but in any large institutional setting, no society can afford the luxury of sorting out, case by case, war stories from heroic tales in order to separate those people who know their own interests from those who do not. The dangers of the misapplication of the principle force us to a rough-and-ready rule of decision, one that is treated more absolute in law than it is in fact.

Accordingly it is only in cases of manifest incompetence that the law resorts to the test of substituted judgment, which requires empathetic evaluations by one individual about the desires of another.[10] Usually any effort to short-circuit individual self-control is sharply rebuffed, even for a patient in constant pain who operates with compromised faculties of attention and judgment. In light of the inevitable nature of these difficulties, those who know that they cannot speak for tomorrow are encouraged to make their wishes known today, and where necessary to leave written instructions that tell doctors what should be done or to create durable powers of attorneys that delegate future medical decisions to certain named persons.[11] Every effort is made to move the decision forward in time and bring it within an institutionalized support structure; no effort is made to force that decision into the hands of the state. No one to my knowledge regards a refusal to accept treatment as an immoral decision, or one that the legal system should second guess. When the proposition is "just say no," the principle of individual autonomy operates at its high level mark.

The entire landscape changes radically when a physician is not asked to honor the patient's "mere" refusal of treatment, but to participate actively in bringing about the patient's death. The autonomy principle still constitutes a useful first step in the analysis, but it no longer dictates the final resting place. Instead of a continuous progression, we encounter a conceptual chasm. The state interest in the preservation of life, which did not override an individual decision to refuse treatment, now rises to a dominant position. No matter how lofty the motives behind the act, and no matter how great the suffering relieved, no person has the right to take his or her own life either by suicide or by the act of an agent.[12] "A physician is prohibited from knowingly and directly causing death, irrespective of the patient's wishes, quality of life, or prognosis."[13] The legal system constructs a vast gulf between refusing treatment and hastening death, even with the consent of the victim. The first is the highest expression of individual self-control; the second is a criminal act, both for the principal actor and, in cases of assisted suicide, for any confederate or accessory.

The fundamental puzzle lies in articulating any rationale that justifies the distinction between these two cases—active and deliberate killing, and the fatal refusal of treatment or support. The quest here is strictly normative. The current law accepts this distinction even though restive juries seem more reluctant to apply it in fact, as the refusal of a Michigan jury to convict Jack Kevorkian for five offenses in three separate trials plainly reveals.[14] But the question still remains, should the law remain in its current condition? My basic conclusion is no. The arguments that can be marshaled in support of the autonomy principle cover all cases in which an individual seeks to exercise control over his own life, whether to prolong it or to end it. Some modest procedural safeguards should surround that decision, but we do not have to linger unduly on this question. The basic position should be that the safeguards that are deemed acceptable in cases where treatment has been refused should be regarded as sufficient in which active euthanasia is sought. It does not matter whether the patient asks to receive an injection of morphine or pentobarbital, or to withdraw feeding and breathing tubes. In both cases, the best set of safeguards is likely to be informal and consultative, as is now the norm in cases to refuse treatment. It will not lie in a procedural thicket, whose major purpose is to destroy the right, not to protect it.

The best way to defend this position is to review the objections to it. These objections fall into two categories. The first line of resistance is designed to show the philosophical incoherence of any system that purports to recognize the right of individuals to take their own lives. The second set of barriers is more practical and is directed toward the likely abuse, especially with the old, the poor, and the vulnerable, if any such right is recognized—no matter how it is administered. In responding to both defenses of the established legal order, the lodestone never shifts: if any given objection is sufficient to defeat a claim for active euthanasia, why does it not also defeat the established practice that allows all individuals to deliberately refuse to receive medical care that might extend their lives?[15] Conversely, if the arguments do not block an individual's right to refuse treatment, it should not block the practice of active euthanasia. Under the revised regime, the delicate line-drawing problems between the two classes of actions disappear because both are subject to the same legal requirements. We need not longer ask whether an additional dose of morphine is to palliate pain or to end life when it may be meant to do both. The overall simplification brought about by eliminating the distinction between active euthanasia and the refusal to deal has a double virtue: it enhances liberty and reduces administrative cost and legal uncertainty. Let us turn to these objections, starting with the most philosophical and working down to the most practical.

A DENIAL OF RESPONSIBILITY

The first line of defense of the current distinction is to deny any human culpability, either of patient or provider, for a decision to refuse medical treatment or life support, made with the certain knowledge that death would ensue. The current position is defensible only by entering into abstruse debates over causation, with an eye to preserving and glorifying the distinction between acts and omissions, or misfeasance and nonfeasance. The persistence of these distinctions in the health area is in odd counterpoint to the diminished role they play more generally in the law of tort. The law today continues to adhere, however uneasily, to the traditional common law view that no person owes a duty to rescue a stranger, even from imminent peril. That view depends on accepting the common law distinction between not-doing, or nonfeasance, and doing-wrong, or misfeasance. But as applied to rescue cases, that line has been attacked as "revolting to the moral sense."[16] As the faith in that distinction erodes, the pressure to create some duty of "easy" rescue intensifies.[17]

In response to this sense of outrage, the more recent tendency has been to invoke a unitary standard of reasonable care under the circumstances for all cases of actions and inaction, so long as it can be said that the defendant owes the plaintiff a duty of care, one that has not been discharged in the particular case.[18] That view is, I think, deficient because it fails to maintain the older distinction between harms suffered by strangers on the one hand, and harms suffered by persons with whom a defendant stands in some consensual or status relationship on the other. Of these relational situations, parent and child is one illustration, and physician and patient is surely another.[19]

A duty to rescue strangers falls within none of these categories. The only case for imposing the duty is that it works for the long-term average advantage of all individuals governed by it. This is a point on which I have doubt, given the willingness of most people to rescue without legal compulsion, but it is surely one on which reasonable minds can easily differ.[20] Whether these arguments against a legal duty to rescue strangers are right or wrong, they say nothing about the obligations between persons who have entered into consensual arrangements, where it is understood that some affirmative actions are routinely required, and the only question is to identify which ones. The physician can cease treating his patient for the same reason he can continue it: authorization by the patient who has the capacity and competence to decide. Consent is the key, as it should be in an autonomy-based system.

In this world, as Glanville Williams and others pointed out long ago, a distinction between not prolonging life and ending life has nothing to commend it from a moral point of view.[21] Can it really make a difference whether the physician disconnects the ventilator or sets it to shut off automatically at some fixed point in time? In both cases, he is responsible if the respirator no longer functions when the patient wants it to; in neither case, is he responsible if the patient has consented to its being turned off.[22] To call turning the ventilator off an "omission" or a bit of inaction, instead of an act, does more than mock the English language. The use of this verbal sleight of hand also makes it impossible to explain why a stranger who "did" that same "omission," that is, who disconnected the ventilator *without* authorization should, and would, be prosecuted for murder as a matter of course. Within the framework of any ongoing arrangement, the question of duty and omission can only be decided with respect to some overarching set of expectations, express or implied, that the parties set for themselves. The knowledge needed to make sense of those expectations does not spring from the nonfeasance/misfeasance distinction, but from an awareness of what course of action will maximize the patient's welfare.

A kindred distinction between extraordinary and ordinary care, which seems to have fallen into disrepute today,[23] has, for all its apparent vagueness, far more to recommend it because it tries to track these social expectations. Thus it is commonplace today for persons to tell their doctors, "you may keep me on a respirator, but you may not engage in any heroics to keep me alive." The "Do Not Resuscitate" order falls exactly into this category. Where the patient has not spoken, a physician who follows this rule of thumb may not perfectly match the patient's expectations, but is likely to approximate them far better than anyone who organized the inquiry around the act/omission distinction. If a patient articulates this line (subject to constraints on cost, already discussed in connection with futility), the physician should honor it both ways: continue routine care but avoid the more invasive interventions.

I am not quite sure why this distinction has fallen into undeserved disrepute, for it is surely superior to the act/omission distinction that continues to be defended today—but to what end? Daniel Callahan, while keenly aware of the difficulties, seeks to revive the distinction by arguing that killing is attributable to human agency; but failing to keep alive is attributable to natural events, namely, the underlying disease condition.[24] But surely we would not allow that version of the causation to dominate if a doctor just forgot to take some standard precaution that could have saved a person from death by disease. If one doctrine is settled in the law of tort, it is that an adverse outcome may have more than a single cause. The defendant can be held responsible if his conduct is "a" cause of the harm, no matter what other facts cooperated in bringing it about.[25] Thus, in the inevitable malpractice action that would follow, the failure to act, the omission, would be the decisive fact, and the inexorable physical progress of the underlying disease condition would be effortlessly reclassified as a "mere condition" that would do nothing to diminish the physician's level of responsibility.[26]

The one evident truth about the distinction between action and omission is that the act results in death even if the patient is healthy, whereas the omission results in death only for a person in a diseased state. The point shows that dangerous acts cut a wider swath than dangerous omissions. We cannot kill healthy persons by denying them the use of a ventilator they do not want and need. But this observation does not prove that it is blameless to disconnect, without authorization, the ventilator that a sick person needs. The spirited enterprise to shape duties of care, both individual or professional, out of whole cloth and to fashion a metaphysics to match cannot solve the action/omission dilemma or invest it with greater weight than it deserves. The patient's permission, not our fine-spun philosophical theories, determines the scope of duty and legitimizes any decision to stop treatment.

If killing a patient with consent is illegal, cessation of treatment with consent should be illegal as well. The distinction between the two cases is, ultimately, not principled but pragmatic. Allowing cessation of treatment protects a huge range of necessary and sensible acts routinely performed by physicians, and in hospitals, without fear of liability. It also has the workaday virtue of avoiding a massive collision between popular sentiment and legal rule. In this regard the act/omission distinction, although less attuned to the wishes of patients, leaves someone more room to maneuver without running afoul of the law: provision of nutrition and hydration is surely ordinary care, and use of a ventilator may be.[27] With this hard-edged distinction between (forbidden) acts and (allowable) omission, the scope of permissible conduct is *increased* beyond what it otherwise would have been. In this metaphysical world, it is better to bend and not break. But these artful compromises are far from ideal. The failure of the act/omission distinction to account for the prohibition on euthanasia forces us to look elsewhere for the philosophical arguments to support the legal prohibition.

A CONSTRAINED DEFINITION OF AUTONOMY

The second conceptual attack on the right to take one's own life relies on a narrow definition of autonomy. The term no longer refers to actions that individuals can take or cannot take at their own will. It now refers to actions that an individual can take in his own interest, so long as that act is consistent with the fundamental and enduring features of human existence. Taking one's own life by one's own hand is against the nature and purpose of life, whose highest aspiration is self-preservation. In this regard, the debate once again tracks the narrow conceptions of autonomy (it does not include the right to sell bodily organs) that has long framed the debate over organ transplants.

This viewpoint has been most clearly developed in Leon Kass's recent penetrating defense of the current prohibition on euthanasia, which begins by noting that the metaphor of autonomy as individual self-ownership has been deeply contested in the philosophical literature.[28] As Kass observes, John Locke, for example, rests his labor theory of value on the idea of individual self-ownership. "Though the earth and all inferior creatures be common to all men, yet every man has a property in his own person; this no body has a right to but himself. The labor of his body and the work of his hand we may say are properly his."[29] At one level, it looks as though this passage marks a strong claim of self-ownership— "every man has a property in his own person." But the context reveals the limited, but critical purposes for which Locke invoked this right. His passage was designed to explain (and it does not do a good job at that)[30] why the addition of labor is sufficient to permit individuals to take tangible things out of the initial commons where they were placed by God and to treat them as though they were their own private property. Locke's passage, less controversially, is also designed to explain why, when individuals add value to what they already own, they are allowed to capture the gain from labor in the form of increased value of the property on which that labor is expended.

Nothing in this passage speaks to the question of whether any individual should be allowed to take his own life, or indeed sell himself into slavery. In fact, on that last question, Locke takes precisely the opposite view: "For a man, not having the power of his own life, *cannot* by compact, or his own consent, enslave himself to any one, nor put himself under the Absolute, Arbitrary Power of another, to take away his Life, when he pleases."[31] The clear image here is that of inalienable rights, of individuals as the keepers of their own lives under grant from God, and who are thus so constrained by the terms of that grant that they cannot sell themselves into slavery. To be sure, people may enter into employment or apprentice contracts for some definite period of time, but even there the master is under a strict injunction not to injure the servant.[32] Kass notes that similar sentiments can be found in the writing of Immanuel Kant: "to dispose of oneself as a mere means to some end of one's own liking is to degrade the humanity in one's person, which, after all, was entrusted to man, to preserve."[33] Again, the settler of the trust is not some anonymous individual but has to be in God, as the creator and grantor of all life.[34]

The limited account of personal autonomy works far better in a theistic universe than a legal one, and nothing that I can say should, or would, influence religious persons to depart from this conception of behavior in their own self-governance. But however strong those arguments bind within the faith, they do not justify the use of state coercion against anyone who departs from those beliefs. In this context, the inquiry must be directed toward the merits of the underlying dispute. What is inherent in the nature of man that allows anyone to brand acts leading to death as unnatural and self-destructive, and as acts inconsistent with his basic nature? But what happens when we deny, in the secular context, the proposition that all human beings hold their rights as limited grantees from some higher authority? At this point, should we follow Kass's narrower definition of autonomy, that speaks of the right to use one's labor to the exclusion of others? Or should we commit to the broader account of self-rule that gives each person full control over all decisions pertaining to the body, including the power to terminate life?

The first foray here is by now familiar. The initial difficulty with Kass's narrower conception is that it does not account for that portion of the modern law that recognizes the right of autonomous individuals to refuse medical treatments or life support devices, even when they are aimed at self-preservation. The principle of autonomy is thus strong enough to allow an individual to turn down even free gifts of assistance to prolong his own life when he wants to end it. We should not impose a set of implied conditions on the scope of individual self-rule in order to constrict the domain of individual choice. Autonomy, then, does not only embrace the right to exclusive use; it also embraces the right not to use the resources supplied by others.

The right to take one's own life, however, surely goes beyond refusing treatment and signals a distinct shift in the balance of power between the individual and the state. Should people be allowed to consume resources to end their own lives, just as they may consume resources to make that life more pleasurable under other circumstances? Here again, the quotations from Locke are not very helpful because whatever the objections to euthanasia, no one could argue that they derive in any way from the condemnation of slavery and perpetual subordination to the will of another that drove his initial account of the "inalienable" right of self-ownership. Euthanasia is not a form of alienation or disposition to others; it is the ultimate in self-assertion, a form of termination of life that in no way leaves any individual at the risk or the whim of another person. Nor does the Kantian concern with individual dignity account for the disparate legal response to refusing care and taking one's own life. Why isn't anyone required to accept treatment against his will to stay alive? Kant's proposition that people are "entrusted to preserve" human life is not consistent with passively allowing our own powers to erode with the passage of time. Trustees have active duties to manage, preserve, and maintain their trust property, which is why they are empowered in the first place. The Kantian conception again fails to distinguish between the two relevant cases—refusing treatment and hastening death. So, what theory might be able to do so?

I think that these abstract inquiries into the nature of man, whether divine or human, shed little light on the appropriate legal responses to the euthanasia question. Instead, we must turn immediately to a more functional account and ask what set of initial entitlements will yield the greatest level of human satisfaction over time, taking into account the welfare of the individual patient and that of all those around him. In this light, the common sense behind the decision to allow people to refuse medical treatment becomes more evident.

Suppose that the legal rule were otherwise, such that refusing treatment and hastening death were both prohibited. Now other people could hold an individual down against his will and administer unwanted treatment, all for his own good of course. The parties in charge of treatment need not respect the preferences of the patient because, as manifested, these have already revealed themselves to be untrustworthy. The legal system must, therefore, designate some other person or group of persons to make the initial, benevolent decision to treat as well as all the subsequent decisions on what kind of treatment and by whom. In the absence of an autonomy rule, how is that person chosen and on what principles does he proceed? The autonomy principle makes labor markets (Locke's direct concern) possible because it allows a single seller and a single buyer of labor to define their relationship without regard to what the rest of the world thinks.[35] To be sure, there are externalities, but, as noted earlier, most of these are positive, especially when the focus is not solely on a single transaction but on an entire system of transactions in goods and services.

The same efficiency in decision making is present when the question turns to matters of life and death. The autonomy principle selects, at virtually no cost, a single person capable of making a decision. It also designates as decision maker that person who, all things considered, has the best information, the largest stake in the outcome, and the best incentives to get it right. The functional case for the autonomy model is evident where the question is "what treatment," for which the duty to disclose requires the physician to convey information that allows the patient to make an informed and responsible choice.[36] A major inconvenience is generated by organizing matters on a model that allows an individual autonomous control over choice of treatment, but imposes collective or physician control over decisions to terminate his own life.

This argument, however, does not clinch the case for active euthanasia. The defenders of the status quo believe that *no one* should ever be allowed to practice active euthanasia, thereby eliminating any reason for the legal system to decide *who* should make the decision in any individual case. That response presupposes that some antecedent *collective* decision can make better tradeoffs than individuals acting in their own self-interest. It is just at this level that the conceptual arguments against the broader account of autonomy falter. In the abstract, all individuals value life and want to preserve it. But that account ceases to be accurate in the extreme circumstances in which these life or death choices are made. Treatment, even free treatment, is often refused because the patient finds it worse to go on than to stop. In individual cases, no vast philosophical contradiction precludes the judgment that my life is better over sooner rather than later, even if active steps must be taken to end it. So long as local knowledge is better than global knowledge, the preferred account of autonomy should encompass all aspects of self-control. The once-universal prohibition against taking one's own life should yield to the necessities of the individual case.

EXTERNALITIES

The analysis thus far has treated individual choice as the touchstone for thinking about death and dying. The effects of euthanasia, however, are not confined solely to the patient. They also touch family and friends and the larger web of social interactions. If euthanasia benefits the patient, do potentially grave losses to these outside parties justify a prohibition on the practice? Two baselines for evaluation should guide the analysis. The first is the normal presumption against a finding of negative externalities in the absence of force, fraud, or monopolistic practices. The second is that the weight attached to externalities for active euthanasia should parallel their weight in cases of deliberate refusal to accept treatment in cases of certain death. These two starting points are headed toward the same conclusion.

As noted earlier, any reckoning of the overall externalities of a social practice must incorporate both positive and negative third-party effects. The chief effects on third-party strangers are emotional and symbolic. Will people decide to follow the example of those who have practiced active euthanasia? But in and of itself that observation tells nothing. If the act done by one person was a good thing, as I have argued it can be, its imitation by others is a good thing as well. The external effects are then positive and hardly a reason for a ban. People, of course, can argue against the practice on the strength of their religious and moral beliefs, but they run the risk that the arguments made in the opposite direction will prove more persuasive. Either way, the fuller discussion over these matters has to count as a good, regardless of which way the debate turns out. We would never regard the sentiments of third parties, positive or negative, as a reason to alter our current views with respect to the right to refuse treatment. We should follow the same course of action here.

A more pressing concern is the effect of any decision on immediate family and friends. In most cases, the individual motivations to seek active euthanasia are likely to be multiple. Some family members might wish for the quick death of a close relative for good reasons or ill, but they are frequently bound by obvious social conventions from stating their true wishes. Nonetheless, sooner or later, the death of a loved one removes a heavy burden measured in time, emotional commitment, and uncertainty. Death serves as a form of liberation that allows family and friends to return to the ordinary rhythm of life after an appropriate period of mourning. The tragedy lay in the original illness, not in death, nor in any considered decision to shorten life. In any event, the toleration of the patient's decision should be well-nigh complete. No third person can override any personal decision to stop treatment or to refuse nutrition and hydration. Yet it is manifest that these decisions have a profound impact on the lives of friends and family members. Why take a different approach here? The dominant interest is the one to decide, and that interest belongs to the patient.

With so much said, what is gained by championing a slow death through starvation instead of a quick and painless death by injection? For the patient, the death could well be painful, especially if conscious. For the family, the death is the increased psychological torment of witnessing avoidable pain and developing a sense of guilt that keeps its hold after death. These psychological sentiments may be compounded by the crushing financial burdens of the final illness. The simple truth is that passive behavior in end-state situations often leaves *everyone* worse off than does the alternative of active euthanasia. Does any ethical theory require widespread suffering for an abstract principle that itself has no conscience and bears no pain?

CHAPTER 14

Physician-Assisted Suicide

AUTONOMY, CONSENT, AND RATIONAL CHOICE

Chapter 13 defended the modest, but controversial proposition that the right of self-determination carries with it the right of an individual to end his or her own life by active means if necessary. From that initial premise, the case for assisted suicide might be thought of as an obvious corollary to the central proposition. Whenever a person is entitled to perform some particular act, the normal rules of agency allow him to hire someone else to do that act for him. Nonetheless many determined opponents of active euthanasia try to undermine that proposition with a second-level argument, namely, that individual autonomy does not carry with it the power to give consent to harms inflicted by others. The point is critical because it insists on a sharp disjunction between individual and cooperative conduct toward that same end. Just this form of argument is advanced by the noted ethicist Daniel Callahan who writes:

> It is, first, a mistake to classify active euthanasia and assisted suicide as acts, solely expressive of individual autonomy, as is now common. On the contrary, because they entail the assistance of another (someone who will kill us in the case of active euthanasia or help us kill ourselves in a case of assisted suicide), they are essentially a form of concerted communal action, even though the community in question may only be two people. That ceases to make them individual acts; they become a form of social action. Second, we have never allowed

killing as a form of contractual relationship between two consenting adults. The killing of another is now justified only in
cases of self-defense, capital punishment, and just war. In none
of those cases is the killing for the benefit of the person killed,
but allowed only to protect the lives and welfare of others,
even if that life is our own (as in self-defense).... Third, even
if I could make a case that I have a right to self-determination
even unto death, it does not follow that my right to kill myself
can be transformed into the right of someone else to kill me.
What is the basis of his right to do so? My authorization? But
what right have I to authorize another to kill?[1]

Callahan is surely correct to observe the leap from autonomy to
consent, and to observe that traditionally consent has never succeeded as
a defense to murder in ordinary cases. To evaluate his argument, therefore, we must first understand the strengths and limits of the criminal
prohibition on murder with consent. The question here surely raises
something of an intellectual puzzle, given the centrality of consent elsewhere in the organization of human affairs.

Consent is normally respected in cases of bodily contact and bodily injury, where it serves much the same office as does a promise to buy
and sell services and goods. The manifestation of consent is the strongest
evidence that the transaction in question is for the benefit of the party
who has consented. It is for precisely this reason that consent is considered so critical within the medical context for everything from routine
physical examinations to major invasive surgery. Where all parties to a
transaction consent to participate in it, the outcome should be a positive
and not a negative sum game—a conclusion that holds as much with
health care as anything else. Why incur the costs of entering a transaction
without the prospects of gain? In virtually every setting, the law goes to
great lengths to protect consent from being undermined by duress, fraud,
incompetence, and undue influence. Therefore, the respect accorded
consent depends heavily on the alignment of individual interests with
social welfare. But why then should the law refuse to recognize consent
as a defense in murder cases? And if consent is irrelevant in ordinary
murder cases, why then any putative exception for active euthanasia?

To begin the analysis, note that the law has traditionally explained
the importance of consent in individual cases in two distinct ways:
observation in the individual case, and inference from background

knowledge about general patterns and motivations of human behavior. Observation, the first method of analysis, involves an inquiry into the subjective state of the individual in question, often by observing overt behavior, to see whether some sign of consent has been given. Where consent has been manifested, we can then conclude, even if we do not quite know why, that from an ex ante perspective the transaction offered the consenting person a net gain. Thereafter, in our descriptive capacity, we could try to identify the costs and benefits of the observed transaction for the actor. Thereafter we can use this information to explain why it was in fact rational for that person to consent, in light of our background knowledge of the economic and psychological mainsprings of human conduct. But even if we cannot understand the reasons for which consent was given in any particular context, our limited knowledge does not count as a reason to vitiate the transaction. Individual actors have better knowledge of their own preferences and may also have gained from experience the wisdom to make decisions that outsiders cannot understand. Manifest behavior thus trumps the rational reconstruction of motives.

Inference, the second method of analysis, starts from the opposite pole: with the global knowledge, first, of the impulse to act from self-interest, and second, from the common understanding that certain outcomes are, or are not, in the interest of these individual actors. If these stylized facts are established with sufficient power, our prior evaluation of the anticipated outcome may be used to falsify a claim that consent has been given in the individual case. The background evaluation could be used to deny the fact of consent at all, or to infer the additional fact that the consent was not freely given, but rather was a product of duress, fraud, or incompetence. Either way, the rational model is used to discredit the claim that consent was freely given in the individual case. Taken to the limit, these general facts could establish that it is *never* in the interests of a rational being to accept a certain state of affairs. Arguments of this sort are found, for example, in Hobbes's observation that no individual could sacrifice his rights of self-defense,[2] or in Locke's view that rational people never would yield to the state the power to deprive them of their "lives, liberties, and estates," which collectively count as their property.[3] In political theory, the rational reconstruction of consent has to do all the heavy intellectual work because no observed transactions can be found in some state of nature to provide individuated evidence that cuts the other way. But even if that evidence were proffered, it would, and should, count for naught if the background conditions were known for certain. Once the probability that consent was not given is one, then we should refuse to credit any individualized offer of proof of consent in the particular case. Just because we cannot figure out exactly where this transaction went off the rails does not mean that the transaction did not go astray. Who would credit the rationality of a sale to a stranger for $1,000 of a beachfront estate worth $1 million? As the older common law judges were prepared to say, the inadequacy of the consideration was conclusive evidence of undue influence or want of capacity.[4]

These two approaches are in constant tension with each other. One starts from our belief in individual self-knowledge and the capacity to achieve them. The other starts from the view that we can detect sufficient regularities in human behaviors to be confident that any gross deviation from the social norm suggests the undetected operation of fraud, incompetence, or undue influence. Given these warring tendencies, the problem in form is identical to the usual Bayesian inquiry that asks of a finder of fact to integrate background information with individual evidence.[5] If the background evidence is certain, the individual evidence should always be disregarded. It is just that level of certitude that led Hobbes to disregard any individual signs of consent in cases of slavery and self-defense. There can never be consent to outcomes that are manifestly against the supreme interest in self-preservation.

In contrast, where there are no prior judgments about the rationality of consent, observation takes a far greater role, as is the case with ordinary commodities in a marketplace. There our background estimations tell us that different people like different things and are willing to attach different values to them. The market, conceived as a system of voluntary exchanges, offers the best way to match individuals with their preferred goods, such that any background assumptions about the choices of rational beings slip into deserved obscurity as a predictor of consumer choices in individual cases. No one thinks that all consumers with $100 should walk out of the supermarket with the same basket of goods. But in situations where the background estimates are certain, as on matters quite literally of life and death, the grander philosophical insight displaces the individualized inquiry. No one can capture the uses and ambiguities of consent by ignoring either of these two polar opposites. Indeed, Hobbes receives the credit for developing *both* concepts of consent, side by side, even though he does not resolve the tension between them.

And tension there is. Thus the full range of intermediate cases are those that have a background presumption of certain strength and some evidence of the individuation of this particular transaction. It is for this reason that many assumption of risk cases in tort are so difficult to resolve on their facts. Thus, in athletic contests, that background norm for liability requires the injured party to prove reckless behavior by the defendant. Ordinary negligence is not enough. Yet in some fraction of these case, some conversations and interactions between the parties suggest that the parties had adopted the more stringent negligence rule. The hard question is whether that individuated evidence displaces the background legal standard.[6] In principle, if we could assign probabilities to both the background rule and the individuated facts, we could apply Bayes's rule and compare the resulting probability with the level of proof required (preponderance of the evidence, beyond a reasonable doubt, and so on) to decide who prevails.[7] In practice, the numbers turn out to be elusive, so the matter is either left to the jury to weigh the two tendencies as best it can. Alternatively, the court may decide, as a matter of law, that the individuated evidence is so strong that it cannot be disregarded or so weak that it cannot be taken into account.

This same tension between observed and inferred consent covers the length and breadth of the law. We could never invoke the image of purely rational beings to tolerate the proposition that all voluntary exchange is theft because we can envision countless circumstances where exchange is for mutual benefit. So we individuate the transactions, with no background norm to guide us. Likewise, as regards sexual relations, the dispute between the radical feminists ("all heterosexual sex is rape" is the crudest form of the proposition) and the traditional law of rape also depends on the strength of the social priors about consent in individual cases. In some presumed world where coercion is everywhere and sexual relations are never in the interest of women, true consent would be impossible and all sex thus becomes rape. The background norm would dominate the idle presentation of evidence about the individual case. It is precisely because most people, both male and female, can see the joint pleasure from most sexual activity that the law has never adopted that extreme position. Now consent must be battled out in individual cases, without setting some automatic presumption against its appearance, and with all the attendant evidentiary and procedural uncertainties found in the hard assumption of risk cases. No matter which way a rebuttable presumption is set, no matter what testimony is credited or not, when the dust settles, we can be sure to find cases where the loser cannot be reconciled to the outcome. All systems of proof have to allow for some degree of error in both directions.

The background norms of rational behavior, however, assume a far stronger role within this framework when the question is whether killing another individual is so contrary to that person's self-interest that the per se bar should be maintained in the face of individuated evidence on consent that cuts the other way. Clearly, this categorical approach sets out the correct rule in many cases: if a person of normal health and disposition were deliberately killed by another person, the background judgments are so strong that individuated evidence would be excluded. We do not believe the scenario in which that deal makes sense to the deceased individual. The Hobbesian norm of self-preservation rings true in the broad run of cases. But not in all cases. The background position can no longer be that consent is impossible to have; rather it is that consent is so unlikely that to introduce evidence in individual cases produces more error than ignoring that evidence altogether.[8] This rule seems perfectly sensible given the massive amount of feigned or improperly procured evidence that could be presented, especially when the decedent is no longer around to explain his side. However, there are limits to this approach. The standard presumption should not be made in the same fashion for individuals hurt in boxing contests, which are often heavily regulated by the state. In these cases, the prospects of fame and fortune could explain why someone takes the risk of death.[9]

When the focus is solely on the subset of cases involved with end-of-life conditions, the background conditions change, and so too our prior estimates of rationality. In situations of constant misery, pain, disorientation, incontinence, nausea, mood shifts, and exhaustion, why should we keep to the priors that are adopted for persons who are in the pink of health? Sometimes it is asserted that the medical powers of palliation are such that it becomes safe to ignore this grim scenario: painkillers and counseling can do the job. But much evidence suggests that the final stages of life are not free of serious pain and discomfort.[10] In this context, taking one's own life begins to make sense, and so too having someone else help with it or even do it. From the subjective point of view, the release of pain could offer a sufficient gain for individuals who prefer death to life. Precisely that outcome happens when patients refuse to accept treatment or support, and that is why physicians who stop treatment are not guilty of some criminal omission that could result in their punishment: the maxim "preserve life" is not transformed into an instrument of torture. If we get beyond sheer assertions of what the law will and will not allow, the ultimate question is whether a rational agent could prefer death to life: anyone who reads the medical description of terminal cases knows to the marrow of his or her being that life may not be worth living, which is why the refusal of further treatment and life support makes sense.

One prop of Callahan's argument, therefore, cannot be sustained: the prohibition on all killings in the criminal law should not be retained in the context of terminal illnesses. But it is one thing to reject a categorical position, and quite another to develop an alternative position. Thus the next question on the agenda asks just how much pain and despair are needed to justify active euthanasia in an individual case. That question is one of degree. Its uniqueness and subjectivity cries out for individual choice and thus precludes collective power in the absence of independent evidence of physician or family abuse in hastening or securing death. The matter of timing is best taken explicitly into account by the person whose life hangs in the balance, and no amount of second-guessing is conducive to good decision making or to anyone's peace of mind.

The other props quickly fall as well. Thus it makes little difference here that the acts in question involve the cooperation of two individuals instead of the isolated actions of a single individual, or that the patient has authorized someone else to do something for him that he is unable to do for himself. A criminal conspiracy normally requires an unlawful means or an unlawful end. Neither is present here. Accordingly the "concerted communal action" that Callahan condemns is no more suspect than a routine joint decision to suspend treatment or terminate life support.

To see why, refer again to the earlier analysis of the logic of voluntary exchange and the possible reasons for prohibiting these exchanges. Cooperation allows two or more persons to reach their individual goals at a lower cost than either would have to pay if acting separately. Once we have recognized that it may be rational for some individuals to seek death in extreme circumstances, why shouldn't they be allowed to do so at the lowest cost to themselves, by whatever means they see fit, and at whatever time they regard as appropriate? Individuals are allowed to perform surgery on themselves, but they are not very good at it, so even trained surgeons prefer to be operated on by someone else. The gains from trade work no matter what ends the contracting parties have in view. Agreements should be restrained only where they seek to obtain an *illegitimate* end, such as the death of a third party, where the low-cost cooperative solution leads to higher levels of *impermissible* actions. But where the ends are legitimate, the answer to the autonomy question provides the answer to the authorization question as well. "But what right do I have to authorize another to kill?" was Callahan's question. The answer is: my self-ownership, when it is authorization to kill *me*.

PHYSICIAN-ASSISTED SUICIDE

A second line of attack on euthanasia and assisted suicide is physician-specific. Leon Kass notes that the issue of euthanasia raises two distinct questions.[11] The first is whether the patient is allowed to take his own life or to ask someone else for assistance. The second is whether it is consistent with their ethical obligations for *physicians* to provide the service in question. On that last issue, Kass insists that the very meaning of what it is to be a physician is, again, to preserve life, so that even if euthanasia were legalized, no physician should participate in the practice. It should, I hope, be evident that any claim of physician autonomy does not preclude those who agree with Dr. Kass to refuse to participate in active euthanasia. A physician should be under no duty to perform euthanasia; nor should public institutions condition physician advancement or hospital privilege on the willingness to participate in practices that they find morally repugnant.

Kass's claim, however, goes beyond protecting reluctant physicians from conscription in an unworthy cause. Rather, his argument explicitly rejects the proposition that the doctor-patient relationship rests ultimately on *contract*, where the physician turns his art to the benefit of the patient as the patient then sees it. Instead the doctor-patient relationship contains within it certain immanent principles and standards of conduct for ethically proper conduct: one of which is the prohibition that the physician should not kill patients—period. His approach thus has a strong Aristotelian feel about it. Physicians must serve certain prescribed ends independent of their own will. To deviate from those ends in the service of a patient is to violate the defining norms of the profession, even with patient consent.

As with all theories postulating a higher good, the source of the external norm is difficult to locate. In most cases, patients go to physicians for health and for cure. Thus the injunction to preserve life is driven powerfully by patient demand. But why should the norm survive when it is flatly inconsistent with the wishes of the patient? Kass himself does not believe that the imperative to preserve life is so powerful as to override the refusal of a competent patient to receive medical care. Why then does that norm become so powerful when assisted suicide or active euthanasia is on the table? One critical element of the doctor-patient relationship is that of trust, and personal trust can arise only where there is confidence that the physician will do the patient's bidding. If Kass's norm were universally imposed on all physicians, how could the bond of trust be maintained? It would surely be a manifest betrayal of trust secretly to provide treatment that a patient has explicitly rejected. Is a relationship of trust advanced or thwarted if a patient cannot be sure that her physician will honor her requests on matters of greatest moment to her?

There is no conceptual warrant to smuggle an account of ethical duties into the definition of a physician. A physician is someone who is learned and skilled in the techniques of medicine, someone who understands the origins of disease and the causes and consequences of various actions on the human body. Treatment is the end of medicine, not by fiat, but because most individuals who consult a physician desire it. The ethical obligations of that office are not inherent in the role or defined independently of the desires of the parties to the relationship. They are chosen in view of the ends that this knowledge serves. A physician who uses his skills to murder is a murderer, no matter what the norms of the profession. But if, as the Dutch experience suggests, patients who desire euthanasia also want a doctor's assistance, their wishes should not be denied for definitional reasons alone.

In sum, then, the legal relationship between patient and physician should be determined by agreement and not by law. Kass may well be able to persuade some doctors and patients that their views on euthanasia and assisted suicide are seriously misguided., but those who are unpersuaded by his arguments should be allowed to practice voluntary euthanasia and assisted suicide. The autonomy principle not only protects patients in their choices; it also protects them in their relationships with third parties, physicians included.

PARADOXES OF TIME AND MANNER

A third and more empirical strand to the debate over assisted suicide, stated in its most general form, asks what we can learn about the practice of assisted suicide from the behavior that we have observed thus far to date. As a theoretical matter, most of the information revolves around the activities of a single physician, the defrocked Jack Kevorkian. Much of the opposition to the practice rests on the assumption that legalization of the practice will result in the repetition of the spectacle of watching his well-publicized 46 cases of assisted suicide from June 1990 and November 1996.

In looking at his record, it is easy to discover ample reason for ambivalence if not outright distaste. Kevorkian's first case took place on June 4, 1990, when he helped Janet Adkins, a 54-year-old woman, commit suicide. She was in the early stages of Alzheimer's disease but was still fit enough to play tennis. She committed suicide with the aid of Kevorkian's crude contraption, which connected her to three bottles on a simple rack. One bottle contained a harmless solution of saline; the second contained thiopental, which was used to make the patient unconscious; the third was a combination of potassium chloride and succinylcholine, which together cause the heart to stop beating. Putting the line into place immediately delivers the saline solution. The thiopental can then be activated by pressing a button, and the combination of potassium chloride and succinylcholine is activated shortly thereafter by a timer. In assisting Ms. Adkins, Dr. Kevorkian had difficulty connecting his machine to her veins, but he persevered and on his fifth attempt was successful. The murder charges against Kevorkian were dismissed in December 1990 because Adkins had activated the button by herself.[12] In later cases, Kevorkian switched his methods, preferring to aid his patients with lethal doses of carbon monoxide. The activities in question resulted in three trials on five counts of assisted suicide, the last two under the Michigan statute passed to deal with his behavior,[13] which was sustained against various constitutional challenges by the Michigan Supreme Court.[14]

My purpose is not to labor the details of the individual trials, but rather to understand the context in which Dr. Kevorkian operates. The Kevorkian saga arises only where euthanasia is illegal *and* some form of assisting, or advising on, suicide is not. The stubborn question of first principle, however, is whether *either* euthanasia or assisted suicide should be illegal? It is surely a black mark against the legalization of euthanasia and assisted suicide that so many people are willing to take their own lives when they still have time to enjoy life's pleasures. One common understanding of this pattern hearkens back to the earlier theme of the irrationality of any decision to practice either euthanasia or assisted suicide: no rational being would choose to die earlier.

Once again, however, the introduction of regulation distorts the choices in question. How would Janet Adkins have responded in June 1990 when she learned that she had Alzheimer's disease (a) knowing that euthanasia was illegal and (b) dreading that she might hang on for years under the grip of that terrible disease? She herself is reported to have understood the point: "if she was going to err she'd rather err on the side of going too soon than going too late."[15] Making voluntary euthanasia illegal necessarily rules out any forward contract whereby she instructs Dr. Kevorkian or anyone else to kill her after her condition has deteriorated beyond a certain point, when she would no longer be able to take her own life, but remains deeply resentful of that fact. Nor could she develop objective standards to guide her physician because he would not be free to abide by her instructions. Still trapped, she could not delegate that decision to any committee, when all of whose members could be charged with a conspiracy to commit murder just for participating in its deliberations.

The upshot is that her domain of choice was restricted by the criminal prohibitions: as the ideal time was precluded, she was left with the unhappy choice of acting too soon or waiting until she could not act at all—when no one else could help her. At this point, her rational calculation forced a comparison of these two imperfect alternatives. Although we can identify the imponderables of both horns of her dilemma, we cannot resolve them in principle. Some people in Adkins's position would decide, like her, that too soon is better than too late, and it is just these few people who choose to sign up with Kevorkian, the only (ex)physician whose personal convictions are strong enough to withstand the blizzard of criticism and prosecution hurled against him.

If the ban on active euthanasia were eliminated, the de facto monopoly of Dr. Kevorkian would be eliminated. Individual patients could still turn to Dr. Kevorkian for help, but more likely they would find some other physician who could help them. Either way, they could terminate their lives at some *later* date consistent with their clearly expressed prior wishes, now that the scope of their legal power over their own lives was no longer ambiguous. The changes in legal rules and market behavior would remove the ghoulish character of the Kevorkian adventure. The phenomenon here is not unique to the area of health law. The prohibition on long-term contracts does not necessarily block the prohibited activity; it could result in arrangements that call for immediate performance. For the afflicted persons, these unhappy compromises are better than going without any assistance, even if they are worse than the arrangements they could craft for themselves in an unregulated market.

This point is capable of some generalization. In his recent treatment of assisted suicide, Judge Posner offers the suggestion that the legalization of assisted suicide would result in fewer and later suicides.[16] His basic argument is that the prohibition against assisted suicide generates a set of unintended consequences when people seek to reduce its impact. So long as individuals can wait before committing themselves to assisted suicide, they will postpone any irreversible decision. Other people will feel less compelled to end their lives by violent means, knowing that they can turn to medical assistance later on. As events unfold, however, recourse to assisted suicide may turn out to be unnecessary, thereby reducing the total level of suicides in question and postponing those that remain.

This empirical point can, of course, be debated because the prohibition on assisted suicide has consequences on physicians and institutions as well as on patients. Even if few criminal prosecutions are undertaken, the isolation that the law imposes on physicians could easily curtail the opportunities for assisted suicide across the board. It is commonplace for physicians to allege that the law has prevented them from assisting in suicides even if the risk of prosecution is slight.[17] When all is said and done, Jack Kevorkian is one of a kind.

It would be a mistake to assume that the case for legalizing assisted suicide depends on this asserted paradoxical effect on overall suicide rates. Even if the rates of suicide go up, the outcome should be welcome if it reduces thereby the needless amounts of suffering that otherwise would attend the end of life. Right now, patients who want to end their own lives face sharp limitations on where and how assisted suicide can be performed. It is ghoulish to watch people running off to remote locations to trigger primitive contraptions that result in their own death. Indeed, the Dutch experience with euthanasia, on which more is said in Chapter 15, strongly suggests that a majority of the people who seek euthanasia want their doctors to perform it even if they are physically able to act themselves.[18] It seems as though the idea of willful self-destruction is easier to accept when the physical deed is performed by another. Yet that alternative is effectively precluded by laws against assisted suicide, which inhibit most physicians, health care providers, and hospitals from engaging in voluntary euthanasia as well as assisted suicide. Even if the law does not prosecute practitioners of assisted suicide, it places the practice on the margins of respectable social conduct and thus makes the last days of suffering more isolated than they need be. Undoing the illegality of euthanasia and assisted suicide takes the process out of the closet and brings it forward into the light of day. Once that is done, assisted suicide could be performed in friendlier and more compassionate settings, and the stigma of breaking the law would be removed from those who embrace it. A welcome change in social practice could, and should, go hand in hand with a welcome change in social perception.

CHAPTER 15
❖ ❖ ❖
Abuse and Overreaching

TWO KINDS OF ERROR

The domain of social issues contains few necessary truths. Neither voluntary euthanasia nor assisted suicide forms an exception to this rule. It may well be, therefore, that both of these practices should remain illegal, but if so, it is not because of the conceptual arguments that were considered and rejected in the last two chapters. Quite the contrary, a successful defense of the traditional position must rest on a different set of considerations that until now I have addressed only obliquely. These can be grouped together under the heading of abuse and overreaching.

The basic concern is easily stated. Sick people are vulnerable people. They are faced with the most gut-wrenching choices of their life just when they lack the strength of will and clearness of mind needed to make them. To allow voluntary euthanasia is to pave the way for greedy people to pressure their elderly relatives to a quick and convenient death. It is to invite harried and burnt-out physicians to kill their patients instead of caring for them. And it is to subject the weakest and least educated portions of the population to manipulation by institutional players capable of dominating their lives. Arguments such as these proved persuasive to the 24-member New York Task Force convened by then Governor Cuomo to review the legal status of both voluntary euthanasia and assisted suicide.[1] They have carried weight with the American Medical Association, which has repeatedly affirmed its opposition with physician-assisted suicide, and to medical associations overseas.[2] They have been reiterated countless times in the press[3] and other scholarly articles as well.[4] The risk of abuse has also been listed as one of the major reasons why voters in Washington (1991) and California (1992) have rejected measures that would allow assisted suicide even under closely regulated conditions.[5]

This theme of abuse never moves far from center stage. As befits its generality, it has a long legal pedigree. Even an ordinary consumer sale is not immune to the charge that the seller used some sharp practice to take advantage of an uninformed buyer. Those fears quickly multiply when an elderly widow, inexperienced in trade, sells her large country estate to an attentive young man for a fraction of its market value. In both cases, a court could minutely examine the facts of each transaction for particular evidence of fraud, concealment, or undue influence. In all cases, the nagging concern is that the skilled malefactor will cover his tracks and thus escape the condemnation he so richly deserves. A broad rule that bans these types of transactions has the evident virtue of controlling these abuses, but that cure in turn may suffer from the greater risk of overbreadth. What sense does it make to prohibit thousands of legitimate consumer sales in order to block one fraudulent transaction? As the background rate of fraud and abuse increases, the error costs of invoking an overbroad rule correspondingly decline. The law, therefore, seeks out settings where general folk wisdom, or, less commonly, empirical research, suggests that the rate of abuse could be high. It might, therefore, be appropriate to regulate the widow's sale of the large estate but not the consumer sale by Sears. Preventing the widow from selling altogether strikes too deeply, so the receipt of advice from an independent lawyer is usually sufficient to rebut any charge of undue influence. However, that rule in turn imposes additional costs on widows capable of transacting for themselves. Thus the hard and fast rule could be reduced to a presumption rebuttable on a showing of her individual competence after the fact, an inquiry that both injects uncertainty and adds administrative costs of its own.

This cycle of proposing and refining remedies for abuse never reaches closure. All sound legal regimes depend on the estimation of the costs of two different types of error. One type blocks voluntary exchanges that should be respected; the other type tolerates tainted exchanges that should be blocked. It is not possible to eliminate both kinds of error simultaneously. Only by pouring more resources into monitoring is it possible to reduce the combined incidence of error, at the cost of diverting resources that otherwise would be available for other activities. The proper social inquiry asks first what level of resources should be committed to controlling abuse. It then asks how much error of each type should be tolerated when combatting one kind of error increases the risk of the other, perhaps to an even greater extent. Greater risks of abuse and overreaching need more resources to combat them, and when the risks become sufficiently large, it is unlikely that the arsenal of available remedies will be confined to case-by-case relief after the transaction is concluded. The new administrative remedies must kick in ex ante, before any transaction takes place at all.

Getting the right mix of remedies is a matter of continuous adjustments and successive approximations. In so fluid a situation, the first step is to set the initial presumption. In general, that presumption should be set against the use of remedies before the fact. Why incur the cost of ex ante remedies when ex post remedies are still held in reserve for the bad cases that do occur? It is risky to ban pornography on the ground that it could cause violence. The violence itself can and should be subject to criminal and civil sanctions. Similarly, when ex ante remedies are required, those of limited focus should presumptively be preferred to a comprehensive ban. Bans should be reserved as a last resort and only for extreme cases. It is better to allow a "cooling-off" period for door-to-door sales or for home mortgages than to ban them entirely. However, even these limited requirements could prove to be excessive and unnecessary. My mortgage broker reports that she has never had a customer who has canceled a loan within the cooling-off period. All that paper work and delay for nothing!

This general approach easily carries over to the risk of abuse and overreaching with voluntary euthanasia and assisted suicide. A high enough level of abuse and overreaching could, in principle, justify a complete ban, given that the cost of abuse is essentially premature death. Broadly conceived, this argument for maintaining the ban of active euthanasia and assisted suicide now rests on a pessimistic evaluation of the motivations and capabilities of the dramatis personae to the typical end-of-life play. It asserts, often passionately, that abuse and overreaching occur so frequently that the entire apparatus of euthanasia must be shut down to curb them. Ironically the argument from abuse concedes precisely what the philosophical objections to euthanasia deny, namely, that people may legitimately choose to take their own lives. Shifting the debate from entitlement to enforcement highlights the preoccupation with a high stakes illustration of the two conventional kinds of error—keeping people alive who want to die, and killing those who want to live. The case for the ban uses the basic tenet of self-preservation to assign greater weight to errors of hasty death. It then claims that the error costs of allowing the voluntary euthanasia and assisted suicide exceed those of banning it, *even if* the practice itself, properly conducted, were morally unquestionable. Intermediate restrictions are similarly eschewed as offering inadequate protection against the greater peril. This chapter examines this argument at the empirical level. Chapter 16 picks up the constitutional threads.

AMERICAN ANECDOTES AND THE DUTCH EXPERIENCE

The conceptual framework just set out does not dictate the selection of remedies against admitted wrongs. It provides no information about the frequency and severity of abuse or about the types of countermeasures that might be arrayed against them. At most it only indicates the kinds of information that must be collected and evaluated before some provisional judgment is made. Frequently that evidence is notoriously difficult to collect. That is especially true in situations like voluntary euthanasia and assisted suicide where the practices have been made illegal for so many years. To be sure, both euthanasia and assisted suicide are practiced covertly and are rarely if ever prosecuted. But one of the collateral effects of the legal ban is to make it more difficult to collect evidence as to the frequency and propriety of the practice. Even if that evidence could be collected, how should it be interpreted when the disputed conduct, as with Jack Kevorkian, is heavily influenced by the threat of criminal prosecution. The mix of patients and physicians is hardly randomly chosen; it would be transformed by hospitable changes in the legal environment.

One way to overcome this dearth of evidence is to resort to anecdotes that verge on fiction. Just that was done in 1988 when *JAMA* published "It's Over, Debbie,"[6] an anonymous (and perhaps fabricated) account of a mercy killing administered by a gynecology resident to a 20-year-old woman suffering the final stages ovarian cancer. The account reads like a fast-paced detective novel, so that it is hard to unpack what actually happened.[7] But it appears that the physician-protagonist had no prior knowledge or even acquaintance with the patient; that he made the decision to kill on the spur of the moment, but in the presence and with the tacit complicity of both the nurse and a friend of the patient; that it was unclear whether consent was obtained for painkillers or lethal injection; and that the dosage of morphine injected was more than needed for palliation, so that death could not be chalked up as the unwelcome side effect of a medically justified act.

As might be expected, the case sparked both indignant commentary[8] and more nuanced responses.[9] Surely, no one can be blind to the hints of uncontrolled discretion and abuse. Ironically, however, it is the current prohibition on euthanasia that precludes candid discussion and forces the case into a "gray market," which Professor Kenneth Vaux, for one, is willing to tolerate: "I argue that while positive euthanasia must be proscribed in principle, in exceptional cases it may be abided in deed."[10] Unfortunately just this netherworld creates ample opportunity for abuse. It blocks any explicit institutional standards to regulate patient care, and it ensures that the dissemination of information about the practice will be haphazard and unequal, as in other gray markets.

The "Debbie" incident thus highlights the abuse question and raises considerations that resonate more tightly with the public at large than any categorical arguments against euthanasia.[11] So where can we turn for information about how the system of active euthanasia works when the cloud of criminal prosecution is lifted? At present, the only available source of information is the Dutch experience, for the Netherlands is the only place in the civilized world that institutionalizes the practice of euthanasia and assisted suicide. To evaluate the risk of abuse in that setting, it is first necessary to summarize briefly the tangled evolution of the Dutch practice.

No formal statute in the Netherlands makes mercy killing a defense to what otherwise would be a charge of murder. Instead, the current non-prosecution practice was reached by a circuitous route. The Netherlands Penal Code contains provisions that prohibit both killing and assisting suicide, even with the consent of the victim. Article 293 reads "He who robs another of life at his express and serious wish is punished with a prison sentence of at most twelve years or a fine of the fifth category" (100,000 guilders, around $50,000). Article 294 on assisted suicide reads: "He who deliberately incites another to suicide, assists him therein or provides him with the means, is punished, if the suicide follows, with a

prison sentence of at most three years or a fine of the fourth category"
(25,000 guilders, or around $12,500).

Neither provision contains any explicit exception for euthanasia or
assisted suicide. Enforced as written, Dutch law prohibits both forms of
conduct. Dutch practice, however, gives prosecuting attorneys in each
district the discretion not to press charges. Dutch judges can read
implied exceptions into blanket statutory injunctions, and the Royal
Dutch Society for the Promotion of Medicine has been able to influence
the interpretation of the law at the behest of its members.

These institutional ingredients proved crucial to the evolution of
Dutch legal position.[12] The saga began in 1973, with a case from the
District of Leeuwarden involving euthanasia that a doctor performed by
injection on his 78-year-old mother. She was incontinent and confined
to a wheelchair with other unstated disabilities and diseases. She had frequently repeated her desire to die and to be killed, if necessary.[13] The
Court did not deny that the state's case fell squarely within the criminal
prohibition, but it fudged the remedy by imposing on the accused physician a one-week sentence, suspended for one year, subject to the understanding that no time would ever be served if the physician remained on
good behavior in the interim.

The case was unique because the defendant was both the physician
and the son of the deceased and the suspended sentence did not amount
to a declaration of legality of the underlying act. Rather, the court simply created an ad hoc exception to a criminal statute that left key questions unanswered. Did the exception only apply to physician-children or
to all physicians? Was the suspended sentence available only in this case
or more generally? The Court thus created its own legal limbo: acts that
were neither legal nor punishable.

Matters remained more or less unchanged for the next eight years,
but the practice was clarified in a case from the Rotterdam District in
1981. On that occasion, the *conviction* of a lay person for assisting in suicide became the vehicle for explaining and expanding the scope of physician protection from prosecution.[14] Thus the Court stressed a long list of
familiar factors: unbearable suffering; conscious desire to die; a voluntary request; time to consider alternatives; the want of any alternative
solution; care to avoid unnecessary suffering to others; decision making
by more than one person; great care throughout the procedure; *and*
actual performance of euthanasia by a physician only. The decision was

painted in broad strokes without any definitional provisions or administrative guidelines, and it left open the question of what body, public or private, should enforce its remaining legal restrictions.

In this uncertain setting, the Dutch prosecutor's office insisted on an administrative review of each reported case of euthanasia, as an obvious check on private abuse. Its administrative response was critical, for although the Dutch courts might not punish, the state's attorney could still prosecute cases of assisted suicide or killing, even with patient consent. No physician wants to be acquitted after the expense and adverse publicity of an extended public investigation and trial.

Events started to move more quickly. In short order, in 1982, yet another case from the district court in Alkmaar worked its way to the Supreme Court in The Hague. The case involved a 95-year-old woman in failing health who had undergone several harrowing episodes and who asked to be euthanized. No particular fatal disease was specified. Two lower courts had insisted on the "material illegality of euthanasia," but the Supreme Court in review held that the lower courts had not looked at the matter from all points of view. It then asked the Court of Appeals in The Hague to decide "from an objective medical perspective, whether the practice of euthanasia could be regarded as one justified by a situation of necessity (beyond one's control)."[15]

On remand, the prosecutor then asked the Royal Dutch Medical Society for its opinion on the practice. The Society responded that active euthanasia had to be evaluated from the point of view of a physician whose back is to the wall. It concluded that the doctrine of force majeure or legal necessity allowed the physician to honor a patient's request for assistance in dying during a last illness. The Society's stated position should raise more than one legal eyebrow. The defense of necessity is properly invoked only when a person takes property from another innocent individual in order to escape the imminent threat of death *to him* by external forces, such as starvation or thirst.[16] These physicians are not subject to that form of risk even if their patients are desperately ill. It will hardly do to stretch the concept of necessity to include psychological compulsion on the physician, as did a 1988 Dutch decision[17] because then all medical decisions are made under conditions of necessity. A narrow defense is thus transformed into a universal state of affairs.

Necessity in this context is best understood as a pretense for a *justification* of the social practice that, by focusing solely on the plight of the physician, neatly sidesteps all the pros and cons of the basic debate. But once the Dutch placed euthanasia into its distinctive legal pigeonhole, necessity quickly disappeared from view when the Royal Society drafted its 1984 guidelines.[18] These guidelines followed familiar lines. Euthanasia should be used only as a last resort when all other alternatives fail. Only physicians could perform euthanasia. A voluntary request is required. The request should be well considered, and the demand for it should be stable and not motivated by depression or family resentment. The request should be documented in writing, if possible. The patient should experience "unacceptable" suffering. Collegial collaboration is required, but review by an independent physician was not. The consult could be with a second treating physician.

The guidelines were silent on two points. They did not mention what techniques of euthanasia were allowed, nor did they instruct on the proper way for filling out the death certificate. On this last point, they hinted that euthanasia need not be entered as the immediate cause of death and furthermore warned that an investigation might be begun "if the doctor does *not* enter a declaration of natural death." These evasive death certificates have remained a matter of critical importance because prosecutorial oversight depends heavily on self-reporting, which in practice often avoids references to euthanasia. Indeed, the legal situation remains unclarified, for in the 12 years since the original decision in Leeuwarden, the text of Articles 293 or 294 have remained unchanged. Efforts to draft exceptions to the basic criminal code to reflect the movement of judicial decisions have gone nowhere, as legislators of all political persuasions seem quite content to leave this hot potato in the lap of the courts.[19] A combination of judicial instruction, prosecutorial deference, Medical Society guidelines, and legislative caution has thus worked, by indirection, a profound and enduring revolution in the Dutch law of euthanasia. By diffusing the responsibility across four major institutions—prosecutors, courts, legislators and physicians—no one need claim full credit or take full blame for the de facto decriminalization of active euthanasia.

But what of the practices that have emerged under this set of incomplete procedures? In a 1987 study, the Dutch government reported about 200 cases of euthanasia each year, which commentators at the time regarded as far too low.[20] The comprehensive survey undertaken by the Committee on the Study of Medical Practice Concerning Euthanasia (the Remmelink Commission) offered more precise figures on the sub-ject.[21] Of the 130,000 persons who died in the Netherlands each year, some 49,000 cases raised the issue of whether to continue or terminate life support, or to increase dosages of morphine to reduce pain. Assisted suicides occurred in some 400 cases. Voluntary euthanasia, defined as "any action that intentionally ends the life of someone else, on the request of that person," took place some 2,300 times, or about 5 percent of the cases of withdrawn treatment. Some 9,000 annual requests for euthanasia suggest that these requests were granted in about one-quar-ter of the cases, hardly death on demand, although others will surely and strongly disagree.[22] The cases where requests were made and granted were the obvious ones: AIDS, cancer, multiple sclerosis, at some advanced stage. In about two-thirds of the cases, life expectancy was under two weeks at the time of the request. In about 10 percent of the cases, life expectancy exceeded three months. These numbers were some-what lower than the extrapolations from earlier studies whose unofficial estimates ran between 5,000 and 12,000 cases per year.[23] They are consis-tent with a high demand for assistance in suicide as well as a high level of abuse, and probably should be read to support the former and not the latter. American data shows much the same story, with AIDS cases hav-ing the highest level of suicide and suicide requests.[24]

Against this background, it is instructive to review the work of Dr. Carlos Gomez, one of the leaders of the anti–assisted suicide movement, on the Dutch experience with an eye to the abuse question. His own judgment, shared by others,[25] is that abuse is extensive and that the Dutch should reimpose the standard prohibition against active euthanasia, just as the United States should retain it. In responding to his criticism, it is important to distinguish between two separate questions. The first is whether the Dutch routinely disregard the formal procedures required in euthanasia cases, chiefly by issuing incorrect death certificates and failing to obtain the mandated review. And, when second opinions are sought, they usually come from preselected physicians who favor the practice and might be disposed to granting the request. The second question is whether abuse took place when these requirements were disregarded, which in turn boils down to: Did the patient voluntarily consent to euthanasia? Or was there familial coercion or physician impatience?

The misdeeds that Gomez recounts are chiefly of the first kind, most notably the failure to report euthanasia as a cause of death. Far from revealing telltale signs of foul play or improper pressure, his cases only reveal a pattern of informal consultation and deliberation, with a minimum of interference by public authorities. Dutch physicians are not euthanasia enthusiasts and they are slow to practice it in individual cases, however much they endorse its possibility as a general philosophical proposition.[26] For example, Dr. Admiraal, a leading proponent of euthanasia, refused "euthanasia to a young woman who was dying from leukemia and whose parents refused to let her [lesbian] lover move in."[27] Physician practice seems to reflect the gravity and irreversibility of the decisions.

Gomez's 26 case histories, with two exceptions match this dominant mood.[28] These cases often involved individuals of advanced age (8 of 26 were over 80; and 7 were between 70 and 79). The three cases in their 30s included two terminal AIDS patients and one patient with advanced ALS (Lou Gehrig's disease). Cancer was involved in about one-third of the cases; 6 had suffered strokes; 4 suffered congestive heart failure; 2 had pneumonia; and 1, age 28, had leukemia. Most patients had received extensive medical care and hospitalization. Where death took place in a hospital, the full record had been reviewed by a terminal care team and a euthanasia committee. Psychiatric care was only ordered when the patient's mental condition was in doubt, but not when the team "knew the patient" and his condition. Consultations with family members were routine when possible; delays of one month or more were taken between the original request and the final action. Frequently the patients had refused further medical care and treatment, and many repeated their requests for euthanasia on numerous occasions. In virtually all cases, euthanasia was listed as a cause of death on the death certificate. Misstating the cause of death is, of course, commonplace in the United States, where the possibility of indictment or prosecution is always in the offing.[29]

With this said, of Gomez's 26 reported cases, only two merit separate comment. In one (Case 20),[30] a 2-day-old infant suffering from Down's syndrome was killed at the insistence of his parents. The child had a stomach blockage that required surgery, and the parents had to care for two other children at home. The consulting ethicist explicitly told the parents that they did not have to approve of the surgery, even though the child was certain to die without it. On any reading, this case is the antithesis of voluntary euthanasia and should have been excluded from this study. The key question is whether the parents have the duty to undertake ordinary surgery to preserve the life of a Down's syndrome child, to which the answer should be, after some misgivings perhaps, an emphatic yes. But, if for some reason, the parents have no duty to keep the child alive, active euthanasia is probably preferable to the slow starvation of a helpless infant.

The second dubious case (Case 22)[31] involved a 56-year-old patient brought into an emergency room with massive internal and brain injuries. The physician in charge decided to inject the patient with fatal drugs before the family could arrive because he wanted to spare them the agony of a lingering death. The difficulties present in this case are also far removed from patient self-determination. It should have been resolved by clear, separate policy that requires the patient to be kept alive so long as the family can be readily consulted before making any final decision. At that point, the terms of the debate shift rapidly if the family demands heroic measures that the physicians regard as futile or worse. But none of those issues is germane to the question of voluntary euthanasia.

The remaining 24 cases in Gomez's sample show systematic departures from the formal guidelines requiring public and independent review.[32] However, that review is not an end in itself because the ultimate question is whether patient self-determination was violated. And no horror stories stand out from either this or other studies. Gomez's own spirited criticism of the practice is largely unsupported by his own data, as some of the Dutch physicians he interviewed pointed out.[33]

All in all, it looks as though euthanasia in Dutch practice operates as its proponents predicted, as the last step in downward cycle when life is no longer worth living. It happens when pain is unbearable, both from the initial disease or from its treatment. It happens when palliation cannot be achieved and when the patient suffers from serious and irreversible medical conditions that impair basic life functions. It comes after all other alternatives are considered and rejected. And, in this environment, why harp on the failure to obtain formal review when the levels of private deliberation and reflection seem sufficient in practice? It hardly seems necessary to insist that patients demonstrate to others that they are overwhelmed by constant and unremitting bouts of illness that leave them fatigued and weary of life.[34] That hurdle is not imposed in cases where further treatment is refused; it should not be imposed here.

Is it so terrible to choose euthanasia because of a deep fear of going on a respirator or other life-support devices?

The difficulty in the Dutch experience does not lie in its outcomes, but in the clumsiness of their formal requirements. Recall that the Royal Medical Society set these requirements not to meet patient demands, but to stave off legal prosecution. The distinction matters. If patients cared about the formalities, we should expect them to be routinely observed. If they do not, we should expect haphazard compliance at best. Indeed, if the guidelines truly mattered, we should expect to find at least one case, and perhaps many cases, where family members protested the killing of a loved one to the prosecutor, the media, or both. But here the record is largely barren of such evidence. The closest that I have seen was reported by Stephen Chapman in the Chicago *Tribune*. "Last year a psychiatrist was acquitted after assisting in the suicide of a physically healthy 50-year-old woman who was distraught over the death of her two sons and collapse of her marriage. He had not even had her see another doctor (much less another psychiatrist) as the guidelines mandate. But the Royal Dutch Medical Society refused to suspend his license."[35] Yet this case did attract a prosecution and a disciplinary hearing, so its distinctive nature was surely recognized. Why then the acquittal and the refusal to sanction? Perhaps the woman was bent on suicide no matter what her physician did. Even if this one incident was botched, it falls so far from the mainstream of cases that it hardly justifies any categorical ban or regulation of active euthanasia. Given the need to balance two kinds of errors, it takes more than a single counterexample to upset an established practice.

What of those people who fear that they will become weak and vulnerable and want to avoid the risk of euthanasia against their will. At first blush, it looks as though they have no place to hide because the formal checks don't work and the informal ones are insufficient. It appears, however, that the Dutch system developed a *private* response, whose importance Gomez underappreciated to protect both individuals who prefer to let nature take its course and physicians who regard the entire practice of euthanasia as a sordid and immoral business. Thus, today, Dutch hospitals and nursing care facilities commonly advertise whether they will practice euthanasia or not. "Even [Dr.] Admiraal [a strong advocate of euthanasia] pointed out to me that some nursing homes now advertise publicly that they do not perform euthanasia, and one of the nursing homes I visited gave me a document that they hand out to the families of newly arrived residents, which declares that the facility does not practice euthanasia."[36]

The importance of this institutional safeguard is that it allows for a *voluntary sorting* of physicians and patients into their desired groups long before they are called on to make any ultimate live-or-die decisions. Physicians who do not want to practice euthanasia can opt out of the institutions that provide it, or, if they choose, enter into contracts that do not oblige them to participate in the process. More important, prospective patients who are opposed to euthanasia can opt into an environment that insulates them from their worst fears, no matter how their terminal illness progresses. The patients who use hospitals and nursing homes that *do* practice euthanasia can then be in an environment that develops internal checks on the practice, which can be improved over the years. The mechanism is cheap to enforce and avoids the pitfalls of collective choice when the law forces all institutions to follow a given path that may be suitable for none.

The sorting mechanism could also help with respect to second-order decisions because, in principle, no single set of rules has to apply to the entire population that is willing to practice euthanasia. Some hospitals require that the patient's request be made when family are not present; others seek the active participation of family members in the process.[37] The former rule can be justified to neutralize family coercion; the latter to prevent lonely and isolated persons from choosing euthanasia prematurely. *Both* sets of rules, operating side by side, may be justified as expanding the role of patient choice, because patients can choose hospitals based on their preference of one set of procedures over another. The richness and variety of private responses should not be regarded as evidence of some deep-seated confusion about the proper setting for hard choices. Rather, it is better understood as an effort to satisfy different segments of the basic population, each with its own distinct set of needs.

Whether this sorting function is sufficient in itself to answer the question of abuse is hard to say. One obvious difficulty is that it does not deal with individuals who are taken to hospitals, perhaps unconscious, for emergency care. Yet here too a private response is possible. In the Netherlands, it has been reported that some people have taken to carrying "passports for life" to make clear their opposition to active euthanasia in any of its forms.[38] Without questions, these cards should be respected by all institutions, like the Do Not Resusicate orders that are routinely requested by the old and infirm. It may also be that these private responses are not quite enough. The Dutch themselves appear to have some second thoughts. They have tightened up their guidelines to require, first, that the treating physician confirm his judgment through an independent opinion and, second, that the patient self-administer the drug whenever possible.[39] The former may be a welcome safeguard, but the latter appears not to be, given that it is unclear which patients can take what actions toward the end of life.

Similarly the American proposals all contemplate an elaborate network of safeguards against precipitate action. A referendum with that objective—Proposition 161 in California, The Death with Dignity Act—garnered 46 percent of the California vote in 1992, but it failed passage largely because of public fears that it lacked sufficient protection against abuse, a subject on which it was far from silent. The bill required that patients make an "enduring request" for assistance in dying,[40] which had to be easily revocable at any time, either orally or in writing.[41] It also allowed physicians to order psychological or psychiatric examinations if they were concerned about the patient's competence to give informed consent;[42] and it further provided that any directive on death "shall be signed by the declarant and witnessed by two adults" who had no familial or financial connection with the patient or his estate, and who are not involved in the medical treatment or operation of any facility in which the patient is located.[43] The proposal, however, was criticized because it did not provide any supervision over the process after the patient had signed the initial consent form.[44]

In November 1994, Oregon voters adopted a more tightly drafted legislation—Measure 16, The Oregon Death with Dignity Act—that allowed competent adults suffering from terminal conditions to request that physicians supply them with medications to hasten death.[45] Under this Act, requests had to be made on two separate occasions: the first time both orally and in writing, and a second time 15 days later, at least orally, subject to the familiar understanding that the authorization could be revoked without question at any time.[46] The original physician is required to make full disclosure to the patient of her condition and prognosis, and of the consequences of taking various forms of treatment.[47] He is authorized to refer cases for counseling if appropriate. The Act only authorizes a prescription and explicitly refuses to allow "a physician or any other person to end a patient's life by lethal injection, mercy killing or active euthanasia."[48] By the same token, it protects actions taken under the Act from being branded as "suicide, assisted suicide, mercy killing or homicide" for any legal purpose.[49] The Act immunizes physicians from liability or professional disciplinary action when their judgments are made in good faith, but does not insulate them from liability for negligence for any other form of professional misconduct.[50] It ensures that various obligations under insurance policies and other contracts are not altered when death occurs as prescribed under the Act.[51] Finally, it requires all the relevant information to be entered into the patient's medical records, a sample of which may be inspected by the health department for the purposes of preparing a statistical report,[52] but no individual files are open to public inspection.

To my unpracticed eyes, this statute seems like an all-too-conscientious attempt to preserve the basic right on the one hand, while combating any risk of abuse on the other. Indeed, to go further, it looks far too restrictive of individual rights of self-determination. At the structural level, it refuses to allow physician injection and thus places a heavy burden on individuals to administer prescriptions when in all probability they would prefer to die in peace. The Dutch experience seems to show that although physicians often want their patients to take charge of their own fates, the majority of patients are reported to prefer active euthanasia over death by drinking some lethal potion.[53] And of the physician-aided deaths, some 85 percent are by euthanasia, whereas only 15 percent are by assisted suicide.[54] (Why force individuals into a choice that they regard as unnatural?) On top of this restrictive right, it also imposes a set of procedural requirements that would be widely rejected as intolerable when treatment is refused or withdrawn. Who could afford to wait 15 days to decide to stop treatment? To sign forms? To undergo psychiatric counseling? To keep official records? So understood, the Oregon Act vastly complicates the process of dying. In all likelihood, few individuals or physicians would want to run the gauntlet that it prescribes.

Opponents, however, have attacked the Oregon Act as far too lenient.[55] Edward Grant and Paul Linton, for example, stress that its good faith provisions on liability and disciplinary proceedings are at variance with the usual standard of reasonable care. Yet the good faith standard is surely dominant in dealing with cases of withdrawn or discontinued treatment, so that the parity of the two cases is effectively preserved. Indeed, the decisions of physicians to assist in suicide have little to do with matters of technique and much to do with questions of judgment, for which the good faith standard is more appropriate.

Grant and Linton also attack the Oregon Act for allowing individuals to make final decisions without first having to consult family and friends. Although the Act allows for that option, it does not compel it (after all, who should be consulted, and when and why?), so the authors fear that elderly people will be reluctant to consult family members who live far away and will thus make their decisions in relative isolation and fear. Grant and Linton also speculate that physicians who are inclined against assisting in suicide will find their resolve weakened once they can no longer point to the illegality of the practice as a reason for refusing aid. But, in this context as well, the abstract identification of these risks is unconvincing without any sense of their frequency and severity. Both types of problems have surely arisen in the context of the withdrawal of treatment, where patients could also be regarded as highly vulnerable, but in practice, neither problem has presented any insurmountable obstacle. It would be helpful to know why they are the source of such acute concerns here. Without some experience, it is not possible to have any confidence on the matter. As a matter of first principle, the argument from abuse in its various manifestations does not appear, as yet and on balance, to be strong enough to justify the ban on either assisted suicide or active euthanasia. The question of abuse may be relative, but not decisive.

CHAPTER 16

Unwelcome Constitutional Complications

CONSTITUTIONAL CACOPHONY

For three chapters, I have struggled with the philosophical and legal issues that surround active euthanasia and assisted suicide. When I wrote the initial drafts of these chapters, I gave little thought to the possibility that the entire issue might become enmeshed in constitutional complications, but times and sentiment have moved more quickly than expected. By mid 1996, it became quite clear that the general maxim of legal practice has carried over to this controversial problem. No matter what the issue, someone, somehow will be able to make a constitutional claim that his position is not only philosophically correct, but constitutionally mandated.

The strength of that appeal depends on the attitudes that are taken toward constitutional interpretation. If the applicable standard asks whether we can trace a continuous line from our early legal practices to the current law, we can reach one result: the prohibition on active euthanasia and physician-assisted suicide remains intact.[1] Whatever reasons were good enough to ensure their initial passage remain, at least for the purposes of constitutional adjudication, good enough to ensure their continued vitality today. But it is not easy to tie constitutional interpretation to a single theory, especially one that places so great a premium on the established patterns of social history. There is always the strong temptation to adopt the opposite tack and to insist that constitutional deliberation be guided by abstract philosophical inquiry that brings to these questions the highest level of available moral sophistication.[2]

Yet moral theories are not easily cabined, and sophistication can be found on both sides of hard questions. Nowhere is this more true than on the matters of death and dying. Because moral arguments of great sophistication have been urged both for and against the practice, it is hardly surprising that the constitutional attacks on legislative enactments and popular initiatives have been launched from both sides, with equal enthusiasm. This chapter examines the recent developments in this area with the knowledge that the matter will, for better or worse, be resolved in a Supreme Court decision that will, for legal purposes, displace the unruly discord in the lower court decisions throughout the land.[3] In analyzing these debates, it is easy to see how the teams divide. The constitutional positions advanced follow continuously from the social attitudes and moral views that the various players have toward the underlying practices. As a good contrarian, I want to depart from the dominant practice. The legislature should take steps to allow both active euthanasia and assisted suicide; as a constitutional matter the courts should not.

The legal divisions are easily summarized. On the one side, Chief Judge Hogan of the Oregon District Court struck down Oregon's Measure 16 for failing to provide sufficient protection for old, infirm, and isolated individuals, who under the measure would have been deprived of their liberty without due process of law.[4] Judge Noonan of the Ninth Circuit followed the same path in upholding the criminal prohibition against assisted suicide as a safeguard against overreaching.[5] But the fortunes of war quickly changed. On rehearing, a long opinion of Judge Reinhardt reversed the decision of Judge Noonan by condemning the ban as an unacceptable limitation on individual choice.[6] The constitutional movement gained additional force when Judge Miner in the Second Circuit struck down the New York assisted suicide statute on equal protection grounds. He could see no good reason why the risk of abuse should be decisive in assisted suicide cases when it is not decisive in cases where treatment is withdrawn.[7]

The pattern of argument in both cases should be evident. Each set of decisions tends to stress one form of error and to minimize the impact of the other. The defenders of assisted suicide stress the errors that occur when individual choice is thwarted; and the defenders of the status quo, when assisted suicide is illegal, chiefly see the risks that could arise when the protections against assisted suicide are overturned. The topic of abuse does not lend itself easily to categorical judgments, either way, when people of good will can have such strong disagreements on the underlying principles and facts. The empirical issue is surely in flux and hotly disputed. And, where the risks are large both ways, judicial deference to legislation looks like an attractive alternative even for those, like myself, who do not treat judicial restraint as the lodestar of constitutional law. Thus it is instructive to look more closely at the weaknesses in both attempts to create constitutional imperatives on the question of physician-assisted suicide.

FOR THE STATUS QUO

Lee v. State of Oregon,[8] which struck down the Oregon Act, approached the reform with the aid of two broad philosophical presuppositions. First, *Lee* assumed that if the right is granted to some persons, it must be granted to all.[9] It thus declared that it suspected that, on its face, the Act limited coverage to "terminable diseases." Second, *Lee* asserted that the physician's role as healer is fundamentally inconsistent with participation in assisted suicides.[10] Armed with these two propositions, *Lee* struck down the Oregon Act both as a violation of the equal protection clause of the federal constitution and for its evident conflict with the federal Americans with Disabilities Act. The Oregon Act was said to fail because it allowed disabled and vulnerable people to be railroaded to their death, without the legal protection routinely available to competent persons. More concretely, the statute was flawed for not requiring individuals to undergo psychiatric counseling before obtaining their lethal prescriptions, and for leaving that decision to the treating physician whose lack of psychiatric training could blind him to the depressive symptoms that could respond to timely treatment. Nor did the Act contain civil commitment provisions needed to protect persons dangerous to themselves; nor did it require consultation with family members or an independent examination of the patient before the assisted was tendered. As the last straw, it protected physicians from ordinary tort liability in negligence. From this record: "The court finds that there is no set of facts under which it would be rational for terminally ill patients under Measure 16 to receive a standard of care from their physicians under which it did not matter whether they acted with objective reasonableness, according to professional standards. This defect goes to the very heart of the state's reliance on a person's consent to treatment."[11]

Poppycock! Many rational persons would be quite happy to waive the protection of tort liability and cumbersome procedures for difficult surgery, so it is not clear why they cannot waive the protection here. Owing to the chilly response that Measure 16 received in *Lee*, its good faith standard of liability may be necessary to secure physician-assisted suicides. More generally, we can hardly brand any given set of safeguards as insufficient simply because we can devise others still more stringent. The ultimate question is only whether the Act tries to balance the two relevant kinds of error. In a world lacking any self-evident meter stick, some degree of deference must be accorded to a legislature that has struggled with setting the balance. It hardly counts as a demerit for the Act to deal only with terminal diseases because these are the core cases in which the practice of assisted suicide has been defended. And it is odd in the extreme to suggest that the assisted suicide statutes would make more sense if they allowed the privilege to extend to everyone *except* the ter-minally ill, as Stephen Carter has recently proposed.[12] The risk of too many false and precipitate deaths surely grows exponentially as we migrate away from the terminal cases. No doctrine of equal protection of the laws should require the state to make the same judgment of cost and benefit in these two settings. The Oregon Act could be attacked logically as going both too far or not far enough; yet it is precisely because both attacks are plausible that neither should prove decisive, especially in con-stitutional discourse.

But what about the other side of the coin, the commonplace statutes that make assisted suicide a crime? Here again, the judicial atti-tudes have split, but in a strange configuration. Until recently, every state that had addressed the question, whether by statute or judicial decision, had accepted the bedrock importance of the distinction between killing and letting die. End-of-life issues do not form a sort of legislative back-water driven by inertia and little else. "Forty-five states and the District of Columbia expressly disapprove of mercy killing, suicide, assisted sui-cide in either their natural death/living will statutes, or their durable power of attorney for health care acts, or both."[13] Washington is one of their number because it blends its prohibition on assisted suicide[14] with its Natural Death Act that ensures all persons the fundamental right to withdraw health care treatment.[15]

This said, Washington's criminal prohibition should be sustained against constitutional challenge, but not for the reasons advanced by

Judge Noonan, who thought it necessary to denounce the proposed reforms in order to give constitutional blessing to the status quo. His claims are far bolder: "Tort and criminal law have never recognized a right to let others enslave you, mutilate you, or kill you."[16] The trio of offenses shows the weakness of linkage—no rational agent desires slavery or mutilation, and none to my knowledge has asked. The bone of contention is mainly on killing for terminal diseases, where rational arguments cut both ways. But undeterred by differences in background probabilities, Judge Noonan holds that Washington's assisted suicide statute "rightly and reasonably draws the line."[17] The term "reasonably" is a fair bone of contention. The term "rightly" says it all. Judge Noonan's decision is, in the first instance, directed with right and wrong, not with the sound distribution of political power. It would have been quite sufficient for Judge Noonan to write a short opinion that stated his agreement with the consensus view that assisted suicide should remain on the list of criminal offenses, so that those who would oppose him in the legislature could side with him in the constitutional debates.

Judge Noonan also attacks the question of abuse, but it hardly persuades to claim that the repeal of the prohibition on assisted suicide will lead to a parade of horribles that venture far beyond the terminally ill to "[t]he depressed twenty-one year old, the romantically-devastated twenty-eight year old, the alcoholic forty year old."[18] Why claim that once the barriers are removed, the floodgates will break? The actual cases that prompted the litigation in *Compassion in Dying* bear no relationship to their hypothetical extensions.[19] They cover the gamut of physical ills—swollen limbs, bed sores, incontinence, constant pain, grand mal seizures, pneumonia, loss of vision, skin rashes, impaired circulation, and panic disorders—all piled one on top of the other, all in terminal cases, and all conditions for which palliative measures are claimed to be largely ineffective in curbing the constant pain and continued degeneration. Lots of physicians are prepared to say that the set of cases that fall into this category is empty, such that with proper pain management, which busy physicians often neglect to provide, the demands for assistance in suicide vanish.[20]

If affidavits in *Compassion in Dying* and *Quill* are true, this confident proposition seems false. Although it is tempting to dismiss cases brought forward for litigation as anything but a random selection, a more comprehensive survey of physician-assisted suicide in Washington

State[21] tends to reinforce the basic insight that demand for assisted suicide and active euthanasia is strong and persistent. Of the responding
physicians, 26 percent (218 of 828) had received some request for assisted suicide or euthanasia, including 12 percent during the past year. The
types of cases involved cancer, AIDS, and serious neurological disorders.
As might be expected, the cancer and AIDS patients, fearing pain, tended to make their requests when they had less than six months to live. The
neurological cases made their requests earlier in the cycle, in part because
of their loss of self-control over an extended degenerative disease. Cases
of heart disease were only sparsely represented in the sample, presumably because they were not associated with the dread of suffering from
other kinds of conditions.

The requests that were made were not uniformly honored.
Physicians were prepared to provide lethal prescriptions in about 24 percent of cases (38 of 156) and lethal injections in about 33 percent of cases
(19 of 58). It is also instructive to note that in the assisted suicide cases,
the 38 cases were handled by 32 different physicians—a far cry from the
lone-wolf Kevorkian situation—which suggests that the willingness to
treat assisted suicide as compassionate care is widespread, but by no
means uniformly held, among Washington state physicians. It is also
worth noting that the requests for active euthanasia, although less frequently made, were honored in a somewhat *higher* percentage of cases (33
percent versus 24 percent), perhaps as a reflection of the more hopeless
condition of the patients that requested care. Finally, the reasons for
declining to assist cut across the full range. In about half the cases where
lethal injections were refused, the physicians announced their categorical
opposition to the practice, but in the other cases, the explanations were
more case-specific: the patient was not terminally ill, the degree of suffering was not too great, or the patient was depressed. More telling, perhaps,
in about 15 percent of the cases, assistance was denied because of fear of
adverse legal consequences. To be sure, doubtful cases arose in practice, as
with persons in the early stages of Alzheimer's disease, but the study suggests that physicians were alive to the distinctions of degree and sought to
do the best they could with the cases close to the line. All in all, the
Washington State study appears to replicate the Dutch experience where
physicians do not routinely accede to patient demands and uniformly
rebuff frivolous requests born of momentary depression and despair.

Much the same can be said of the strange pattern of behavior that
has emerged in the Northern Territory of Australia, whose "Rights of the

Terminally Ill Act" went into force on July 1, 1996. The Act contains provisions not unlike (but less stringent than) those in Measure 16 and has met with fierce resistance, medical and religious,[22] inside Australia so much so that outsiders who have *flown* to the Territories to gain the benefit of the Act have, to their bitter personal regret and financial ruin, not been able to find *any* treating physician or psychiatrist, both of whose authorizations are required to activate the statutory right.[23] It is hard to imagine that individuals who have made this type of arrangement are so decrepit that they would not have opted for other solutions if they had been persuaded that palliation could reduce their pain to acceptable levels. In cases like this, the determined response of those *traveling* to obtain assistance does not easily square with assertions of abuse or overreaching.

Viewing the evidence as a whole, it is odd to condemn a practice for leading to a set of consequences that no one supports but that has yet to occur. Perhaps later yes, but not now. The system of balancing may be an imperfect art, but doubts in close cases do not imply that all requests are seriously out of order. It is hard enough to find consensus in this area, and where it is found, it should not be lightly tossed away.

FOR CONSTITUTIONAL CHANGE

Noonan's success in *Compassion in Dying* was short-lived, for it was reversed the next year by the Ninth Circuit sitting en banc. Judge Reinhardt's long and impassioned opinion has to count as a rhetorical masterpiece that exhaustively covers the entire controversy over assisted suicide. The decision has been forcefully attacked as bypassing the political process and ignoring the importance of judicial restraint.[24] The seriousness of the charge invites a close look at the decision.

Judge Reinhardt started from a very broad definition of individual autonomy, namely, that every person has the right to control the timing and conditions of his or her own death. Stated as an abstract proposition, the statement seems true enough. The question is whether the philosophical generalization can survive the particularistic attacks mounted against it. For Reinhardt, this broad liberty interest, in turn, carries with it the right to the assistance of a physician in committing suicide.[25] The claims here are intimate and personal, and are, in his view, every bit as persuasive as those that are raised in claiming the right to have an abortion, protected under *Roe v. Wade*,[26] or, as in *Loving v. Virginia*,[27] to overthrow the antimiscegenation laws that once barred interracial marriage.[28]

Reinhardt is careful to treat autonomy as a protected interest, but not as a constitutional absolute. The second half of his argument concludes that no state interest, including abuse and overreaching, is sufficient to dislodge this claim.[29] All of these concerns could be met by a set of lesser means, including many that sound suspiciously like the safeguards incorporated into Measure 16.[30] In essence, Reinhardt took the position outlined earlier: whatever the risks of physician-assisted suicide, they arise in equal measure with the withdrawal or discontinuation of treatment. If these shoals can be successfully negotiated in the one case, they can be negotiated as well in the next, without the ban.

It is troublesome to disagree with a constitutional decision that makes so many excellent intellectual points. Even so, the difference between constitutional law and sound policy has to be taken into account, even by those, like myself, who do not worship at the shrine of judicial restraint. Thus it surely counts for something that an unbroken tradition has prohibited assisted suicide. To counter this unbroken legal tide, Reinhardt adds a learned chronicle of the equivocation in social attitudes toward suicide from Biblical times to the present.[31] But this latter-day version of the Brandeis brief reveals a clouded history that runs the gamut from the glorification of suicide as a rational act of the will to its condemnation as a crime that denies its perpetrator, with a stake through his heart, a decent burial. The same history shows no explicit legalization of physician-assisted suicide. It just as easily could have been penned by the judge who believes that, on this question at least, the legislature should police the boundary between the respective domains of individual choice and social control. And it was, in Judge Beezer's dissent.[32]

My position on this matter must be distinguished from my views of the takings clause, where I have advocated extensive judicial supervision over legislative activity that curtails the ordinary use and disposition of private property.[33] In the property setting, I do not think that it is possible to confuse the ownership of land (where the controversy rages) with its bare possession. It also embraces the question of use and disposition. In that regard, it closely parallels the definition of individual autonomy, which covers not only the right to be let alone by others, but to make positive choices about the use of one's talents, the conduct of one's own life, the risks to be run, and ultimately whether to live or die. If the attack on assisted suicide depended solely on a shrunken definition of individual self-control (such as that advocated by Leon Kass), then a good deal could be said against leaving the matter to public control. But the interest is broader than this.

With private property as with personal liberty, the inquiry does not end with the identification of a protected interest of the individual. Into the balance must fall the state's interest in limiting that choice, which under police power can include the prevention of harm to others, be it by killing or by committing ordinary common law nuisances against others. If the case for criminalizing assisted suicide rested on the proposition that taking one's own life counted as a harm to others, I should be quite content to strike it down, just as I would strike down any statute that declared the construction of an ordinary single-family home as a nuisance.[34] For what it is worth, this same logic applies under the first amendment guarantees of freedom of speech where elastic definitions of public or private nuisances may not be casually invoked to justify restrictions on speech.[35]

These assisted suicide cases, however, do not resemble the takings cases on that score either, for surely the end that is undertaken—the protection against abuse and overreaching—is legitimate. Everything turns on the choice of means. In the present context, I find that the stakes are high both ways, but it is far from clear that either form of error should be given greater weight than the other. As such, the issue of assisted suicide resembles the question of what kinds of remedies, both forward and backward looking, can be used. It is often unclear whether certain conduct will amount to a nuisance. Thus the inquiry here resembles that raised in deciding whether it is permissible to enjoin a halfway house before the occurrence of actual assaults or vandalism in the neighborhood, which is a type of zoning case in which a fair degree of legislative or administrative discretion is appropriate. The nature of this dispute—how to deal with two forms of error under conditions of uncertainty—exerts the decisive influence on the constitutional standard. In one way, though, the decision over assisted suicide is more stark than those under the takings clause because the intermediate solution, take and pay, is systematically foreclosed. It is quite inconceivable to think that the state could ban assisted suicide so long as it was prepared to give money recompense to individual recipients.

Likewise, the precedents on abortion and antimiscegenation laws are hardly dispositive in this case. The antimiscegenation precedent is easily dismissed. In *Loving*, the prohibition against marriage to a person of one's own choice was justified, at most, by a claim that these laws were necessary to preserve the purity of the races, a claim so weak that no one could credit it on rational grounds. But the case draws its real power from the potent combination of choice in marriage and the desire to curb explicit racial classifications. Lest we move too rapidly from this stronghold, ask first whether the autonomy claim without the race claim would be decisive in cases of incest, of polygamy, and of same-sex marriages where the reception, both political and constitutional, has been far less celebratory. Once again, I have much sympathy for two of these claims (polygamy and same-sex marriage), but a good deal of work needs to be made to persuade others to follow suit. No matter how these are resolved, none of those prohibitions raises, at least in stark form, the issues of abuse and overreaching so central to the debate over assisted suicide.

The abortion cases hardly offer a better precedent. The strongest objection to the legalization of abortion is a direct application of the harm principle made famous by John Stuart Mill: liberty may control in its domain but it ends when harm to others begins.[36] That objection has powerful weight whether we defend the constitutional right to have an abortion as an autonomy (or privacy) claim, or whether we recast it, more dubiously, into the mold of sex discrimination. Viewed as an issue of autonomy and choice, I wish that this first part of the original *Roe* principle were applied with the force it deserves in order to strike down so many of the restrictive rules that govern employment because there is nothing about autonomy that limits its gravitational pull to intimate associations. But today any contracts between self-sufficient adults in competitive markets are often looked at, with far less cause, as prime targets for state regulation. Excoriating *Lochner v. New York*[37] for striking down a 10-hour maximum hour statute for bakers is a routine exercise that delights our Supreme Court and most constitutional law professors who champion the modern labor laws, antidiscrimination laws, and safety laws. So why think that the assisted suicide cases deserve a different fate, when the doubts about abuse and incompetence loom far larger?

Ironically the Millian principle does have real bite in the abortion cases. Disputes abound over how broadly harm should be defined on such matters as economic competition or the failure to rescue.[38] However these are resolved, no one could define them so narrowly as to exclude the deliberate killing of another human being. At this point, the abortion debate assumes an unhappy all-or-nothing quality that resists easy compromise. If the fetus is regarded as a person, its killing has to be regarded as a form of homicide, although perhaps not murder, given the set of possible excuses and justifications (for example, health of mother, birth defects, and rape). But even with these qualifications, abortion by this test could be subject to some form of state sanction, whether through direct regulation or the criminal law. In contrast, if the fetus is regarded only as an indistinct blob of protoplasm, it is far more difficult to impose any limits on a woman's choice to terminate pregnancy.

These third-party interests are not at stake in the assisted suicide cases, so in one sense the constitutional case against criminalizing assisted suicide is *stronger* than that against criminalizing abortion. I remain, therefore, utterly puzzled that Yale Kamisar, who has fought for nearly 40 years against the legalization of assisted suicide, could pronounce himself on conventional grounds as "pro-choice" on the abortion question.[39] As a matter of first principle, it is precisely because *Roe v. Wade* did so little to answer the question of "what (or when) is a person?" that it remains a ripe target for intellectual counterattack more than a generation after it was decided. The outcome of *Roe* may please the committed advocates of choice, but its utter lack of principled argument leaves the opponents of abortion entirely unpersuaded. Thus it lays an imperfect foundation on which to build a constitutional right to assisted suicide.

Roe also operates at cross-purposes with the assisted suicide cases, which are concerned with the question of abuse. On this score, however, the second generation of abortion cases should give little comfort to those who think that the abuse and overreaching issues are not ideal grist for some constitutional mill. Questions of whether parental notification should be required of minors, whether they should be required to sign informed consent forms before having an abortion, whether they should be required to wait some short period after initial consent, and whether they should receive counseling or psychological examinations have all been subject to litigation. The defenders of the original liberty interest in *Roe* have proved resistant to the introduction of the same types of safeguards that are often proposed for assisted suicide cases.[40] And they are not without reason because the addition of procedural safeguards is often little more than a backdoor attempt to reduce the exercise of a right that is in fact opposed on much broader philosophical grounds.

The twists and turns of this argument will not come to an easy resting point. Indeed, the outpouring of writing on assisted suicide reads like fast-breaking war bulletins, so quickly does the battlefront change. The inability to come to cloture on what procedures should apply, and why, is not a sign of healthy constitutional adjudication. Broad constitutional initiatives should not be undertaken on the installment plan. We should not guarantee a right today that is subject to definition and implementation by a set of regulations and procedures to be fabricated tomorrow. There is evidence of movement on assisted suicide in the political process and little reason to believe that the spasms of constitutional litigation will generate a better set of results than the rough and tumble of legislative initiative and social experimentation. After all, *Compassion in Dying* and *Quill* do not preclude political action; it positively invites the legislature to determine what safeguards should be put into place once the basic criminal prohibition has been blown away. Many think that the question of abortion would have been resolved more amicably had the court not intervened. The same can be said, before the Supreme Court speaks, about the controversy on assisted suicide.

Finally, notwithstanding their doctrinal boldness, Reinhardt's opinion in *Compassion in Dying*, and in Judge Miner's equally elegant decision in *Quill v. Vacco*[41] suffer from a certain lack of courage, or at least rigor. In their effort to take on assisted suicide, both judges ducked grappling with active euthanasia.[42] The difference between the two practices is easy to state. With assisted suicide, the physician provides the patient with a prescription of a deadly medication that the patient (if able) takes by herself. With active euthanasia, the physician administers the medicine to the patient, with her consent. In essence, both judges sunder in two the standard language of the assisted suicide statutes—"to cause or aid." Their constitutional sense strikes out the second verb, while consciously bypassing the first. Why?

The easy answer is that the plaintiffs framed their challenges in that narrow fashion. But once again, why did they do so? And why did two judges who roamed the intellectual landscape find themselves bound by the litigants' decision? The opponents of physician-assisted suicide such as Yale Kamisar[43] and Grant and Linton[44] have long insisted that there is no principled difference between these two practices because both actions exalt the consent of the patient over the state's interest in preserving human life. Many supporters of assisted suicide candidly, and correctly, embrace that same assertion to the opposite end.[45] The assisted suicide acts also agree in their equivalence by subjecting both to identical sanctions. What subtle ground of distinction could undermine this well-established and fundamental equivalence, either way? By standard common law principles, the consent to another's act treats that act as though it were done by the party who gave the consent, unless that consent were vitiated by duress, fraud, or incompetence. So stated, causing and aiding look to be two sides of the same coin. They hardly lie on opposite sides of some deep constitutional divide that only the foolhardy would attempt to span.

No practical reason, therefore, helps to salvage the first half of the prohibition, while dooming the second half to its well-deserved rest. Judge Reinhardt notes with evident uneasiness the possibility that a patient who attempts suicide with the assistance of a physician could botch the attempt and find himself in greater pain, but without the means or ability to finish his plan.[46] Physician-administered medicines work in a far more humane fashion. So why is Reinhardt reluctant to say that the same set of concerns that leads to the invalidation of the "aiding" part of the statute also marks the "causing" part as well? This riposte is especially troublesome because Judges Miner and Reinhardt both place so much stock in denying that the distinction between aiding suicide and withdrawing treatment can survive rational discussion (when religious and medical leaders are willing to stake their all on it). Yet that gulf seems wider by both history and logic than the distinction between causing and aiding suicide, which are closely entwined as a matter of history, logic, and statutory command. The question squarely raised is one of clear principle and needs no further litigation for reflection and deliberation. Both Miner and Reinhardt flinch at the moment of truth, and neither explains why he succumbs to that sudden burst of timidity.

The problem here is especially difficult for Judge Miner because he rests his opinion in *Quill* on the equal protection clause.[47] Impressed (but only after a fashion) with the uniform historical opposition to assisted suicide and active euthanasia, Judge Miner refused to follow the lead in *Compassion in Dying* and held that, under the due process clause, no person has a liberty interest in assisted suicide.[48] Well enough. But that history counted for naught under the much weaker and less plausible equal protection claim that Judge Miner embraced (and which Judge Reinhardt only endorsed in passing).[49] But these equal protection concerns formed the centerpiece for Judge Miner, who detected a fatal imbalance in allowing some individuals to have a peaceful death, while others were denied that outcome because of the unavailability of physician-assisted suicide.

Yet that claim fares, if anything, even worse than the deprivation of the liberty interest. Sick people do not enter the hospital divided into two classes: those whose terminal illness will linger on and those whose terminal illness will dispatch them quickly. Rather, all terminal patients enter the hospital uncertain as to the future course of their disease. Under the current legal regimes, they are all told that they are entitled to receive palliative treatment at any time and to call, without question, for the withdrawal of life-support mechanisms. They are also cautioned that active euthanasia and assisted suicide are unavailable to them. Wherein lies the illicit classification of persons on which any equal protection claim rests? We do not have here a case of discrimination by race or by sex where the die is, quite literally, cast at birth. All we have is a set of protocols that apply to all persons equally. To treat this distinction between treatments as tantamount to a distinction between persons is to expose virtually every distinction articulated by statute or at common law to a potent but formless equal protection challenge. Is it possible to impose liability for deliberately killing a person if the deliberate failure to rescue a person in need is not actionable? If we provide some remedy against physical harm, must we supply the identical remedy against economic harm as well? Clearly this enterprise is subject to risks that are evident in the case at hand. After all, Judge Miner and Judge Reinhardt direct all their fire to the line between aiding suicide and withdrawing treatment, while evading the more tenuous distinction of causing and aiding the death of another person. A jurisprudence that is this selective in its targets at birth cannot command our ultimate respect. The short truth is that on matters this contentious, some measure of reluctant deference is appropriate.

Just that approach was taken, in an oblique sort of way, in Judge Calabresi's concurrence in *Quill*.[50] Taking an acknowledged leaf from his earlier writings,[51] Judge Calabresi argues that this case calls for a "constitutional remand" to the legislature to reconsider its ban in light of the swirl of developments in both constitutional law and social practice. In essence, he would strike the statute down, subject to the understanding that if it were reenacted in the future with a fresh set of reasons, he would reconsider its constitutionality under standard legal principles. The deft effort to avoid the ultimate judicial responsibility might work in an area characterized by desuetude, but it hardly fits the case of assisted suicide, given the huge volume of legislative activity and intellectual turmoil in New York and elsewhere over the question of death and dying generally and of assisted suicide in particular. In 1990, New York passed legislation that allowed proxies to make health decisions for incompetent persons, but it cautioned against any implication that it advanced the legalization of assisted suicide or euthanasia.[52] Then the 1994 Task Force unanimously rejected the proposed legalization for all to see. Calabresi dutifully notes both events, as well as other parallel developments. So what reason is there to require the legislature to restate reasons that have already been articulated by those who endorse the status quo?

Note, too, that the constitutional remand does not simply give the legislature an opportunity to state its reasons for the ban; it also shifts the burden of going forward, perhaps decisively. With assisted suicide today, as at Normandy in 1944, the initial advantage lies with the defense. In a system of checks and balances, power is dispersed between two legislative branches and a governor armed with a veto. Each legislative house contains a rabbit warren of committees that must be negotiated before any bill gets turned into law. At present, the legislative burden falls on those who want to legalize physician-assisted suicide, voluntary euthanasia, or both. Calabresi would shift that burden, raising the possibility that the statute, once dispatched, would never be reenacted. And for what?

The arguments for and against assisted suicide have been canvased exhaustively, and for every assertion, there is an equal and opposite one. We don't need strategic remands that invite the possibility that a statute will be scrubbed from the books without any authoritative determination of its unconstitutionality. We need to recognize that it hardly makes a difference whether we start down the road of due process or of equal protection. In both cases, credible arguments for keeping the ban have been made by the proponents of the statutes, and flawed, if powerful arguments, have been made the other way. In that kind of setting, the claims for deference are at their highest. When this issue finally is decided in the Supreme Court, I, for one, would welcome a short decision to that effect. From the skeptical response that the Supreme Court gave in oral argument to pleas that it strike down the assisted suicide laws on constitutional grounds, it looks as though this will prove to be the case.[53]

❖   ❖   ❖

CHAPTER 17

Incompetence

WHO DECIDES? WHAT DECISION?

The many twists and turns in the heated debate over euthanasia and assisted suicide all rested on the optimistic assumption that individuals are normally competent to regulate their own affairs, even—or perhaps especially—on matters of life and death. But the people whose lives hang in the balance all too often lack the intellectual powers and physical stamina to make the decisions required of them. All too often the dilemmas in medical ethics start where rational economic theory leaves off, with the task of deciding what should be done by, for, or to incompetent persons. Health care providers must deal with infants and other impaired individuals who have never had the capacity for choice. They must respond to the demands of persons who even in the best of times have only limited capacity to understand complex arrays of available alternatives or to give informed consent to them. They must cope with persons who have suddenly lost mental capacity because of traumatic injury, stroke, or the wear and tear of long illness. And they must fashion rules for dealing with people locked into a permanent vegetative state.

In all these cases, the "they" cannot remain nameless abstractions searching for a concrete identity: *someone* must decide whether to prolong life, whether to cease active support, or whether or not to kill. In a world in which consent does not justify suicide or active euthanasia, this last option is removed from the table because if people are not allowed to kill themselves or to have themselves killed, certainly no guardian could arrogate that decision unto himself without their consent—ever.

The permissible options would then fall between continuing and withholding treatment. But suppose, just suppose, that the arguments made in Chapter 16 are sufficient to carry the day, so that active euthanasia may be practiced on, say, the Dutch pattern, or even under some more restrictive rules. Although assisted suicide is no longer an option because the patient is incapable of acting for herself, the expanded set of choices includes taking active euthanasia for people who are helpless to defend themselves, helpless to care for themselves—and helpless to end their own suffering.

Revulsion and uneasiness are surely the appropriate initial reactions to any proposal to end the lives of helpless individuals by a deliberate act. Individual consent is a powerful barrier against abuse, and one that is not easily overcome in practice given our strong instincts for self-preservation. But now, necessarily, other individuals must make the critical decisions. In the so-called "easy" cases, the decision maker, however chosen, works to follow the course that a once-competent person has charted in anticipation of her eventual incompetence. Often this precise mandate conceals an illusion because the directive often requires the decision maker to use his best judgment and not to follow some inflexible command formulated without knowledge of precise future circumstances. These advance directives or authorizations are of no use for people who are incompetent from birth or who become incompetent before they could plan for their stunted and unwanted future.

Once we leave this miniature command and control economy, the basic instinct to preserve life does not mesh well with the realities of that life as we see it. We know that many people would, and do, choose to refuse medical treatment and many (if fewer) people would choose to accept active euthanasia if only allowed to do so. Many people have no chance of regaining the use of their higher functions; sometimes the continuation of life imposes heavy emotional burdens on other people who can neither ease nor ignore the plight of a loved family member. Note that Karen Quinlan lingered on for several years *after* her parents won their protracted legal fight to disconnect her respirator. Yet before she died, her father, having fought so long and hard to remove Karen from a respirator, was "amazed" at the suggestion that he would cut off her nutrition and hydration.[1] The question of what should be done evidently has two components. The first is *who* shall be entrusted with the power to decide, and the second is *what* decisions should be made.

The legal battles in this area have all coalesced around the question of whether family members have a right to terminate life-giving support mechanisms for an incompetent person, including the withdrawal of nutrition and hydration. In *Cruzan v. Director, Missouri Department of Health,*[2] the Supreme Court answered that question in the negative, at least as a manner of federal constitutional law. Nancy Cruzan lay in a Missouri state hospital in a permanent vegetative state, the result of an automobile accident. Her parents, as her guardians, requested that the hospital employees withdraw nutrition and hydration, which would result in her eventual death. Citing the state's interest in the preservation of life, the state employees refused that request. The Missouri Supreme Court recognized the constitutional right (both state and federal) of a competent person to refuse treatment, a right it derived from the common law doctrines of informed consent. But that court then denied that this right extended to the care of an incompetent person in the absence of any clear and convincing expression by Nancy of her desire not to be kept alive in a comatose state.[3] The court, therefore, held that so long as the state bore the full economic costs of Nancy's care, and so long as the respirator imposed no additional burden on her, the operative legal presumption remained: preserve life, regardless of the quality of life of life preserved. Judge Robertson was explicit and candid: "The state's concern with the sanctity of life rests on the principle that life is precious and worthy of preservation without regard to its quality. This latter concern is especially important when considering a person who has lost the ability to direct her medical treatment."[4]

Starting from this premise, the Missouri Supreme Court held that the use of the respirator therefore would be continued, notwithstanding any psychological pain that her parents would have to endure, knowing that they had maintained bedside vigils for over five years and might have to do so for the rest of Nancy's natural life, perhaps for 30 years or more. The state Court's decision was heavily influenced by its reading of the Uniform Rights of the Terminally Ill Act (URTIA), which allows competent patients to stop any medical procedure or intervention whose sole purpose is to prolong the act of dying.[5] Yet the same Act does not list nutrition and hydration in the class of medical interventions subject to termination, and Missouri's version of the Act, like so many others, states emphatically that the statutory provisions "do not condone, authorize, or approve mercy killing or euthanasia nor permit any affirmative or deliberate act or omission to shorten or end life."⁶ The state court thus upheld the wishes of the hospital employees against those of the family. Continuing along this path, the United States Supreme Court refused to recognize or create a federal constitutional right for an incompetent, especially because the Court had not authoritatively established the analogous constitutional right for *competent* individuals.

I will not address the issue of incompetence in constitutional terms at any great length because I think that the sensible attitude easily follows the broad outlines of Chapter 16. The question here is of sufficient delicacy on a matter, individual competence, that has long been close to the state power to regulate. Once we recognize that competent individuals should not have constitutional entitlements for physician-assisted suicide or active euthanasia, it quickly follows that these same rights (if they be rights) cannot be accorded to incompetent individuals. On the other hand, if the pattern established in *Compassion in Dying* and *Quill* holds fast, active euthanasia is off the table for incompetent persons just as it awkwardly remains off the table for competent individuals. Either way, the question of what should be done for, or to, incompetent individuals remains a legislative choice. Rather than couch the arguments in the rarefied terminology of a liberty interest under the due process clause, or an equality interest under the equal protection clause, it is better to address the merits of the claim in plain English and let the constitutional discourse fend for itself.

Because incompetent persons cannot defend their own interests, other persons must be appointed to represent them. In deciding what they should do, one possible approach is to ask what the incompetent person "would have" decided to do, or have done, for herself if she could have been a disinterested witness to her own future fate. By that standard, should the initial presumption be set for or against continued care, and, either way, what kind of evidence is needed to override the presumption? The Missouri Court in *Cruzan* held that the universal imperative, choose life, regardless of its quality, continued to bind unless overcome only by clear and convincing evidence.

Both parts of this dominant approach are vulnerable to counterattack. Why, in particular, set a tough presumption when the refusal of treatment is commonly accepted by people whose prognosis is more favorable than Nancy Cruzan's? The maxim, preserve life, only makes sense when the expected utility of that life *to the holder of that life* is positive. But when, in our best judgment, that utility turns negative, the case for that presumption withers, especially because the incompetent person might have wanted to avoid imposing burdens on family members and perhaps even public funds. Nor can this presumption in favor of continued treatment be justified as a way to prevent the strong and powerful from taking advantage of the helpless. The permanent vegetative state is so radically discontinuous from other ailments and maladies, and so irreversible, that it falls into a separate category governed by its own rules. A rule that said "allow death in a permanent vegetative state" could easily be adopted without sliding down some slippery slope, so close is the permanent vegetative state to clinical death. So long as the parents or guardians can veto the withdrawal of life support, what is there for the state to fear? Popular sentiment recognizes that some fates are worse than death: Nancy Cruzan's is one of them. (Ask this question: Given her present condition, could you sensibly wish that she had not survived the initial accident?) The command "choose life" cannot rest on mere affirmation when there is so little to live for.

But if the Missouri Court set the presumption correctly, what evidence can rebut it? As Professor Nancy Rhoden clearly noted, only two responses are possible, and neither will usually work.[7] The first possibility is to override the presumption by subjective or objective evidence of the wishes of the incompetent person. A subjective approach tries to ferret out considered personal statements about what should be done if tragedy should strike. In *Cruzan,* for example, the Missouri Court easily brushed aside as "unreliable" her own casual remarks that she would not want to be kept alive unless she could live a halfway normal life.[8] Alternatively the objective approach speculates about what most (reasonable) people would do if placed in her situation. But now there is no way to split the difference because if these speculations override the presumption of continued treatment even one time, they must do so every time. That outcome is good as far as it goes, but in reality it functions as a disguised way of undoing the "choose life" path for incompetent persons.

The second approach, championed by Rhoden, forsakes these individual judgments and allows the family to chart its course of action, regardless of the intentions, supposed or real, of the incompetent. We need not go quite this far because it is possible to hold that the family judgment controls only when evidence of subjective intention cannot be reliably collected. But in its stronger form, the best interests test puts the position of the family on her welfare (and its own welfare) ahead of that of any intermeddler, including the state as represented by the hospital employees. The guardianship arrangement is never painless even in the best of times because, even though the arrangement has obvious fiduciary elements, a family guardian is *not* a business trustee paid for its services.[9] And most decidedly, the family is *not* some disinterested entity whose only job is to maximize the welfare of its ward. In daily life, for example, parents are not *always* required to put the interest of a minor child first at the expense of all their own food, clothing, and shelter. The most that can be asked is that they accord the child's interests a dignity at least equal with their own and sacrifice some parental enjoyment to protect their children from exposure to danger and privation. The implicit goal is not simply maximum welfare for the child, but a more uniform distribution of wealth and advantage across the family. Because the family guardian is part trustee and part beneficiary, a conflict of interest is built into the relationship at the ground floor. We tolerate this conflict when the guardian chooses what kind of treatment should be provided for a minor child, or whether treatment can be stopped altogether. Is there any reason to displace this arrangement when the stakes are higher and the conflicts more stark? No doubt the family mechanism will work less efficiently in this setting than with smaller conflicts, but perhaps its rate of decline will be matched by substitute institutions.

One hard case in which to test the conflicting intuitions is *In Re A.C.*,[10] a painful decision that required the court to decide, first, who has the right to choose treatment for a pregnant woman who is near death while carrying a viable fetus, and, second, what procedures should be made to implement those choices in the event that the woman becomes incompetent. On the first of these questions, the court opted without hesitation for honoring the intentions of the woman, no matter what the consequences for the fetus. In this situation, her choice was to defer having a cesarean section that was likely to kill her, but save her baby, in the hopes that she could live long enough to hold her baby in her arms before she died. The mother was in her twenty-sixth week and hoped to carry the baby for another two weeks before having a cesarean, even though her choice reduced the child's chances of survival. But when she failed rapidly in the interim, the hospital obtained a court order that allowed the cesarean section against her apparent wishes, only to have both baby and mother die shortly after the operation. It was not clear whether an earlier operation, in fact, would have saved the baby's life.

The situation raises a manifest conflict of interest between mother and child. It is easy to construct examples to say that the mother should never trade off her own last fleeting wishes against the diminished probability of survival for an innocent child with the prospect of living a normal life. Doubtless just those calculations moved the trial judge to order the invasive procedure, if necessary, against the mother's wishes. After all, would *you* trade a 50 percent chance of survival for your unborn child against a few hours of additional time for your own life? Or to remove the element of egotism from the equation, suppose that you had a fixed amount of money that could be used to purchase either two weeks of additional life for an adult woman or a full normal life for her newborn infant. No compromise solutions are possible. Assume that you cherish both persons equally. No matter how wide your allotted discretion, your only responsible choice (and I say this with knowledge of the Americans with Disability Act) is to spend all the resources on the child who has the prospects of a normal life. It would be an abuse of discretion to do otherwise. If so, how could you argue in principle that this woman made the right choice when she acted as an interested party?

There is, of course, a difference. In the one case, you hold a fund that could be spent one way or the other. In the second case, a mother must sacrifice her physical integrity in order to have any chance of saving her child. Of course, the entire issue will be clouded by uncertainty: the mother just might hold on long enough to deliver the child, who might die if the operation were done today, and so on. If there were ever the possibility to second-guess a parental decision, given the harm to others, this case is it. Nonetheless the court in *In Re A.C.* came down firmly the opposite way, holding that the mother's autonomy right trumped, notwithstanding her fiduciary duty and the manifest conflict of interest with her child. As if to hammer home its point, the court insisted that her right was of "constitutional magnitude."[11] The interests of her offspring were not sufficient to overcome her right to make the critical decision. Indeed, even after she became incompetent, the court took the view that the inquiry into substituted judgment did not allow the state or her husband to do the best thing for the joint welfare of mother and child, which would have given paramount weight to the unborn child. The guardian's sole duty was to find out what the mother's desires were in light of *her* own values and concerns. One might suppose, therefore, that once the mother knew that she could never hold her baby in her arms, she might now have consented to the cesarean so that the baby might live. But the court's test required everyone else to defer to her intentions, and it precluded all covert efforts to balance her interests against those of her child. For the court, the invasive nature of the procedure dictated the conclusion.

But why defer to her wishes after she becomes incompetent? In my view, the new guardian—probably her husband—should not be bound by the decisions of the mother in this case. To be sure, if she were not pregnant and requested that no active euthanasia be practiced on her person, that decision should be regarded as airtight, even if the state or family decided not to support her with their own resources. But here we have a woman whose own judgment gave scant protection to the welfare of her offspring. Her decision is to be respected so long as she can make it, but only grudgingly, and largely in the hope that persuasion will in most cases lead her to sacrifice her own transient interest for that of her child: she could hardly be insensible to the relative magnitudes of gain and loss. But once she is incompetent, her husband, as the next guardian, has two wards and hence conflicting obligations to both her *and* her offspring. He should not be required to abandon his task in order to effectuate her dubious decision; he is obligated to do the best he can to balance the interests of both persons in his charge. Just letting her hang on and die in the ordinary course of events now carries with it the death warrant to another innocent life. Why that second interest should be ignored as some incidental effect is quite beyond me. The only way to make sense of the situation is to allow the guardian to choose between two claimants and to take whatever steps are necessary to preserve the one whose interest is greatest. He should order the cesarean, but his decision should be protected whether he orders it or not. The mother was not a perfect decision maker when in control; her husband will not be either. But the task of any set of rules is to simplify decision making and reduce error; it is not the dangerous pursuit of perfection. The internal norms within a family, aided by physicians and counselors, are the best we can expect. Don't ask for more.

In Re A.C. is a unique case because the mother's health was at risk along with that of her child. Yet outside the obstetrical setting, parents are often forced to make decisions, both small and great, for the benefit of their children. In principle, we would want more care and attention to be paid to the larger decisions than to the smaller ones, and normally the differences in magnitude will be registered, not by any shift in control away from parents, but by their greater care and attention to the choices at hand. But it is hard to gainsay that, as the stakes get larger, the conflicts of interest get larger as well. A decision to care for a sick child carries with it obligations far heavier than those borne by parents whose children enjoy the blessings of good health. Any temptation to use the higher stakes to enforce greater judicial control should be stoutly resisted. We know, going in, that the autonomy principle cannot receive perfect respect in any regime of substituted judgment. State intervention may have the laudable objective of softening the pronounced conflict of inter-est that grips all parents faced with life and death decisions for their chil-dren when the choices the parents must make are major sacrifices. But even if we cannot expect parents to act in a remotely disinterested way, it would be far worse to allow state officials to keep a suffering child alive indefinitely, knowing that the parents will be drawn close by a siren call, unable to disengage themselves emotionally from the fate of their child. Accepting the conflict of interest between parent and child is the lesser evil.

To put the point in high relief, compare the position of the parent with that of a person deciding whether to undertake a risky therapy that promises either material improvement in the patient's condition or death. Embracing the treatment option drives the probability of main-taining the status quo sharply downward. But so long as people make this choice in their own lives, they should be able to make them for their children or wards. It is too heroic to require parents and guardians to maximize longevity without regard to quality of life, as Judge Robertson would have us do. Our imprecise techniques of judicial review make it unwise to invoke any standard more intrusive than "abuse or neglect" to override familial decisions. In practice, that standard leads to a hands-off public response because neglect in this context means abandonment and indifference, not a decision not to treat.

The upshot is a twofold procedure. Whenever the incompetent has been able to make clear a course of action (for example, no heroic mea-sures), it should be followed, (subject to the exception in *In Re A.C.* when needed to save the child). Whenever the incompetent has not or could not have done so, familial judgments are preferred to judgments by the state.

This pattern of authority should carry over even if the guardian refuses further treatment or withdraws a respirator, or even nutrition and hydration. These last alternatives hold no pretense of improvement, but only of certain death. But the alternative is to force expensive and unwanted treatment in all cases unless some independent party satisfies itself about the soundness of the original judgment, a task that will take time to complete and will require costly and painful public review. We cannot pretend that conflicts of interest do not exist, but we must learn as well that a sound legal system cannot demand their ruthless elimination.

BABY DOE

The importance of family discretion over incompetence is strikingly revealed in *Bowen v. American Hospital Association*,[12] which struck down the Baby Doe regulations issued under the Rehabilitation Act of 1973. The basic statutory provision gives the federal government power to protect disabled persons from discrimination at the hands of parties who have received federal assistance.[13] Pursuant to this statutory mandate, HHS introduced several regulations designed to ensure that handicapped infants received the same level of medical care routinely offered to infants without handicaps. Toward that end, the regulations adopted rules that required the posting of notices in critical places (for example, neonatal wards) containing information on where and whom to call whenever someone believed that a handicapped infant had not received the same type of medical treatment as normal children. The regulations authorized expedited access to patient records to determine whether the charges could be substantiated. They allowed persons unrelated to the child to initiate proceedings, also on an expedited basis, to ensure that these children received suitable medical attention, even against the wishes of their parents and their own physicians. Finally, they required state child protection agencies to prevent those instances of medical neglect, broadly defined, of which they were made aware. The system was designed to achieve only one result: to ensure that any child, regardless of its condition, received all possible medical assistance to ensure its survival. To achieve this end, the United States was prepared to displace the parents as guardians of their own children.

The United States Supreme Court held that these regulations fell outside the powers delegated to HHS under the Act. So long as the parents did not consent to any treatment or procedure, the child was not denied treatment "solely by reason of his handicap," but rather by reason of parent choice—a thin distinction that exalts parental consent in the teeth of an antidiscrimination statute that appears to make other considerations paramount. To see why, recall that the Baby Doe regulations were not directed solely toward the exclusion of handicapped children from treatment programs. They were also directed against all forms of discrimination, including the lobbying by hospitals and physicians to withhold care to handicapped children. So why not enjoin that improper official behavior even if the parents chose to undertake lifesaving treatment?[14] If the state power extends this far, the snooping and external intervention are now justified to protect the parents from receiving the "wrong" message before making any life and death decisions. Moving forward, why not aggressively displace the parents as guardians if they practice some statutory neglect or abuse by failing to treat their handicapped children as required under the Rehabilitation Act?

Our primary purpose in examining *AHA* is not mainly to decide whether the Baby Doe regulations were rightly interred under the Rehabilitation Act, but whether state intervention in these life and death cases makes sense. Again it is critical to make distinctions. One of the underlying suits in *AHA* sought to force the parents to allow an operation to remove an esophageal obstruction from a Down's syndrome baby—a procedure that is routinely done in normal children. The question presented is the same one that Dutch authorities faced in dealing with euthanasia. Here the child has the potential for living a sentient life like that of other Down's syndrome children without the blockage. We would not and should not allow the parents to kill a Down's syndrome child that had no such blockage, so why should the parents be allowed to hide behind the blockage and refuse treatment? The case is one of omission and not action, but it is an omission that counts, given the special obligation of parents to exercise ordinary care for their children. It is a sufficiently clear-cut situation that the hospital should be authorized under state law to perform the operation, and parents who prevent it should be charged with some form of homicide.

But what of Baby Jane Doe, whose parents refused to allow complicated and prolonged operations to be performed on their daughter who was born with spina bifida and subject to several other serious conditions that would have prevented her from ever having a normal life?

Their decision was reached only after consultation with social workers, religious advisors, and physicians. Neither Lawrence Washburn, the officious intervenor in this case, nor William Weber, the guardian ad litem, had any personal knowledge of the family situation, but they requested the state to order the operations, without so much as first finding out the facts. Preserve life, again, was the motto. The New York Court of Appeals had the good sense to damn with suitable understatement Weber's "sometimes offensive" behavior, the additional, unnecessary anguish that two weeks of litigation through all three levels of the state court system had inflicted on the hapless parents.[15]

If parents are not given control, "Baby Jane Doe" will be a routine occurrence, but some way must be found to distinguish between acute spina bifida and an esophageal blockage that is removable by routine surgery. On this matter, the rough-and-ready line between extraordinary care and ordinary care provides the best test because it allows parents not to subject an infant to painful and delicate surgery whose successful outcome could bring in its wake a life of pain and subsequent rounds of fruitless medical treatment. In these agonizing circumstances, no possible gain comes from state intervention that disrupts the anxious deliberations already taking place. Whenever extraordinary treatment is required, parental decisions should be final. By keeping the lines of authority clean, the parents will know that the responsibility is theirs and will have the incentive to consider the matter with the seriousness that it deserves. The solution is not perfect, but it is less flawed than its rivals.

EUTHANASIA AGAIN

The cases just considered provide yet another opportunity to examine the gap between the refusal to accept treatment and active euthanasia. The Missouri Court in *Cruzan* refused to attach any weight to this distinction, notwithstanding its bedrock significance in the law governing competent persons. Quite the opposite, the Missouri Court forbade the removal of support systems in precisely the same way that it would have forbidden active euthanasia. In principle, the first half of its argument is correct—namely, its belated recognition of the essential correspondence between these two types of choices in end-of-life situations. The second half of its decision in *Cruzan* is wrong because it decides both cases the *wrong* way. The parents should be allowed to decide, perhaps after taking consultation (which they would seek in any event because time is not of the essence), on whether or not to continue respiration, nutrition, and hydration. Once parents are vested with the power not to prolong life, then what possible social gain justifies requiring a helpless person to die slowly by thirst and starvation to the immense discomfort of everyone around her?

If someday active euthanasia is made available to competent people who are terminally ill, and if parents or family still have the best chance of making the right decision, then, with assisted suicide not physically possible, why not perform active euthanasia as well? The risk of abuse is effectively constrained by limiting that option to individuals who are in a permanent vegetative state or who have slipped into a final coma. Likewise, advance directives offer an additional check against unwanted active euthanasia. Although no one can command the active support of others, anyone can command others not to kill them and can select guardians and institutions who will honor those wishes, just as people in the Netherlands can select hospitals and long-term care facilities that follow the end-of-life practices they prefer. No one should be comfortable with this solution. However, the source of discomfort is not from making the wrong choice, but from the inescapable burden of having to make some choice. Here, as elsewhere, why have confidence in the state as a decider?

Consider how these arguments about active euthanasia apply in both *In Re A.C.* and *AHA*. Simply put, the guardian has to make a set of choices that no one welcomes and no one can escape. In *In Re A.C.*, the husband (and father) should have the power to ignore the wishes of the mother in order to preserve the life of the child. The parallel discretion with active euthanasia differs in only one regard. When the incompetent has forbidden active euthanasia, there is no life or death conflict of interest that allows the guardian to disregard her wishes. He need not spend his own resources to preserve her, but he must excuse himself from the situation, however painfully, if he cannot respect her declaration against active euthanasia. However, if the incompetent is shown to have been silent on the issue, the animating principle throughout is one that minimizes state intervention. When therefore the incompetent who falls into a permanent vegetative state has been silent as to his future prospects, all decisions of life and death, including that of active euthanasia, should be left in the hands of the guardian. Social sanctions are appropriate, but legal ones are not if it means that people like Nancy Cruzan will be forced to linger on in half-life indefinitely.

This issue also arises in *AHA*, once it is conceded that the parents fall under no duty to undertake extraordinary measures to preserve the life of their child. If additional surgery is not worth the candle, then why balk at active euthanasia if it is honestly invoked to avoid the pain and suffering that would otherwise follow? The fate of the incompetent should lie exclusively in the hands of her guardian. In responding to the Down's syndrome case, state intervention was justified for the same reason that the parent could be barred from killing their young child: the act/omission distinction does not carry any dispositive weight in settings rich in affirmative duties. Once the condition of the child or ward is hopeless, the guardian should be able to control the fate of the ward. If the refusal for treatment is acknowledged, active euthanasia may achieve the same end with less suffering and cost all the way around.

As in so many other situations, the question of abuse must be faced But the conditions that call for judgments by parents and guardians are well defined, and the bonds of natural love and affection restrain parental and familial choice in these cases, where often the difficulty lies in persuading parents, husbands, and wives to let go even when the case is hopeless. Although the stakes are surely high, the proper legal response seems tolerably clear. State intervention must be used to preserve lives known to be worth living, but it should be rejected as a tool to preserve lives haunted by pain or doomed to eerie silence. Imperfect utilitarian judgments as to the prospects and quality of life are inescapable whenever life and death decisions are made, for ourselves as well as for others. That issue cannot be glossed over with unthinking categorical rules that ignore evident, perceived differences in prognosis and expectations. When life is hopeless or inert, the guardian may not have the duty, but surely has the right, to see that the life ends; and if active euthanasia is the best means to achieve that end, so be it.

CHAPTER 18
❖ ❖ ❖

History, Doctrine, and Evolution of Liability

STRANGERS AND TRADERS

Conflicts in the domain of choice are not confined to the dramatic debates over organ transplantation and euthanasia. Our legal system has also had to confront the more prosaic but highly contentious controversies associated with the allocation of risk for mishaps that arise in providing health care services. The responses to this issue straddle the uneasy boundary line between tort and contract law. Viewed in one way, the topic involves legal liability for bodily injury and for death, and thus the topic looks like a branch of personal injury law. Viewed in another way, the parties can allocate any risk of loss from poor treatment by agreement, and thus looks like a branch of contract law. The controversy focuses on the dry but critical issue of classification: does consent dominate injury, or injury, consent. Over time the tort, or regulatory, side of the system has gained strength relative to the contract side.

Today the physical nature of the harm invites the indelible stamp of the tort law. That development may be politically inexorable, but it is also intellectually mistaken. The first side of the autonomy principle protects both individual choice and freedom of association and contract. It organizes matters of liability as much as questions of transplantation or assisted suicide. The central thesis of this chapter is that the historical ambiguity in the legal response of medical injuries should be resolved decisively in favor of the contractual solutions that are routinely frowned on in modern public debates over liability and that are accordingly excluded by operation of law.

To understand why contract should dominate tort on liability issues in health care, we must retrace briefly the function of tort and contract in responding generally to bodily harm or property damage. The history of tort is as old as the law itself. Bodily security is the first task of any civilized society worthy of its name. But bodily security from what? If we ask what kinds of conduct hold the greatest peril to bodily security, deliberate aggression by strangers jumps to the top of the list. Everyone who is not family or a trading partner is a stranger. But the companionship of family and friends and the indifference of most strangers offer scant compensation if even one sworn enemy may with impunity use force against our person or property. No subtler reason is needed to explain why the first historical mission of the tort law was to devise remedies to protect everyone from strangers: actions for trespass to the person, goods, and land; remedies against squatting;[1] and nuisance law for the nontrespassory interferences with property.[2] To be sure, the sharp dichotomy is softened in these land use cases when we have permanent relations with neighbors who are legal strangers. In the context of medical injuries, however, that intermediate category is of no relevance and will not be discussed further. In fundamental opposition to the stranger cases stand the hotly contested issues of product liability and medical malpractice, which were simply not on the radar screen during the formative periods of the common law. They were not, for example, so much as mentioned in Oliver Wendell Holmes's learned dissection of tort and contract found in *The Common Law*, published in 1881, even though by then these topics were at the edges of common law litigation. These stranger cases are easy to solve at the doctrinal level, but today they are often governed by the criminal law. In an age when violent crime is perhaps the number one social issue, too many aggressors also prove insolvent.

Bodily harm can, of course, also be inflicted by friends as well as by strangers—by bad surgery or dangerous drugs as well as by muggings and robberies. As a broad empirical generalization, however, most individuals can limit the harms that their trading partners inflict on them. In a world bereft of legal recourse, they need follow only the simple expedient of choosing their doctors and suppliers well. Even today's legal remedies are so costly and imperfect that an owner is better able to protect her valuable possessions by choosing a reliable storage company than by turning to legal remedies after her possessions are lost, stolen, destroyed, or sold. Trustees and guardians for family fortunes are not picked at random from a telephone directory; they are chosen for their intelligence, character, temperament, and loyalty. Indeed, the major problem in relations of trust is to get people to undertake the job in the first place. To help coax them into service, liability is usually limited to cases of gross neglect, willful default, or conscious misappropriation, leaving untouched the workaday performance of trustees. Typically the legal rules serve as a useful backdrop and guide for routine practice. They are invoked only infrequently when the usual set of social sanctions breaks down. Doctors and pharmaceutical houses are not quite trustees and guardians, but they share with them one key characteristic. They are selected by the people who use their goods and services. The risk of deliberate harm is rare and harshly punished when it occurs.

Although the concern with harm starts with deliberate injuries, it surely does not end with them. On this score, at least, we can state one instructive parallel between stranger and consensual harms. A bullet is equally deadly when fired by accident or mistake as by malicious intention. Accidental harms may not present the level of social risk that makes deliberate harms the prime target of the criminal law, but the proper treatment of this class of harms has surely been the focal point of the tort law. In stranger cases, with only a little exaggeration, the major aim of tort liability is to set the rules for compensating accidental harms. In this context, a running but inconclusive debate has spanned the centuries, one between theories of negligence and theories of strict liability—an issue on which Holmes had a lot to say in *The Common Law*.[3]

The basic groundwork needs to be briefly restated. Under negligence, a defendant is liable for inflicting harm only by failing to take reasonable precautions to guard against its occurrence.[4] For those harms that are wholly innocent—that is, those that no exercise of reasonable care can prevent—the risk of loss remains with the initial victim. The defense of negligence system is that the freedom of action it secures to all people is well worth the small residual risk of suffering from some small risk of accidental harm.[5]

The rival strict liability theory also holds defendants liable when accidents occur through their negligence, but in addition it throws on them the more onerous burden of liability for harms *not* avoidable by their exercise of reasonable care. The theory avoids the difficult question of having to define with precision and in advance what level of care is reasonable under the circumstances. It sidesteps that burdensome task from the conviction that each individual will in fact have greater freedom of action if protected from any use of force, regardless of the motive or diligence of its perpetrator. The compensation that each receives for being held liable for unavoidable harms is a like remedy in the event of a parallel harm inflicted by others. The conclusion is said to follow: "It is an elementary principle in reference to private rights, that every individual is entitled to the undisturbed possession and lawful enjoyment of his own property."[6]

The difference between these two theories often turns out to be small in practice and is well illustrated by the hypothetical case of the man who lifts his stick in self-defense and strikes an innocent bystander standing behind him. The strict liability theory holds the assailant liable for the harm even though he had good reason to raise his stick in self-defense; it does not ask whether it was possible to look before swinging or to alter the path of the blow.[7] The negligence theory excuses this defendant if, under the circumstances, he had done all that the plaintiff could have asked of himself. Thus the plaintiff could only hold him liable if it were possible to identify some untaken precaution that at low cost could have reduced or obviated the risk of harm in question.[8] Over the years, I have tended to favor the strict liability approach across the board for strangers on the ground that it is cheap and certain application.[9] But even under strict liability, a plaintiff can be denied recovery either in whole or in part by putting himself in harm's way, as by running in front of a moving stagecoach, or even perhaps by storing his flammable goods on his own dry land very close to the railroad tracks where it is exposed to sparks from passing trains.[10]

In addition, the standard tort tradition allows the defense of assumption of risk, which first came into prominence with industrial accidents in the late nineteenth century.[11] Assumption of risk provides the necessary link between tort and contract. We can pick an employer just as we can pick a trustee. In its simplest and most powerful form, the plaintiff explicitly assumes the risk of an accidental harm to obtain some equal or greater benefit in exchange. The wisdom of that decision cannot, moreover, be assessed solely by looking at the litigated cases where the employee's gamble fails. It must be examined in light of the full cohort of transactions, most of which resulted in successful outcomes for the risk-bearing individuals (now happily debarred from becoming plaintiffs) in transactions that might never have been formed if the risk could not have been assumed in the first place. Once assumption of risk takes some physical injuries out of the domain of tort and into the domain of contract, two recurring questions remain. First, what risks are allocated to whom? Second, does some imperfection in the contracting process, or perhaps even the contracting terms, render the agreement suspect?

ACCIDENTS WITHIN CONTRACTS

A LARGE MENU OF CHOICES

This switch from stranger to trading cases precedes the modern development of medical malpractice or product liability law. In classical Roman law, one question was whether an artisan called upon to repair a delicate vase could be liable for damage in the event that it broke.[12] The strict liability rule would make the repairman the insurer of his own labor, but that would require its owner to pay an extensive premium to guard against accidental breakage. Virtually all owners would rather run the risk than pay the premium, so the default rule starts from a middle position that holds the artisan responsible only for work that is poorly done, with a lower price that reflects the implicit risk assignment. To be sure, a finding of liability requires someone to decide whether the artisan observed the traditions of the craft, and often they decide by contract to cast the full risk of destruction on the owner, without any chance of compensation. Contracts do not have to follow slavishly any allocation schemes appropriate for strangers. In the case just given, the artisan under all scenarios takes far fewer risks than the stranger operating under a strict liability rule. From these simple considerations is born the customary standards of professional care.

That same contracting logic carries over from the repair of vases to the care of people. Bodily harm in medical malpractice and product liability cases is rarely deliberate. Even assault and battery cases typically arise out of unauthorized treatment undertaken by mistake although for the benefit of the injured party.[13] Accidental harms are therefore the norm. Yet the basic insight about trading partners remains: the best protection against the risk of loss lies in the selection of the providers of care. The suppliers of drugs happily warrant their purity (but not their efficacy), so that the same transaction has components of both strict liability and of negligence. But treating physicians violently resist assuming any liability for the bad outcomes of competent care, let alone for natural diseases or injuries that could be mistaken for the consequences of human events. The general norm under contract, therefore, has long been a split regime, with liability only for professional negligence. Once again, the rule can trace its origins back at least to Roman times.[14] To be sure, a strict liability rule could make a physician or hospital attentive to the treatment of those patients that come into their care, but it has (empirically) the greater vice of leading physicians and hospitals to withhold services in the first place. They do not believe that they can charge in fees enough to cover what they must pay in damages and defense costs. Accordingly, the contractual pressures lead away from the strict liability in stranger cases. It is rare, to say the least, to find any case in which an express warranty for cure is granted,[15] and courts are hesitant to infer that response from the ordinary course of dealing.[16] The stakes may be larger with human beings than with delicate vases, but in neither setting do the parties at the time of contracting prefer a strict liability rule.

Although the contextual dominance of the negligence principle relative to strict liability seems assured, the route to that result shapes the subsequent trajectory of the law. One path holds, first, that a negligence principle is best for stranger cases, and then applies that "universal" principal to harms arising out of consensual arrangements. Measured by this standard, the negligence standard does far better than the rival strict liability (or express warranty) rule, which, owing to its polar position, is far less malleable in its articulation and application.[17] The upshot, however, is to blur the line between tort and contract by adopting a negligence rule because it meets some independent and *public* standard of substantive justice, and not because it meets the wishes of the parties to the transaction. Thus contract arguments are kept outside the discourse.

Historically the development of medical malpractice did not quite follow this model; contract elements were blended early on with tort ones. Once again, the overlap was evident in Roman law.[18] The common law scarcely differed. In one notable early case, *Slater v. Baker,* the defendants insisted that the plaintiff could not bring a contract action because the right form of action was for trespass vi et armis (by force and arms), normally reserved for harm to strangers.[19] But the offended court held against both defendants (a surgeon and an apothecary) on the ground that their rash and ignorant behavior was grist to a contractual mill: "although the defendants in general may be as skilful in their respective professions as any two gentlemen in England, yet the Court cannot help saying, that in this particular case they have acted ignorantly and unskilfully, contrary to the known rule and usage of surgeons."[20] Subsequent cases affirmed the general proposition that allowed the plaintiff the option of suing either in contract or tort. The unsuccessful defendants argued vigorously that their commercial dispute should not be governed by tort principles: "This case is distinguishable from that of an attorney or a surgeon, for in them there is a duty implied by law; here the duty depends wholly on the contract, and the remedy therefore ought to be in contract alone."[21] No one doubted the mixed status of the attorney or the surgeon.

The early history then reveals a willingness to impose public duties on physicians and surgeons by virtue of their status and thus takes a more permissive stance toward regulation than I am urging here. These historical attitudes, however, did not precipitate any medical malpractice crisis in the eighteenth or nineteenth century. For centuries, a negligence rule was perfectly serviceable in medical malpractice cases: after all, malpractice means, "bad practice," to which the rule was directed. *Slater v. Baker*, for example, instinctively veered to a standard that stressed customary usage and practice of physicians.

It is easy to exaggerate the level of precision involved in a bad-practice rule. After all, negligence covers most of the enormous ground between an express warranty on the one pole and a total waiver of liability on the other. The law finds a lot of running room between these two extremes, and the earlier negligence cases tended to locate negligence closer to gross negligence or recklessness than to strict liability. The law thus set, without any undue equivocation, an external standard that in the main the profession found easy to meet. Professional negligence generated some systematic discussion before 1960—the date that marks the onset of modern malpractice law—and most of that literature harped on either the dominance of customary care[22] or reiterated the basic proposition that neither bad outcomes nor mistakes in judgment are tantamount to medical negligence.[23] Judges conceived of liability rules as only one tool among many (for example, reputation and peer pressure) to enforce medical norms. Early malpractice action picked up the near-egregious outlier, but little else. The engines for medical advance lay not with the stick, but with the carrot, by the individual dedication to professional excellence and by institutional efforts to train medical personnel. This model worked pretty well in the aggregate until its legal underpinnings started to unravel. The medicine of 1960 featured advances undreamed of 100 or even 50 years before. These advances were not driven by the weak stick of medical malpractice, but were drawn forward by the strong pull of better health and longer life.

Within that earlier framework, the great virtue of medical malpractice was that it did not block advances that could only be obtained by taking prudent risks. For all its commendable strengths, one weakness in the standard tort model of medical malpractice proved, however, to lead to its eventual undoing: rigidity. The subtext of the tort model is that legal standards may be altered *only* by law, not by the parties. Let public satisfaction give way to public suspicion, and the legal rules will follow suit. This sentiment clearly predates the modern revolution in medical liability. Its most notable statement is Judge Learned Hand's oft-quoted attack on customary standards in a case where a tug was alleged not to have the receiving radios required by a modern merchant marine: "a whole calling may have unduly lagged in the adoption of new and available devices."[24] From that premise, it is one short hop to judicial regulation: "[The calling] never may set its own tests, however persuasive be its usages. Courts must say in the end what is required; there are precautions so imperative that even their universal disregard will not excuse their omission."[25] So the law moves a long way from *Slater v. Baker*, all under the guise of a uniform negligence standard. Once courts take their aggressive supervisory role, no feedback mechanism can work to correct defects in the system: courts cannot move or experiment as quickly as private parties with alternative approaches. The tort-like approach first generates the wrong norms and then freezes them into place.

The alternative approach, therefore, rejects the view that medical malpractice is an extension of the negligence law in stranger cases. Instead, it places assumption of risk and freedom of contract at the fore in shaping legal rules.[26] No longer is the primary job of the law to keep people apart. It seeks to develop optimal rules for risk sharing between parties to a joint venture. To be sure, the default rules for some joint ventures will be simple. If two people form a partnership, the default presumption calls a pro rata division of expenses and profits:[27] what other default rule works in complete ignorance of the skills and aspirations of these parties? Yet actual partnerships often deviate from this simple default rule precisely because the contracting parties have far greater information about their *asymmetrical* abilities and weaknesses. Partnerships can and often do require different contributions of capital and labor, and these are matched by unique splits of profits and losses. Corporations often have complex capital structures to reflect the subtle allocation of risks. There is no reason to reject, and every reason to foster, these deviations from the standard default norm. The specific information available to the parties allows them to tailor their agreements in ways that no default provisions can hope to match.

THE WORKERS' COMPENSATION PRECEDENT

The same principle applies to private contracts that allocate the risk of loss in workplace settings. The usual common law rules for personal injuries require the plaintiff to prove negligence and the defendant to prove contributory negligence. The rules also allow some guarded use of assumption of risk (usually in the form of a willing encounter of a known hazard when there is opportunity to avoid the peril). In principle, this system could apply to all personal injury cases, including industrial accidents and medical injuries. Yet the history of the industrial accident law shows the enormous peril of assuming, even on the assurance of eminent authority,[28] the efficiency of this system for all firms, regardless of their internal organization, labor, and product mix. The lack of any litigated cases in which employers and employees have contracted out of the tort system hardly establishes superiority of common law negligence.[29] The substitute agreements used arbitration, not litigation, in both rails and mines toward the end of the nineteenth century.[30] Most critically, these arrangements did not refine negligence principles; rather, they self-consciously displaced them in favor of rules that gave workers broader coverage in exchange for a waiver of full tort damages. Liability reached all accidents arising out of the course of employment, without having to prove negligence, and by refusing to allow the employer's conventional defenses of contributory negligence and assumption of risk. The substitute agreement became the prototype for the mandatory systems of workers' compensation law that came of age in England in 1897.[31] It migrated on a wholesale basis to the United States a generation or so later.[32]

This alternative approach did not cover all industrial accidents, and for good reason. The basic logic behind the voluntary workers' compensation program rested on a multitude of beliefs: that the direct monitoring of the conduct of other parties was a partial substitute for a tort suit; that team production often made it difficult to pinpoint the cause of an accident; that litigation to the hilt was expensive and foolish when the outcomes were uncertain; that delay hurt both sides; that low damage awards (that is, below the ordinary tort damages) gave the worker an incentive to take care, even when recovery was virtually guaranteed; that limited compensation awards, independent of fault, encouraged employer accident prevention; and that the stabilization of compensation rates facilitated joint programs for insurance and savings.

These factors need not have constant weight across firms, even firms in the same broad industry classification: monitoring ability and team production often varied widely across firms. Hence the older common law rules of individual responsibility exhibited a greater tenacity than they did in those mills, mines, and railroads where monitoring was more feasible.[33] Even so, the exercise here is not to predict the proliferation of contractual regimes for responding to industrial accidents. Rather, it is, first, to point out that divergent solutions in different settings may make sense, and second, to rebut the common charge that the inequality of bargaining power between employers and workers led to domination and exploitation.[34] Under that theory, we should have observed large firms contracting out of *all* liability instead of assuming a liability that in some cases could be more onerous than that in the common law. Rather, the better explanation tracks the general justification for contractual freedom. These compensation benefits worked to the mutual benefit of both sides. By expanding liability in some dimensions (basic coverage) and reducing it in others (defenses and damages), the parties hit on solutions that the law could neither invent nor impose.

This capsule history of workers' compensation law is instructive, not only for its contractual origins, but also for its subsequent statutory history. What was a sensible contract for some parties became, by legislation, the legal norm for all. The parties thus lost their ability to contract out of the system. Yet its success depends, not only on the basic form of its protection, but also on its levels of compensation and its modes of adjudication: choose the wrong levels with the right rules and the situation could still disintegrate rapidly, as it sometimes did. Today workers' compensation schedules differ widely from state to state, often in response to partisan political pressures instead of a disinterested search for the optimal compensation levels. Once again, rigidity takes a good voluntary form and robs it of its effectiveness by removing the power of correction from the people with the best relevant information: the parties to the deal.

THE EVOLUTION OF MEDICAL MALPRACTICE LIABILITY

The evolution of medical malpractice and product liability (as with prescription drugs) tracks the history of the workers' compensation laws several generations before, but with far greater dislocations. As has been noted, from its earliest days, medical malpractice straddled the borderland between tort and contract. Starting around 1960, the judicial expectations for malpractice cases began to rise. It is quite difficult to point to any single case or any single issue as the "cause" of the medical malpractice crisis, but it is hardly necessary to do so because a great systemwide result need not have one single great cause. We can, however, usefully identify some reasons for the expansion of liability and show how these changes fit into the overall picture. The simplest approach is to track the standard elements of the tort of negligence: duty, standard of care, breach of duty, causation, and damages.

DUTY AND IMMUNITY

The first element of the common law negligence requires that the defendant owe the plaintiff a duty of care. On this front, there was little if any shift for individual physicians because duties arising out of professional relationships have long been a legal staple. Nonetheless, it is easy to detect a major shift in the treatment of the charitable immunities of hospitals and other institutions that supplied care, often without charge, to indigent patients—a development largely completed before the 1960 benchmark.[35]

Toward the end of the nineteenth century, courts held, first in England[36] and then in the United States,[37] that charitable organizations enjoyed immunity from suit by virtue of their status alone. One ground for this decision was to prevent an improper diversion of the assets of charitable organizations to the payment of tort judgments. This "protection of the funds" theory fails one easy test. In stranger cases, why should a gift to a charity by A allow that organization to take or destroy, without compensation, the property of B? Surely no one who establishes a trust fund wants his resources to go to strangers. Surely the trustee would rather see the money paid out to the intended beneficiaries, the patients victimized by physician malpractice, if it had to be paid out at all.[38] Yet in this context, those wishes should not be respected because the correct legal rule never allows actions of private benevolence to extract a subsidy from unwilling outsiders. Most of the earlier cases that dealt with charitable immunities made just that distinction by refusing to extend the immunity from suits by patients to stranger situations.[39]

The older view on charitable immunity rested on a second theory that better accounts for the distinction between patient beneficiaries and strangers, the so-called theory of implied waiver, which in principle could apply to both paying and nonpaying patients.[40] That theory has been neatly summed up as follows: "that the beneficiary by accepting the tendered aid impliedly agrees that is all he may accept and waives any right of recourse for wrong done, while strangers do not do so."[41] The employer was vicariously liable only when the employee worked for its financial benefit, but this theory had no application to nonprofit charities, even in their dealings with paying patients. Generally that argument excused the charitable institution from liability even when its senior staff had carelessly selected its treating physicians or nurses.[42]

This doctrine of waiver is open to the charge that the principle is "entirely fictional," in part because it cannot deal with infants, the insane, and unconscious persons. Even for competent individuals, it assumes a level of knowledge and awareness that about the terms and conditions of service that most lack. In these cases, though, the doctrine can be speedily refurbished. Infants and the insane have guardians who choose physicians and make other arrangements for medical care. Their power of guardianship surely includes the right to waive liability for the benefit of their wards just as they can waive it for themselves. The waiver approach works when the recipients of treatment are protected by competent parties who can learn of the basic rule without real difficulty, as by prominent notices posted in hospital. The charitable immunity is neither covert nor subtle: in any case, better notice is a sufficient response to the problem of unfair surprise.

Once these matters are addressed, the waiver theory marks the critical conversion of charitable immunity from a defense based on status to one based on contract. No longer did charitable immunity function as an iron barrier against individual recovery, but rather as a *default* rule that the benefited institution could waive. The law never *required* the charitable institution to claim its institutional immunity, but allowed it (if it so chose) to waive that immunity, even selectively, for charitable cases but not for paying patients—a position that drew a sharp judicial rebuke.[43] Alternatively the institution could also maintain its immunity from liability for both paying and nonpaying patients[44] in order to avoid the burden of classifying patients who make partial payment or who receive charitable support from other institutions, for example, churches or friendly societies. Likewise, the charity could waive the immunity only with respect to actions of wilful default, or for ordinary negligence only to the extent of its insurance coverage.[45] Other variations and permutations are possible. In a universe of voluntary transactions, the law has no reason to require institutions to adopt a position on waiver that either is consistent over time or across patients. If powerful administrative, marketing, and reputational constraints cut in that direction, the uniform policy will emerge voluntarily.

The key point is that so long as charitable immunity is waivable in whole or in part, it is at bottom a doctrine of contract, not status. The law could easily dispense with presumptive immunity so long as it allowed charitable institutions to re-create that immunity by contract. The ability to set terms goes hand in hand with the ability to refuse to extend charitable care—a clear part of the original immunity design that has been effectively curtailed today.[46] Indeed, one reason why charities have lost their ability to control terms is that first courts, and then legislatures, regulated them loosely on a common carrier model: once they are required to take business, they can no longer be allowed to set the terms of their engagements. But that shift to social control marks a serious erosion of their independence and their effectiveness.

Charities should have total institutional freedom to decide where and how to allocate their resources. In this regard, they should have the same set of rights once enjoyed by ordinary profit-making firms, but which again have been compromised by legislation. It does not follow that charitable organizations should exercise their powers like profit-making institutions or act in ways that are as capricious or foolish as the law would allow. The basic point is that internal norms and reputational sanctions should do a far better job of setting the priorities for charitable institutions. Charities are organized to give away medical care, and they should not be ordered to defend medical malpractice actions when that same money might be better spent on expanding facilities for the care of others. Does it really make sense to compensate one person huge sums of money for *admitted* medical negligence if it impairs the ability to provide life-saving services to a dozen others who lose, not because of negligence, but because there was no room at the inn?

The attack on charitable immunity begins by assuming medical malpractice liabilities sound in tort, the stance the California court took in abolishing charitable immunity in 1951.[47] At the time of the initial abrogation in liability, a general sense of optimism held that negligence law afforded an institutional defendant ample protection, and that insurance, generally available at low cost, could insulate any charitable institution from financial risk.[48] That prediction was true when made, given the obstacles that lay in the path of a successful medical malpractice action. Early on, the courts thought they could detect something undignified or improper about seeking any kind of waiver from liability. "Few hospitals would announce a policy of requiring such a waiver as a condition of entrance, and few patients would enter under such a condition unless forced to do so by poverty."[49]

That sentiment, however, did not embody a universal truth independent of time and circumstances. Indeed, it quickly became very bad prophecy because by the mid to late 1950s, the general climate had surely started to change when waivers were routinely sought by hospitals that had come to fear medical malpractice liability and were routinely granted by patients in need of medical care. Now the contracts were individual, explicit, and clear, so that the courts could no longer defeat their application by an appeal to common practice or by making some strained, but clever, interpretation of inexact contract language. Now that the stakes were raised, the judicial response was to invalidate contractual disclaimers of liability on grounds of public policy.

The California Supreme Court decision in *Tunkl v. Regents of University of California* formed a critical cog in the overall process.[50] The challenged exculpation clause provided (for services rendered in 1956) that in consideration for the receipt of medical services, "the patient or his legal representative agrees to and hereby releases the Regents of the University of California, and the hospital from any and all liability for the negligent and wrongful acts or omissions of its employees, if the hospital has used due care in selecting its employees."[51] The Court hardly tarried over the factual point of whether the plaintiff was competent to sign the release, on which the hospital prevailed. Rather, it directed its fire to the main issue and struck down the exemption clause on the grounds that it offended public policy by exonerating the defendant for the negligence of its servants during the course of their employment.

So why invalidate this contract? The problem is by no means a small one because most risk allocation by contract is routinely allowed. Ironically *Tunkl* followed the earlier cases in hewing to the idea that medical care was different, only this time, far from treating nonprofit institutions as benevolent Samaritans, the court saw only the danger of economic exploitation of the sick, defenseless, poor, and uninformed. The previous beneficiaries of charitable care became, in the eyes of the court, its prey. To reach this view, the court in *Tunkl* adopted a flawed if popular line of reasoning: Was the contract in question "affected with the public interest" so as to be a fit subject for regulation? The court concluded that the contract was so affected, thereby rendering it a fit subject for regulation. The key passage of the opinion appears in the endnotes,[52] but its essentials are easy to summarize. Medicine is an essential service rendered in time of great need to individuals who have no other choice of services and who therefore must yield to the decisive bargaining advantages of hospitals.

Professor Glen O. Robinson has decisively demolished the economic underpinning of the decision.[53] The critical question is never the size of the institutions, but the number of viable alternatives for services of any given type to patients in both local and national markets. Even charities have to compete, especially for their paying patients. So long as some individuals search the market for the best mix of quality and price—a common result when elective services are involved—then why believe that only courts in malpractice cases can devise the ideal terms and conditions for rendering services? The problem of surprise can be dealt with by the sort of notice and disclosures routinely given today. The question of emergency care can be handled either by advance contract (as with individuals who sign up with health plans of one sort or another), or by offering individuals in need of emergency services the same terms and conditions granted to paying patients. The relevant question is never whether the individual wants to get rid of the exculpation clause after injury manifests itself. Rather, it is whether, before the fact, the person prefers the service with the exculpation clause to no service at all. If he does, the contract is to his benefit, and he should be held to it like any other.

It is often said that exculpation clauses should be struck down because patients lack accurate information about the rights they are asked to surrender.[54] That argument is overstated because although these clauses may be unwelcome in the abstract, they are easy to interpret. In addition, when routinely required, they bind the knowledgeable as well as the ignorant, allowing the latter to free-ride off the intelligent judgments of the former. So even if poverty and ignorance go hand in hand, the proper response is not to invalidate the clause but to insist on its uniform application to all persons regardless of economic conditions—a nondiscrimination approach that most institutions should find reasonably easy to live with.

However, even that solution seems more invasive than necessary because most individuals do not negotiate their own contracts for medical services. Rather they rely on representations by employers, unions, or insurers—informed entities capable of deciding whether a waiver is worth its price. True to *Tunkl*, the California Supreme Court enforces arbitration clauses on just this ground.[55] But again no negative inference can be drawn when these intermediaries are absent. If learned institutions make accommodations on liability to economize on costs ex ante, why deny unorganized individuals that same benefit? Here again it is best for all individuals to sign exemption clauses that parallel those offered to members of organized groups. Why tilt the scales in favor of one form of social organization relative to another when the individual member can happily free-ride off the greater knowledge of the group?

Tunkl also made the apparently innocuous suggestion that any person should be able to pay extra for protection against negligence. After all, making that option available at a standard price negates any objection to the contract based on superior bargaining power. Options of this sort are offered in other contexts in which courts have generally held people to their exculpation clauses.[56] But the converse does not follow. Options to purchase additional insurance may be offered when a firm has extensive control over a well-defined contingency. Thus it is often easy to purchase insurance that pays x dollars for goods lost in shipment. The shipper's strong control, the easily identified insurable event, and the limited liability taken in combination reduce the ability of any insurance to game the system.

The situation, however, is quite different in the market for medical malpractice protection. Now the liabilities are unliquidated and will vary enormously from customer to customer: individuals about to undergo dangerous procedures with a high risk of failure; individuals with large outside incomes; individuals with an appetite for litigation or good access to lawyers will all gravitate toward the additional protection. Owing to these skews, the insurance can only be priced with difficulty. Even then, the insurer takes the risk of a common mode failure, namely, an adverse change in the legal environment that simultaneously boosts the risks on its policies. The economics of insurance does not imply that some insurance policy will be available for every conceivable loss. It only states that insurance contracts will emerge when they work to the mutual advantage of both sides, ex ante, taking into account the full panoply of risks: adverse selection, moral hazards, and common mode failures.[57]

Forcing medical providers to supply insurance protection will drive them into losing contracts and will create some measure of redistribution within their customer base—those who value the insurance feature will gain at the expense of those who do not. Cutting out the liability in tort—or limiting that liability to some fixed schedule—helps prevent that covert redistribution through the tort system. It also creates a uniformity of conditions that prevents any form of favoritism to some patients at the expense of others. Systematically requiring a built-in coverage option may work to the detriment of both patients and providers.

One further limitation in *Tunkl* deserves brief comment. Its exculpation clause only dealt with the liability of a charitable hospital. It did not touch the liability of ordinary physicians and staff. Some of these individuals might have claimed charitable immunity, at least when they provided free care for patients. But most professionals collect a salary or fees so that the charitable component of their work is less evident for them than it is for charitable institutions. But it hardly matters. In principle, the freedom of contract arguments should apply to both settings, so that institutions can protect their employees from suit, even if only to insulate themselves from obligations to indemnify. Once charitable institutions were stripped of their ability to protect themselves by contract, their employees lost protection as well. The rules on liability for institutions thus quickly became the norm on liability for individuals: no contracting out of negligence.[58] At this point, the evolution of the entire law of medical malpractice shifted from the private to the public side. It is necessary to mention briefly some of the doctrinal shifts on other issues that followed in its wake.

STANDARD OF CARE

One consequence of the tort regime is that it tightens the standard of care in medical malpractice cases. The sharpest upward twist comes from the occasional case that refuses to treat the customary care of trained physicians as conclusive evidence on the standard of due care.[59] But holdings of this sort, although generating enormous publicity, are few and far between. They do not account for most of the shifts in liability or for the veritable explosion of medical malpractice cases since 1960. Instead the salient changes occur more subtly. What were once easy cases for defendants become hotly contested issues. The hotly contested cases now become easier for the plaintiff to win.

Exactly this type of silent evolution has taken place. The early cases of professional negligence tended to involve obvious breaches of care, such as not removing broken needles, which then caused major infection.[60] Over time, the required level of skill and judgment crept up as more decisions departed the realm of honest but mistaken judgment to enter the headier domain of culpable negligence, or at least a reasonable jury could so find. So the tipping point moves from blunders in routine surgery to the failure to make a timely decision to perform a cesarean section on a diabetic woman whose offspring is then born with serious birth defects.[61] No clarion call announces these major shifts in standards, but the differences persist, and to lawyers and insurance companies in the trenches they strongly influence the terms of settlement. A standard borne of a suspicion of professional power and arrogance is quite different from a standard borne of deference to professional expertise and good will. Yet no formal declaration signals the changed approach that evolves gradually within the interstices of the reasonable care standard. The incremental nature of the changes makes it difficult to identify the patterns of overt mistake that could prompt legislative intervention or give some direction as to the precise form it takes.

Everyone supports a standard of reasonable care, but everyone interprets it just a little bit differently.

CAUSATION

The next element in the medical malpractice case is causation. On this issue, we no longer face the push/pull type of connections so applicable in cases of trespass to strangers. Even cutting an artery or severing a nerve is likely to be a known risk of a skillful operation, which would have been disclosed to a patient before proceeding. Yet sometimes the mishap could occur through negligence, leaving a great deal of running room to decide whether the artery or nerve could have been spared by the exercise of reasonable care. No grand principle forces itself to the fore; but recently it has been easier for a plaintiff to win on cases of this sort. In particular, the courts have shown a greater willingness to apply the principle of res ipsa loquitur—literally, the thing speaks for itself— whereby the burden of proof is shifted to the defendant) even when there is a substantial chance that some natural process, some action by a third party, or some unreasonable conduct by the defendant is responsible for the loss in question.

The canonical form of the res ipsa loquitur doctrine specifies three elements that must be established before the burden of proof is shifted to the defendant:

1. The event must be of a kind that ordinarily does not occur in the absence of negligence.

2. The event must be caused by an agency or instrumentality within the exclusive control of the defendant.

3. The event must not have been due to any voluntary action or contribution on the part of the plaintiff.[62]

The requirements aim, by a process of elimination, to make it more likely that a cause under the defendant's control actually caused the harm in question. The third requirement is usually of little consequence in medical malpractice cases, given the passive nature of the plaintiff during surgery or treatment—although it surely can arise if the question is whether a patient has followed restrictions pertaining to diet, smoking, exercise, or medical regimen.

But far more critical issues arise with respect to the first two elements. Given that medical mishaps are common, both with and without negligence, the parties can always clash on the first element. With harm to strangers, it may make sense to erode the negligence requirement by reversing the burden of proof. After all, the de facto strict liability regime that emerges is independently justifiable, as discussed earlier in this chapter. But in medical malpractice cases, the erosion of the negligence requirement pulls us further away from the social optimum of not imposing liability on providers who comply with customary standards of care. The boost to hapless plaintiffs comes at the high price of allowing too many dubious claims to go through the system.

The second element is equally problematic. Medical treatment is typically characterized by joint control: hospitals, physicians (including those who used equipment on previous occasions), nurses, equipment, and drugs are all involved in complex surgery.[63] Pointing one finger at all parties simultaneously is at best a mixed blessing. Although it occasionally helps the deserving plaintiff who cannot identify the one wrongful defendant, it also ropes into litigation many parties who ought not to be there at all, thereby substantially increasing the costs of running the system without necessarily improving its reliability. In sum, these cases are far removed from those where an inference, first of control and then of negligence, is drawn from seeing a barrel roll out of the defendant's loft during ordinary business hours.[64] A shift around the edges reverberates through the system. The issue of causation arises in every litigated case, and its effects are synergistic with increases in the standard of care. If each expands by 20 percent, the overall estimate of liability increases by 44 percent, a very noticeable effect, even before changes in damage awards are factored into the equation.

DAMAGES

The third element of the basic medical malpractice cause of action is damages, whose effect on litigated cases is the easiest to quantify. Sociological explanations roll off the tongue as to why damage levels in tort actions increase more rapidly than inflation: bodily dysfunction and disfigurement are not common phenomena today and thus bring greater notoriety and instinctive disdain than in years past; expert witnesses are able to calculate the full present discounted value of lost earnings and medical expenses; expenses of care outpace inflation because of the general upsurge in medical costs and because of advanced medical heroics that can prolong life in a severely disabled condition in ways not possible a generation ago. But whatever the explanation, it is quite clear that damages are on the rise. The evidence is well summarized by Paul Weiler in reporting the results of the RAND Civil Justice Project on jury awards in Chicago and San Francisco:

> The respective average jury verdicts (in constant 1984 dollars) in the two cities rose from $50,000 and $125,000 in the early sixties, to $600,000 and $450,000 in the early seventies to $1.2 million in each city in the early eighties. Admittedly, the absolute amounts paid in these two cities as a result of jury verdicts are not representative of settlements nationally, and even in these jurisdictions jury verdicts are often cut back by trial judges and appellate courts. Nationally, however, the average medical malpractice settlement more than doubled from under $12,000 in 1970 to over $26,000 in 1975, then jumped to $45,000 in 1978, nearly doubled again to $80,000 by 1984, and topped $100,000 by 1986—an aggregate increase far in excess of inflation.[65]

Similar figures with similar import are found in other studies that have traced the rise of medical malpractice insurance, first through the crisis in the mid-1970s and then in the second crisis of the mid-1980s.[66] The expansion in damages is real.

For these purposes, the full impact of the changes in the medical malpractice rule has to take into account changes in *both* the frequency and the severity of medical malpractice actions. Here the effect of the changes in legal doctrine and jury behavior are cumulative and synergistic. The tougher scrutiny of defendant's behavior on the standard of care issue and the more generous inferences on questions of causation combine to increase the likelihood of success from a suit. The larger damage awards increase the payoffs from establishing liability. To find the full impact, we must compare expected costs of liability under the older, pre-1960 system with the expected costs of liability under the newer system. On this score, it is relevant to note the very sharp increase in claim frequency over the relevant period: from one claim per 100 physicians in 1960 to 17 claims per hundred in 1983, down to 13 claims per 100 physicians in 1988 (after the tort reforms of the mid-1980s). Small changes in all the same direction can add up to very large consequences, and these in turn are reflected in the total level of insurance premiums, which marched inexorably upward $60 million in 1960 (divided roughly evenly between hospitals and physicians) to $500 million in 1974, to $1 billion in 1976 (the year of the first crisis), to $2.5 billion in 1983, and to $7 billion in 1988.[67] It does not take elaborate calculations to see that the hundredfold increase in (nominal) premiums, is roughly offset by the hundredfold increase in anticipated liability, precisely what has happened through this period.[68] The efficiency of these changes is the topic for Chapter 19.

CHAPTER 19

The Efficiency of the Liability System

WHAT HAS JUDICIAL INNOVATION WROUGHT?

Chapter 18 detailed the remorseless expansion of tort liability system over the last 35 years. It also attributed that expansion to the judicial regulation that stripped providers of medical services of the ability to inculcate themselves from liability by contract. So understood, the causes of the medical malpractice revolution are prosaic because no coordinated plan ushered in the new system with full awareness of its consequences. Instead, change proceeded incrementally and on a piecemeal basis. Often the balance of advantage shifted when the plaintiff who lost at trial was able to persuade the appellate judges to authorize a new trial under a more favorable set of instructions. No court ever stood back and performed a cost/benefit analysis to evaluate the consequences of the entire set of innovations. Were these innovations large or small, wise or foolish, or even internally consistent? Nor could courts figure out the interconnections between present changes and future developments. No court that championed the abrogation of charitable immunity for hospitals in the 1940s and 1950s had the slightest premonition of the legal revolution in tort liability that would come a generation later. Ironically it is sometimes easier to transform the world by inadvertence than by conscious design.

If Chapter 18 described the origins and scope of the malpractice transformation, this chapter seeks to make sense of its effects. It does so in two stages. First, it examines how the expansion of tort liability squares up against the three key objectives of a tort system: corrective justice, compensation, and deterrence. It then samples some of the vast amounts of accumulated evidence on the overall efficiency of the current system.

JUSTIFICATIONS FOR TORT LIABILITY

CORRECTIVE JUSTICE

The earliest debates over the tort law were cast in the language of corrective justice—rendering to each person his due.[1] The basic story is that P and D are strangers. D commits some act that upsets the appropriate balance with P, and P demands redress for that loss. The concept works best when D has taken something from P that can be returned in its original condition: redress is thus coterminous with restitution and a return to the status quo ante. Strict liability works well in this context, for D should not be able to keep what he has taken from P, even if he honestly thought it was his.

The carryover of corrective justice to medical malpractice liability looks plausible insofar as it preserves the procedural setting for restitution. A single injured party claims redress from a single wrongdoer and not from someone who is causally responsible for the harm. However, the carryover of corrective justice is undermined by two salient differences. First, because medical malpractice cases involve death or injury, it is impossible to return "the thing" to its owner. The issue is no longer restitution, but compensation for a wrongful act. Second, because the death or injury did not take place between strangers, P may well have assumed the risk of adverse consequences in order to obtain treatment. Unless we can divine which risks were assumed by P and which were retained by D, an unvarnished conception of corrective justice does little to unsnarl this tangle of issues, notwithstanding its impeccable Aristotelian origins. The conception of corrective justice is not strong enough to bind individuals who wish to deviate from it. Therefore, unless we are prepared to place inordinate weight on the idea of "wrongfulness" to resolve the underlying substantive questions, the manifest gulf between malpractice and stranger cases blocks any extension of that theory, to our contested terrain. In the end, the issue of consent, express or implied, dominates that of rectification. Corrective justice thus plays only a small role in thinking through medical malpractice liability. Most people, therefore, instinctively turn first to compensation, and then to deterrence.

COMPENSATION

Compensation for serious personal injury fares little better as a social justification for creating medical malpractice liability. Other mechanisms, including ordinary medical, hospital, disability, and life insurance are surely superior for that end. The compensable events that trigger coverage under first-party systems are far easier to identify because they are tied only to a publicly observable adverse outcome and not to a particular origin of that outcome, namely, substandard care. First-party insurance, moreover, allows each person to specify in advance specific compensation levels, which can vary by choice from person to person. Medical malpractice insurance does not allow that degree of individuation and is more difficult to price because its liabilities are unliquidated. First-party insurance is cheaper to run, more precise in reaching its objectives, and covers a far broader class of compensable events than medical malpractice insurance. If individuals were given a fixed pot of money to divide between coverage under these two systems, we can be confident that few, if any, would tie their purchases of medical, disability, or life insurance to the vagaries of the medical malpractice system.

The common response is that these first-party systems are woefully inadequate to deal with compensation for disabilities. For example, relatively little private first-party disability insurance is available, and by one estimate it covers only about $5 billion of the $100 billion in uncompensated lost earnings.[2] Nor could this market be expanded substantially owing to the unending difficulties in policing its coverage provisions. Yet the point, however true, hardly justifies using medical malpractice to fill the void. Huge portions of the uncompensated lost earnings go to persons with no tort remedy against anyone, either for medical malpractice or for anything else. These people have to cope without damage awards, which would have to expand some thirtyfold to meet disability losses comprehensively. No alteration in the doctrinal nuances of medical malpractice can make the slightest dent in dealing with wide-scale disabilities. The various programs of public and private support that are today cobbled together have to stand on their own.

DETERRENCE

The only useful function for the liability system is deterrence: a damage award after the fact reduces the likelihood of future, similar adverse occurrences. The gain does not come from the transfer payment itself, but from the prevention of future injuries through higher care level. If these loss reductions exceed the administrative costs incurred to secure them, the system achieves a worthwhile objective. In some abstract sense, it hardly matters who gets the cash because the deterrent effect on physicians and hospitals bites so long as they pay when they misbehave. For all sorts of sufficient practical reasons, however, liability works best when damages go to the injured party, who is thereby given a powerful incentive to assemble the information and to cooperate with a lawyer in pursuing the underlying claim.

The critical question, then, is whether the system is nimble enough to achieve this deterrent effect. On this issue, the outlook is decidedly bleak. The major difficulty does not lie in choosing the appropriate substantive standard—that of customary care. Rather, it is the more prosaic issue of whether the legal system should limit recovery to cases of real medical malpractice. What, in other words, is the error rate associated with the operation of the liability system? When that error rate becomes too high, the deterrence function crumbles.

To see why, assume for the sake of argument that the selection of winning tort cases is random: liability for careless acts is no greater than liability for careful ones. At this point, a hospital or physician gains no additional benefits from the taking of care. On net, therefore, they are worse off because care requires them to incur additional costs. Liability operates as a tax that falls on good and ill alike. Physicians who take risky cases know that they will pay heavily because liability only depends on the rate of injury, not on how well they perform. The astute plaintiff's lawyer will press forward on big cases first because by definition they will promise the highest rate of return. For the same reason, physicians and hospitals in turn will avoid the very cases where their intervention is most needed. If liability is random, it is wiser, and cheaper, to set it at zero. Why incur administrative expenses solely to transfer cash between randomly paired individuals?

Fortunately it seems quite unreasonable to assume that the legal system is so poor a filter that all big ticket cases are equally welcome to a skillful lawyer. Plaintiffs' malpractice firms spend a good deal of time reviewing the records before deciding whether to accept or decline individual cases. We can safely assume that their exercise of professional judgment allows them to intelligently identify prospective winners and losers. Similarly insurance companies are also repeat players capable of learning from their collective experience, and they too do not naively equate expected liability with severity of damages. Indeed, one careful study on the progression of tort claims through the legal system indicates that the selection pressures do operate as claims proceed through the system. The weak cases tend to get weeded out, the strong cases tend to be settled, and the tough cases in between breed conflict and litigation.[3] A similar study some ten years later indicates that informal dispute resolution often conveys sufficient information to facilitate a settlement in line with legal risk.[4]

The question remains: What comfort can be drawn from studies that confirm the economic model that parties can bargain in the shadow of the law? The local efficiency of the settlement process does not show the social soundness of the system within which settlement takes place; nor does it show that negligence liability effectively deters medical malpractice. After all, the parties follow, but do not determine, the shape of the shadow. If judges and juries give an extra plus to plaintiffs in big ticket cases so long as the plaintiff can produce a credible expert witness, the settlements will reflect those realities. The settlements will not reflect the judgment of independent experts who favor the defendant. If random imposition of liability undermines deterrence, lesser biases impair its effectiveness. A false ruler on liability corrupts outcomes at trial thus distorts how litigants settle their disputes before trial. Settlement does not correct the imbalances within the legal system; it reflects them. The rational behavior of individual litigants within the system neither promotes nor guarantees the rationality of the system as a whole.

It is, moreover, likely that these biases are built into the legal system. One piece of evidence is that, given liability, the level of damage award tends to vary with the type of defendant.[5] Thus a broken bone case fetches far more in damages from a corporate defendant in a product liability case than from an individual homeowner sued in his personal capacity. More generally, "medical malpractice awards against doctors are almost 2.5 times as great as awards against other individuals in average case types, and awards against hospitals are 85 percent larger."[6] These medical injuries may be properly ranked for given classes of defendants, but the entire scale could be skewed upward for some classes in a manner incompatible with deterrence. Astute bargaining does not eliminate this bias.

A second source of uneasiness is the large variation of malpractice awards within states. The formal characteristics of the negligence suits are determined by uniform statewide standards. But even within a state, liability costs, and hence insurance premiums, vary markedly by county. Thus verdicts in medical malpractice for Chicago hospitals are far higher than comparable awards for the farming counties of Illinois; and the same holds for Detroit and Michigan; Los Angeles and California; Miami and Florida; New York City and New York. The persistence and magnitude of these regional variations are not matters of chance, nor are they matters of principle. Rather, they might reflect a sense of distrust and alienation that inner-city jurors have against the great research institutions and the prominent physicians who work within a stone's throw of the ghetto. Or they might reflect a more receptive attitude toward pain, money, and insurance than that found in rural settings. No one quite knows. It is not necessary to identify the source of this pronounced skew. It suffices to point out its negative consequences for a theory of deterrence.

Following cases through the legal system, therefore, provides no substitute for a direct look at the facts of the underlying cases to see if their ultimate disposition jibes with some independent estimation of their value. On this score, the findings on global deterrence are pessimistic. One example should suffice here. In their study of medical malpractice litigation in New York for 1984, Paul Weiler and his associates made their own independent assessment of the medical records of a large sample of hospital admissions.[7] They found that one in every 27 hospitalizations showed evidence of medically induced or iatrogenic injuries. Of these, they estimated about one in four could be attributed not merely to physician intervention, but to physician negligence. As we might expect, the figures show that university and teaching hospitals have a higher level of adverse events than community hospitals (4.1 versus 2.3 percent of cases)—a result that is consistent with the more difficult cases that migrate in their direction. The study seems on firm ground when it also finds that university and teaching hospitals have lower rates of negligence: only 10.7 percent of the adverse consequences in university and teaching settings were attributable to negligence, versus 26.9 percent for nonteaching hospitals. So far so good. What is so troublesome about the study, however, is its rough working estimation rate of negligence for all hospitalizations. "Extrapolating our New York population estimates to the nation as a whole implies that every year there are more than 150,000 fatalities and 30,000 serious disabilities precipitated by the medical treatment in this country."[8] If only one-quarter of these incidents were attributable to negligence, we should expect 45,000 major cases each year. At $1 million a piece, the total bill would be around $45 *billion*—a figure that overwhelms the current system.

Clearly something has to give because, if the study is correct, the true crisis is that we have too few law suits, not too many.[9] The immediate task would be to respond to a silent social crisis of momentous proportions. A more dispassionate view of the entire issue suggests, however, not that the tort system functions well, but that the assertions of a malpractice crisis could easily be overstated. Consider three major difficulties in the Harvard study.[10]

First, the stipulated definition of an adverse event makes little or no effort to control for the severity of adverse consequences. Over half of the adverse events were minor in nature and, after a one-month period, produced no side effects. Thus the results pool outcomes that should receive fundamentally different legal responses. Small cases should be subject to informal redress; only large cases should enter the legal system. It would be wrong to try to reform the legal system to assure recovery for the smaller cases.

Second, the evaluation of the underlying data presents a formidable task, given that over 30,000 closed files in nonpsychiatric cases needed to be evaluated. The original screening was done by teams of trained nurses and medical record analysts, which immediately raises the question of whether different teams in fact applied the same protocols even if in theory they followed the same verbal tests. The initial task was to identify first cases that showed signs of an adverse event and then to find the subset of those adverse events that could be attributable to physician or hospital negligence. Any protocol that employs as many as 18 separate criteria for adverse events alone is suspect, as is the broad definition of what counts as an adverse event—anything from falling off a hospital bed during recovery to heart failure on the operating table.

The situation hardly gets better when two trained physicians reviewed the cases that the initial review team culled out for further consideration. The rate of disagreement between the two physicians was often very high. That disagreement should be expected given that complex hospital cases give rise to outcomes that have multiple causes, only some of which are medically induced. But the "go slow" sign should have been hoisted when the second team that reviewed a subset of 318 cases found the same *rate* of adverse events and malpractice, but *identified* different cases as falling below the applicable standard of care. The lack of correspondence is to have confidence in *neither* set of judgments.

Third, the claim of pervasive physician malpractice should be reflected in the suits brought for litigation. Here plaintiff's lawyers have an opportunity to sift through the evidence and pick those cases that present the strongest evidence of malpractice. Yet the same panels that found physician malpractice to be pervasive in general practice made a very low estimate of negligence in the claims that were actually brought, finding it in only 8 of the 47 cases that resulted in claims.[11] Of the cases where serious harm was attributed to negligence, only 1 in 3 resulted in tort payment.[12] The others either languished or were prosecuted without a favorable settlement or verdict. Alas, mismatching was also found in the other direction as well "because the claims that were in fact filed were as likely to have *no* negligent injury behind them.[13] The system seems broken from both ends.

It is, of course, dangerous to generalize from a single study, but a systematic overview of the deterrent and compensation effects of all forms of tort litigation has verified the pattern that the Harvard study detected in New York. In a recent study, Donald Dewees, David Duff, and Michael Trebilcock compiled the available American and Canadian data to show that it is exceedingly improbable that medical malpractice liability has any significant deterrent effect.[14] The level of medical malpractice in Canada is no higher than in the United States, even though Canadian claims number about 20 percent of American ones (with both rising), and the Canadian medical malpractice premium totals only 10 percent of the American levels. The best explanation of this comparative data seems to be the intrinsic inability of the system to sort and process claims correctly. Although medical malpractice and automobile collision cases are both said to be species of negligence liability, the fundamental differences in their daily operation dwarf the superficial fact that both are housed at the same common law tort address. It is one thing to decide which car had the green light by mechanical rules that verge on strict liability.[15] It is quite another to speak of medical care in the same breath, when even its customary standards of care exhibit none of the precision of the rules of the road.

The unreliability of the medical malpractice system is further compounded by the costs of its operation. Because there are no highway rules to guide the inquiry, cases turn on the application of difficult standards to uncertain facts. The costliness of that system is then evident from a gross, if elementary, statistical summary: "of the claims dollar, 57 cents is spent on processing costs and 43 cents is paid to victims, of which 20 cents goes for pain and suffering and 23 cents for financial loss. . . . Of the financial compensation, 11 cents is expended for items already covered by collateral insurance sources, leaving just 12 cents spent on the actual financial losses of injured victims."[16] These numbers dramatize the heavy drag that pervades the system, but in and of themselves they do not supply any conclusive evidence of the social loss from its operation. If the deterrent effect of the malpractice action (which depends on high reliability) reached sufficient levels, the heavy deadweight transactions costs could repay themselves handsomely. Yet it is precisely because deterrence is so uncertain that these costs loom as just an additional, avoidable cost of running the system. Difficult tradeoffs are necessary when proper incentives come only at the price of high administrative costs. But the social decision is easy when high administrative costs do little to advance deterrence,[17] which seems to be the situation here. It is often said, rightly, that you cannot beat something with nothing. But when judged by the usual concerns of deterrence tempered by administrative costs, the available evidence offers little comfort to the status quo and does nothing to preclude scrapping the system altogether.

MEDICAL MALPRACTICE INSURANCE AND DEFENSIVE MEDICINE

What then should be made of this double failure of compensation and deterrence, especially when compounded by high administrative expense? One tactic is to ignore it and focus instead on the cost and access to the medical system as a whole. Thus Paul Starr, one of the architects of the Clinton health plan, has written: "Since malpractice insurance represents less than 1 percent of health costs, it cannot possibly be a primary cause of the growth in expenditures."[18] An enormous increase in premiums starts from a minuscule base, so that the entire cost of premium is tantamount to only two or three months of ordinary increases in overall medical expenditures. Yet Starr's optimistic analysis moves too quickly. His focus on the total premium understates the influence of medical liability on the overall performance of the health care system.

The first and most obvious point is that insurance premiums do not give an accurate measure of the total level of systemwide exposure to liability. Instead they only form its lower bound. A fuller accounting would, for example, factor into the equation the costs of seeking and opposing legislation to change the law. Countless reform proposals precipitate extensive legislative battles that are fought out in the trenches case by case, with lobbying, organizational efforts, and even grass roots campaigns. Liability can be a major issue in elections for state judges. The perceived stakes are too large to ignore in any social calculation.

Interested parties also make expenditures to adopt liability risks that they are unable to change. Physicians and hospitals must organize their operations in order to minimize the threat of liability. Planning, education, and supervision are routine matters before the first dollar is spent on insurance. These programs cannot come cheaply when the same issues must be addressed for thousands of institutions and for hundreds of thousands of physicians. These expenditures must mount up into the billions, even though they cannot be isolated to any specific budget line.

Second, the cost of medical malpractice law is not limited to the malpractice liabilities of individual professionals, but also includes the costs of hospital care, including those for malpractice coverage of staff physicians, interns, and residents. The basic insurance package ran about $9 billion in the early 1990s and is doubtless more today.[19] In addition, self-insurance covers a large fraction of liability exposure for hospital and other institutions, and for good economic reason. Under the standard contract, the insurance company picks up both the costs of indemnity and defense. Indeed, the traditional insurance arrangement uses the indemnity obligation (that is, to pay settlements and judgments) to bond the quality of the legal defense that the insurer provides. If the insured is liable for indemnity only, the insurer that pays only defense costs has an incentive to "dump" cases by settling too quickly in order to economize on its defense costs. If the insurer is responsible only for indemnity but not defense costs, it will be tempted to spend the insured's dollars on defense to reduce its own liability. Putting both costs on the insurer, therefore, minimizes that conflict of interest and induces the insurer to minimize the sum of the two expenses.

This transfer of indemnity and defense costs makes sense when medical malpractice suits are a comparative rarity. It is difficult to develop any in-house expertise when a serious claim comes along only every couple of years. The package of defense and indemnity is farmed out to a third party whose expertise can minimize the total losses, at the cost of establishing a tricky cooperative relationship with the insured. This approach hardly makes matters perfect, however. The insured may still be liable for some portion of the risk because of deductibles and coinsurance. Excess carriers will come into the picture when the losses are very large. An insured also bears certain reputational losses from settling dubious claims, for example, bad publicity in the general consumer market. The insured's employees must fight through hours of deposition at the insured's expense. The upshot is that as claim frequency increases, these conflicts become more acute. At some point, the frequency of suit becomes high enough for firms to find it cheaper to manage the risk directly. The preferred pattern of coverage is large chunks of retained liability with only excess coverage from outside sources. The 1 percent dollar figure, therefore, does not begin to capture the full costs of running the liability system, let alone the collateral costs that are not registered in the liability system.

It is difficult to find systematic data on this question, but the figures for the operation of the University of Chicago Hospitals give some sense of the costs for medical malpractice that can be incurred by a large, urban organization with extensive tertiary care obligations.[20] The University's hospital system generates roughly $500 million in revenue both for hospital and physician services, and it pays out (in figures typical for Chicago hospitals) $30 million overall a year in direct medical malpractice expense, which includes about $26 million for physician and hospital malpractice (with the former being the larger component by about a 3 to 1 ratio), about $1.5 for direct internal administrative costs (claims recordation and evaluation), and about $2.5 for excess insurance. These numbers (which are actuarially audited) set a minimum base of at least 6 percent of revenues for medical malpractice, of which less than 10 percent is for insurance purchased in the open market. A more accurate accounting would add back in the costs of general administrative over-head, so that a better estimate of its costs may be a half of a point higher.

The deeper question is what to make of these figures. Initially they are driven by several factors that are not replicable in all tertiary care institutions: high-risk obstetrical practice and emergency room treatment typically consume a very large portion of the premium dollars, and these costs vary from institution to institution and from place to place, depending on patient mix. But problems of this sort are common to most medical centers that serve the inner city.[21] The numbers also reflect the jury behavior in Cook County, which for any given injury is far more generous with its damage awards than the collar counties bordering Chicago whose hospitals compete with city hospitals for some fraction of their business. In addition, the premiums were higher in Illinois before a state statute (itself challenged on constitutional grounds) imposed limitations on pain and suffering of $500,000.[22] But it is hard to believe that any major institution has total liabilities that are as low as Starr's inviting 1 percent of revenues figure. The real number could easily be twice and perhaps three times as large, although it is difficult to say.

Wholly apart from the size of the medical malpractice burden, its inconsistent incidence generates social costs that are not recorded on any individual ledger. The competition for medical service takes place in state-wide and, increasingly, in national markets, so that the absence of a uniform regime on liability clearly distorts the competitive process. The systematic shift in liability regimes hampers the ability of consumers to compare the service they receive in different locations. The inability to control this risk by contract gives a systematic advantage to institutions that operate in favorable local environments, or impose some limits on liability or damages, or both. The shifts in investment and business brought about by these differences are impossible to estimate, but it is worth noting that I know of no institution that seeks on a voluntary basis to waive any statutory or common law protection it already enjoys. The clear implication is that liability under the present tort system is excessive.

The potential for tort liability also induces behavioral changes, changes that usually travel under the name of defensive medicine.[23] The phenomenon is both ubiquitous but nonquantifiable. Virtually everyone agrees that because hospitals and physicians are exposed to threats of liability, they incur expenses—keep more expensive records, conduct tests, order extra procedures, and maintain internal supervision—that they might not have incurred if the rules of liability were otherwise. The patient and insurance companies will acquiesce in these practices for a simple economic reason. Once the liability rules are fixed, it is best to spend additional dollars on loss prevention until, at the margin, that dollar yields the same return as the dollar spent on liability insurance. But which expenditures count as defensive medicine cannot be answered in the abstract. Take a large increase in the percentage of births by cesarean section. Is it a function of better medical care or of a fear of liability for vaginal births? But what of the risks of liability for a defective child born from a cesarean? One of the most common counts of medical malpractice is for cerebral palsy, said to result from medical malpractice (poor monitoring, delay, and so on), even though more than 80 percent of the cases have genetic causes.[24] Nor can one exclude the possibility that physicians will take *counterproductive* steps to reduce their liability. Cesarean sections, for example, are associated with longer periods of recovery for the mother, higher incidence of infection, some probability of secondary complications, and reduced opportunities for mother-infant bonding.[25]

The choice of tests and procedures is so obscure that no one can have confidence in the usual figure that says that just as 1 percent of total medical expenditures are attributable to medical malpractice, so only about 3 percent of total expenditures are attributable to defensive medicine.[26] The anecdotal evidence from a biased sample of physicians suggests that higher rates are possible. "A 1987 survey of practicing obstetricians by the American College of Obstetricians and Gynecologists found that 46 percent were performing routine fetal monitoring, 41 percent reported a change in their clinical practice because of the medical-legal environment, 33 percent cared for fewer or no high-risk patients at all, and 12 percent were no longer practicing obstetrics. The widespread use of routine EFM [electronic fetal monitoring] is a form of defensive medicine: it reflects the perception among many clinicians that fetal monitoring and a timely cesarean section can keep them out of court."[27] Surveys of this sort are notoriously unreliable in measuring the response of these practices to liability pressures, as opposed to, say, a patient population with more high-risk pregnancies—teenagers and women in their late 30s and early 40s. But even with malpractice costs hovering at between 2 and 3 percent of the national health bill (recall that for physicians it is closer on average to 4 percent, with wide variations across locales and specialties), if total expenditures on defensive medicine are two- or threefold that level, the numbers start to look much more impressive, perhaps closing in on 10 percent of the total medical bill, with potential for undetected growth over the long haul.

Even that number contains a good deal of rank speculation. Many of the observed changes may well have some residual benefit, albeit it one lower than the associated costs. Surely better record keeping, more tests, and more patient visits are not usually counterproductive in their own right. Nor is there any reason to be believe malpractice expenditures in an ideal world of voluntary contracts would equal zero. They clearly could be positive, and perhaps significant as well. Before the celebration begins, recall the sobering studies that cannot pinpoint the useful deterrent effect of malpractice laws. The label "defensive medicine" gains in plausibility: medicine practiced to ward off liability even though it produces little independent patient benefit. There is little cause for optimism and rejoicing. The question of what should be done is the subject of Chapter 20.

❖   ❖   ❖

CHAPTER 20

The Reform of the Liability System

TORT REFORM

For the past 20 years, highly charged battles over tort reform have been waged on many fronts: state and federal, public and private. At any given time, the professional medical society and the trial lawyers, to name only the most prominent participants, can be found in sharp confrontation on some legislative initiative. The amount of resources invested shows that the general level of academic satisfaction with the current system does not stop a political movement driven by the main institutional players. Indeed, the level of committed resources is one useful measure of the level of discontent with, and dislocation of, the current tort law. Although product liability reform has often foundered on the simple proposition that legislators are more responsive to the demands of in-state plaintiffs than out-of-state defendants, the same is not true in medical malpractice areas. Professional and institutional defendants are all powerful local players whose patient base includes persons from out of state. Although national reform of the medical malpractice system has not borne much fruit, at the state level at least, these reform efforts have surely proved both frequent and successful.[1]

The level of passion and movement in tort reform does not offer, however, a reliable measure of the soundness of the proposed structural changes. In law, as in medicine, identifying some general malaise may be easy, but it is far more difficult to diagnose the underlying condition or to prescribe its legislative antidote. Tort reform (like the opposition to it) is typically driven by partisan and parochial interests that are more interested in reducing their particular burdens than in finding the optimal level of malpractice liability. These proposed cures need not be as bad as the disease, but by the same token, they may miss many important improvements. Just that pattern characterizes the reforms presently on the table. Because the particular issues have been canvassed in considerable detail elsewhere, I shall provide a general critique and not a detailed or textual criticism of any particular statute.

TINKERING

One tactic is to tame the present system by making incremental alterations in its key components. A statute can reiterate in no uncertain terms that the standard of customary care governs in medical malpractice cases,[2] or it can limit the application of res ipsa loquitur to cases that do not call for delicate medical judgments—leaving hot water bottles on patients until they scald and the like.[3] These legislative initiatives reverse judicial expansions of liability. At the margins, they will make some difference, but their overall impact is limited. First, it is far more difficult to pass these statutes in large states where liability is extensive and the plaintiffs' bar—and the truth be known, the defendants' bar as well—are well entrenched in their respective malpractice fiefdoms. In addition, broad statutory pronouncements are not ideal for policing the behavior of judges and lawyers in courtroom settings; there is too much "wiggle room" for elaboration and invention at the edges. Statutory changes of liability rules have a short built-in "half-life" before judicial indifference, hostility, or application start to chip them all away. These may change the balance somewhat but not in any decisive way.

LIMITATIONS ON DAMAGES

A more decisive remedy is to attack the awards of damages. The hard-edged quality of these rules is more difficult to evade in trial and thus more difficult to ignore in settlement. A clear numerical formula does not present any of the interpretive inherent in a statutory reform on causation and care. A damage limitation is less subject to implicit nullification by judges unreconciled to the legislative interference with their common law prerogatives. The key question is what form this intervention should take.

The strongest possible line of intervention is also the simplest: a direct cap on damages. One comprehensive approach limits total liability for the three main heads of loss: pain and suffering, earnings, and damages. But the dominant legislative approach takes the somewhat less ambitious tack of applying (a lower) cap only to pain and suffering, say, around $500,000. Both sorts of caps have always met with a stony judicial stare and have been held unconstitutional in some states, but sustained in other states.[4] Their difficulty stems from their incredible crudeness. The ideal trimming of damage awards would take a very different course. One immediate possibility is to remove smallish claims from the tort system, where the administrative costs are likely to be a large portion of the amount transferred. But any cap leaves these awards largely untouched. A second desirable feature might be to reduce tort awards in large cases by some proportionate amount, so that the suits for the greatest loss do not suffer the greatest contraction. A $500,000 dollar cap on pain and suffering does not touch a $400,000 award, but it does eviscerate 90 percent of the value of a $5,000,000 judgment. The cap thus alters the relative value of the recoveries in a jarring fashion. The alternative approach is to set some maximal figure for the most severe hypothetical case and then to scale down all lesser judgments in some proportionate amount. But that scale is far more difficult to construct and implement than a simple cap. The legislative reform sacrifices legal precision on the altar of administrative convenience and enforceability, with at best mixed results. It is the obvious product of distrust with the day-to-day operation of the legal system. The cap leaves no discretion for courts and juries. It thus avoids the risk that injuries will be rated more serious than they are in order to boost up the total award to what it would have been before the reforms.

A second approach to damages requires that large individual awards take the form of "structured payments," whereby the plaintiff does not recover damages in a lump sum to be invested over a lifetime. Rather he receives periodic payments that cease on death.[5] One nice feature of this system is that it can exploit differences in subjective discount rates. If individuals have a lower discount rate than institutional defendants, the simple stretching out of payments makes both sides better off than the lump-sum payment. The low discount rate gives the income stream a higher value for the plaintiff than it has for the defendant. A second reason for structured settlements is to shift the risk of uncertainty.

The individual receives a larger payment for the years that he or she is alive and in need of care, but leaves less by bequest to the next generation, a result that could again be beneficial to both sides.

The difference between lump-sum and periodic payments is relatively small if the future payments are fixed in amount regardless of the health or condition of the injured party because then all that is at stake is differences in discount rates. The difference between these two methods, however, is very large indeed if the amount of the payment turns on the plaintiff's future health. As against this form of periodic payment, the lump-sum settlement does not weaken the incentives of an injured person to regain his health or to take steps to mitigate other losses. The money is paid regardless of health, so the individual can maximize health without forfeiting income. Lump-sum payments are thus frequent in common law settings where the defendant undertakes no post-judgment supervision of the injured party's rehabilitation. In contrast, workers' compensation law often relies on periodic payments, but only because the employer supervises and reviews the treatment and rehabilitation of the injured employee. That system can be carried over into the tort arena, but only with some difficulty, if because the supervision costs are likely to be higher because there is no prior relationship between the parties. To the extent that legal rules *allow* for structured settlement, they are all to the good. To the extent that they *require* them, the impact is likely to be negative. If there are any gains to periodic payments, the parties should be able to obtain them through settlement. They do not need the compulsion of the law to alter their arrangements.

A third, and less draconian, approach to the damage question sets off the collateral benefits that injured plaintiffs receive from other sources—social security and first-party health plans—from any medical malpractice award. If the medical malpractice system itself operated in a rational fashion, the reduction in rewards would undermine the beneficial incentives that the tort system imposes on health care providers. In principle, therefore, it is eminently sensible to avoid the double payment to injured parties by coordinating benefits through subrogation contracts that are fully enforced by the courts. These agreements could authorize the first-party insurer to recover, either from the tort defendant before payment is made or from the tort plaintiff afterwards, the full costs of medical expenditures. One question that arises is what should be done when the money paid is insufficient to cover both pain and suffering and lost earnings on the one hand, and out of pocket medical expenses on the other. Once again, that question should normally be sorted out as a matter of contract. My own guess is that most contracts, if freed of the fear of judicial invalidity, would give first priority to the tangible medical expenses, which are normally the greatest concern for accidents and illnesses alike. Subrogation, if fully enforced, could reduce the total pressures on the insurance system without distorting any incentives on health care providers. Unfortunately the current system does not appear to be moving in this direction, for the dominant view allows the injured party on "equitable principles" to keep tort damages up to the full level of pain and suffering, even if the contract provides otherwise.[6] The only setoff is that a court will examine the settlement between the wrongdoer and the victim to be sure that pain and suffering damages are not inflated solely to defeat valid third-party claims, which is good as far as it goes—but it does not go far enough.[7]

In practice, the analysis is more complicated because the malpractice system does not fare well in terms of deterrence. If it did, reducing tort recoveries by setting off collateral benefits might return the system to equilibrium. In principle we could gravitate to a system that *both* limits the amount of recovery to a tort plaintiff *and* protects the subrogation rights of third-party payers against that reduced award. But once again, it is best to negotiate these matters in advance to avoid the vagaries of case-by-case adjudication. The current statutes, however, show little solicitude to the subrogee. Instead, they either reduce the award by the amount of the collateral benefits, or, in the alternative, allow the defendant to inform the jury that such benefits exist, so that it may make whatever adjustments it sees fit.[8] It is, of course, difficult to know whether this reform improves or hurts overall social welfare, but these provisions seem to have some teeth and, according to one estimate, account for about a 15 percent reduction in insurance premiums.[9] Oddly enough, the same result appears to hold whether there is an automatic reduction for collateral damages or a simple mention to the jury of that award.[10]

PANELS

A third modest proposal allows a full-dress trial of a medical malpractice claim to take place only after the case has either gone to mediation or been reviewed by a panel of experts. These preliminary canters rarely have any binding authority and surely add an element of cost of their own, so that they create few net gains overall. Requiring arbitration for all cases would generate greater cost savings. For familiar reasons, that result is best achieved through private contract, not through judicial or legislative command.

ADMINISTRATIVE REVIEW

One obvious inefficiency with the current medical malpractice system is the cumbrous judicial trial of individual cases. The American Medical Association (AMA) has suggested substituting a specialized administrative tribunal, staffed in part by physicians. The tribunals would first resolve individual claims. The information discovered in the process would then be fed back into an overall database where it could be used to evaluate the performance of individual physicians.[11] One obvious criticism of this proposal is that it takes the current medical malpractice system as a given and does nothing to correct its doctrinal errors. But in reply, it should be possible to blend a shift in forum with needed changes in the substantive rule. One obvious advantage of the AMA proposal is that it might reduce the inconsistent outcomes among jury decisions. However, it has met the strong resistance (as we would expect) from trial lawyers and has thus far not commanded any support. Its political failure is, however, a sign of its underlying merits, not its fatal structural weaknesses.[12]

REGULATORY ALTERNATIVES

The common law system links deterrence to compensation. That system has the virtue of placing an enforcement right in the hands of the individual who can pursue it most vigorously. Yet when individual actions fall short, that linkage becomes a drawback to any scheme that seeks to deter accidents. The ill-chosen plaintiff is not in a good position to oversee complex forms of behavior. The ostensible advantage of regulatory arrangements is that they allow, when appropriate, for separation of deterrence from compensation—itself a mixed blessing. Good regulations can improve overall performance, but bad regulations can cut off access to medical care. The ordinary licensing of physicians may be used to maintain minimum standards or to exclude qualified competitors by treating them as unqualified practitioners. National testing, for example, might be a useful substitute for malpractice litigation by cutting out newly minted physicians who do not meet established standards. But even those physicians who pass through this basic test are not of uniform quality, and their skills levels are likely to diverge further with the passage of time. An entry control is just too crude and incomplete to displace case-by-case malpractice litigation.

A second stage of licensing, however, involves the revocation or suspension of licenses for physicians who do not continue to meet the practice standards of the profession. These disciplinary proceedings are met with fierce resistance in individual cases. It is generally agreed that strong defense wins out over tentative offense,[13] so that short of drug or alcohol use or serious misconduct, discipline does not weed out unqualified physicians.[14] Informal means (referrals and the like) may be more effective. Patients have little incentive to report physicians to supervisory boards—what's in it for them? Not unnaturally, physicians find it distasteful to sit, often without compensation, on disciplinary panels for friends and associates and to expose themselves to potential suits for tort damages.[15]

THE HEALTH CARE QUALITY IMPROVEMENT ACT OF 1986

Aims and Objectives   The current system of liability and discipline also fails to generate information that follows individual physicians, who today are able to start over fresh in some other location. If a hospital disciplines a physician, its main incentive is to remove him from the staff, not to pursue him to the ends of the earth. But its limited interests leave others at risk if these physicians are hired elsewhere without full knowledge of their background history. To economize on these substantial transactions costs, in the Reagan years, Congress passed the Health Care Quality Improvement Act of 1986 (HCQIA)[16] to help disseminate the information from malpractice litigation and disciplinary proceedings.[17]

Under HCQIA, the Secretary of the HHS[18] set up an information clearinghouse, the National Practitioner Data Bank (NPDB), to gather information about the competence and performance of individual physicians and other health care providers. Consistent with its basic purpose, all settlements and judgments in medical malpractice cases must reported to HHS. The report must contain the name of the physicians charged, together with a statement of the amount paid, the affiliated institutions, and the key acts or omissions that were the basis of the action.[19] In addition, State Medical Examining Boards must report various licensure actions—probation, suspension, revocation, reprimand, and reinstatement—taken with respect to an individual physician.[20] Similarly hospital discipline boards must report the outcomes of investigations and settlements that deny or limit the clinical privileges of individual physicians.[21] The NPDB then makes this information available on a routine basis to state licensing boards.[22] All hospitals must check this registry before hiring a new physician, and they must check the NPDB for current mental and dental staff on a periodic (two-year) basis. In addition, they may check with the NPDB at any time.[23] HCQIA does not state what a hospital or licensing board is supposed to do with the information once it is acquired, but hiring or retaining a physician without checking the record can open the institution up to a medical malpractice action. The hospital that does not request this information when it is available "is presumed to have knowledge of [it]" for (it appears) any and all purposes.[24]

HCQIA's manifest purpose is to compel the dissemination of information of bad news that physicians would like to keep dark. The statute denies public access to these files once the information is assembled. But why limit its use? Even if individuals cannot process the information sensibly, consumer groups and other watchdogs can; and if they misuse or misstate the information, others can still check back against the original records or, in extreme cases, sue the users of that information for defamation or misrepresentation. It is awkward to insist that the risk of misinterpretation is so great that the information should only have selective distribution. However, given the likelihood of error, it is also risky to spread it around as well. A tough call.

Yet with all this said, the dissemination is no better than the information that it contains. HCQIA thus multiplies the influence of any disciplinary investigation or medical malpractice action by making it a permanent part of a physician's employment record. If that information is unreliable, its broad propagation serves only to magnify the severity of the original error. With high levels of error in medical malpractice litigation, and major variations in standards across region, and perhaps across cases, neither a jury determination of liability, nor a settlement short of liability gives reliable information about physician competence. The results of disciplinary proceedings should probably be accorded somewhat greater weight. But on balance, the result is probably the best that can be hoped for: suppression of unpleasant information is probably worse than allowing its full dissemination.

The reporting requirement under HCQIA also influences the way initial disputes are settled. Before the Act, the stakes in any disciplinary proceeding were, at a guess, roughly the same for the institution and the physician. Afterwards, one side of the balance changes because now the physician has something extra to lose from an adverse termination: his bad record will now travel with him throughout his career. At the same time, the institution has no greater interest in discipline than before. That change in relative stakes should lead physicians to contest charges more vigorously than before, which should in turn reduce the number of cases that an institution is prepared to bring and reduce the percentage of cases with findings and sanctions adverse to the physician. It, therefore, becomes more convenient for institutions to let physicians quit and to make bland assurances that service during employment was satisfactory. In addition, we should expect physicians to insist on a larger control of the defense of medical malpractice litigation because they now bear greater collateral consequences to their reputations and employment prospects, even if their employer or insurer covers all the financial costs of the suit. The willingness to settle should diminish and proceedings should on average be more drawn out. It is not clear what will happen to the reliability of the result.

Whatever the doubts, however, it appears that utilization of the system is high. In its first year of operation (September 1990 to August 1991), the NPDB reported 1,968 licensure actions, 790 clinical privilege actions, and 11,721 medical malpractice reports. About 782,000 queries were made of the system of which about 6,500 resulted in a "match" that turned up adverse information about the individual in question. About 10 percent of the reports were disputed by individual physicians, and of these, less than 1 percent required formal intervention by HHS. It is not clear what percentage of these inquiries were made on a discretionary basis and which were required. Nor is there any clear knowledge of whether the information was put to good use. Nonetheless, as government initiatives go, this one seems more promising than most.

Privilege   The judges and juries who decide medical malpractice cases are protected from suit by an absolute privilege. The sole remedy of the disappointed litigation against a miscarriage of justice is an appeal.[25] The use of disciplinary hearings in lieu of medical malpractice suits brings the question of privilege to the fore because private bodies of this sort usually receive only a qualified privilege against suit. That protection is extended for the obvious reason that no individual will serve on such a panel if exposed to suit by the disappointed physicians subject to discipline.

The work product of these panels is, however, no better than the individuals who compose them, so one could ask whether this qualified privilege is sufficient for the task, or whether the same absolute privilege from suit accorded judges and juries (and for that matter all participants in a trial) should be carried over to the nongovernmental systems of adjudication relied on in disciplinary proceedings. In my view, the absolute immunity should be extended to these administrative proceedings, as was frequently done more than a generation ago.[26] Yet the reluctance to extend absolute immunity beyond the official sphere derives from one conspicuous and unmistakable cost: malicious individuals can now profit from their own lies. More recent decisions have therefore limited public officials to qualified privileges that allow suits for false and malicious conduct.[27] From there it is an easy step to conclude that individuals who are not hemmed in by the official sanctions can receive no greater privilege.

The crude empirical judgment of someone deeply suspicious of government—me—is that the absolute privilege is critical to protect those who act *in good faith* from being hauled into court. A simple privilege against suits for negligence will do little good in disciplinary settings when all deliberative sanctions are so easily characterized as malicious. Every report *to* a public official or disciplinary body and every decision made *by* a public official or disciplinary body will contain damaging statements. All witnesses and decision makers know of the explosive nature of their charges. A qualified privilege that allows suits for malice only may work for automobile accidents or even for medical malpractice cases, where instances of deliberate wrongs are so unusual and difficult to sustain. But within the deliberative and testimonial realms, that qualified privilege affords little security. No iron wall separates knowledge from intention, or intention from malice, at least with the clarity that will support summary judgments for defendants. Preliminary litigation over the scope of privilege question imposes a tremendous cost in both time and emotional energy, not to mention hard dollars. Financial insurance, even if complete, covers only out-of-pocket expenses; it does not make a panel member indifferent to being sued.

If these disciplinary bodies were created by the state, I would accord them the same absolute privilege given to judges and juries. But a prolonged discussion of the ultimate virtues of this system is hardly necessary because the case for an absolute privilege is stronger with practicing physicians disciplined by their hospital boards than it is for citizens brought before some public tribunal against their will. The absolute privilege will simply be one of the terms in the standard physician contract. The necessity for decision is thus recognized in advance by the persons who appear before these bodies. Defamation of strangers is as much a tort as is trespass, and one for which the usual mechanism of self-defense—counter the false speech with the truth—is often inadequate, given that a lie travels more rapidly than the truth. The same can be said for the various torts of combination and interference with trade, especially by questionable means.

Physicians and hospitals, however, stand in direct relation to each other from the beginning. They can defend against the charges in the forum in which they are made, so that counterspeech is a more effective weapon than it is in stranger contexts. The individuals to whom the statements are made are under a duty to check their truthfulness, and they will hear other witnesses who can comment on any previous testimony. False statements before these bodies carry risks, of which punishment for perjury is only one, for the people who make them; reputational losses from making false charges are likely to be even greater. The institutional setting thus provides an extra layer of protection that is missing in stranger cases.

Given this background, if employment contracts require physicians to waive a right of action against members of disciplinary boards, so be it. If the calculations made about the leakiness of the qualified privilege are correct, these will be reflected in the standard contract terms. To be sure, this absolute privilege may be hedged by limitations that require a preliminary investigation before proceedings are begun or that require certain procedural safeguards. The hospitals that create absolute immunity for themselves and their staff may have to make still further accommodations to attract staff in the competitive marketplace. Again, so be it. The contract mechanism, applied institution by institution, will outperform any public rule, given the greater knowledge and the better incentives available to them. There is, moreover, no necessity that all institutions reach the same conclusion. Local knowledge could easily justify local variations that would be difficult, if not impossible, to explain to outsiders.

This approach is foreclosed, however, by the conventional wisdom that sees contract as the tool of oppression and exploitation. HCQIA does not so much as mention the contract approach, but instead adopts, as a matter of public policy, its own form of immunity to complement its information gathering function. The basic provision states that members of professional review bodies "shall not be liable in damages" for their actions as board members,[28] but it rightly allows a correction of findings if warranted on the evidence. The unanswered question is whether other forms of suit could overrun the immunity created by the statute. Civil rights claims for discrimination are not precluded by the section, and although private antitrust actions may not be brought against panel members, as was possible before the Act,[29] those serving on panels are still at risk for suits brought by the United States or by the Attorney General of any particular state.[30] Finally, the protection can be lost if the procedures themselves are regarded as deficient under the circumstances,[31] or if there is some question as to whether "reasonable efforts were made to obtain the facts of the matter."[32] The full set of complex provisions reads like Swiss cheese, but it is unclear whether the legal compromise makes business sense relative to the simpler and more secure absolute privilege.

Beyond Discipline   One difficulty with disciplinary proceedings is that they are limited to cases of misconduct. They do not give any systematic overview of the effectiveness of routine treatment that does not flout ordinary misconduct standards. These variations in outcomes above the mischief level cannot be reached either by malpractice actions or disciplinary procedures, but require some systematic form of periodic review that is not triggered by public scandal or patient complaint.

There is every reason to believe that there are enormous differences in the level of productivity, however defined, of individuals who operate well above any malpractice threshold. What is the overall level of performance, given the book of business? How accurate is diagnosis over a class of cases? What is the cost per unit of care? The quality of the care delivered? Lost time in hospital? Unnecessary surgery? Because these variables are measured solely to determine future practice patterns, the focus is on overall effectiveness with an eye toward *business* decisions over personnel and organizational structure. This approach seems to offer greater gains in quality control and thus goes far beyond the information contained in the NPDB. Major quality assurance companies are already in operation, and these market players should be able to assemble more extensive databases at lower cost than any government registry that limits the kind of information collected and the purposes for which it can be used.

NO-FAULT INSURANCE

The last major proposal for malpractice reform would replace negligence liability with a system of no-fault insurance that the state organizes and sponsors.[33] The ostensible exemplar of this approach is the workers' compensation system,[34] which basically covers all accidents and occupational diseases arising out of and in the course of employment, without regard to the employer's negligence or the contributory negligence of the individual employee. Plans of this sort have been on the table for over a generation, but adopted nowhere, either by legislation or by contract, with the sole exception of their limited use for certain obstetrical injuries. Their basic idea is that negligence rules should be displaced by some form of (limited) compensation scheme for all injuries arising out of and in the course of medical treatment, again without regard to physician or patient negligence.

The strengths and weaknesses of these plans have been covered elsewhere, so it is only necessary to explain why these plans have encountered such widespread skepticism even though workers' compensation is in place throughout the United States. The explanation lies not in the broad linguistic parity between the two systems but in the details of their operations. Workplace accidents rarely require the infliction of one harm in order to avoid a second. The path to safety lies in institutional procedures that keep individual workers out of harm's way or protect them adequately when undertaking dangerous tasks. The financial pressures to develop powerful risk control mechanisms independent of the compensation system are very great because employers have to pay handsome risk premiums to attract workers to dangerous lines of work. In most industries, therefore, the compensation system is stable because the number of serious injuries is small relative to the wage base. The exceptions only arise when the compensation net is spread too wide, as when it covers ordinary diseases of life (for example, heart attacks) that may not be work related, or psychological illnesses ostensibly brought on by bad working conditions.[35]

The medical no-fault system has none of these favorable features. All forms of surgery and chemotherapy deliberately inflicted some harm on a patient to forestall greater harms. In this environment, the *frequency* of compensable events under any broad no-fault principle would be very high relative to the levels of patient care. It is quite inconceivable to require payment for the routine harms from surgical or medical treatment. It is also quite unnecessary to provide any. The in-kind benefits from medical treatment provide all the compensation that is needed. These benefits have no direct parallel in the employment setting.

The illustration of routine injury from surgery and drugs alone persuades just about everyone that a no-fault system for medical accidents has to be more narrowly conceived than its now-distant relation is for industrial accidents. But how does the necessary narrowing of the principle take place? No single form of words can do the trick. It is surely not sufficient to say that severe side effects of ordinary surgery or treatment should be covered but that smaller ones should not. The frequency and severity of these side effects would close every cancer clinic and cardiac surgical unit in the country. So the new definition of the compensation event must stress something untoward or unexpected about the outcome, a definition that itself leaves a great deal to the imagination and one that slides by degrees into garden variety negligence. It is for just this reason, for example, that the New Zealand no-fault scheme defines "Personal injury by accident" to cover "Medical, surgical, dental, or first-aid misadventure."[36] And the judicial explication of that term stresses "that unexpected and abnormal consequences may follow to a greater or less degree depending upon the simplicity or sophistication of the treatment being undertaken." With that said, "the normal range of medical or surgical failure" no longer counts as a misadventure. The court then found coverage because the defendant physicians did not close off the plaintiff's fallopian tubes because of "a mechanical and remediable fault."[37] In medical cases, the shift from fault to no-fault amounts to changes in terminology, not in operative standards.

The same analysis applies to another common class of malpractice actions that do not translate easily into a no-fault world: missed diagnosis, which, if made in a timely fashion, could have increased the probabilities of survival. These lost chance cases make sense within a negligence framework because only a missed diagnosis can trigger liability, namely, those where the diagnosis could have been made with reasonable care.[38] But once the negligence element is removed from the case, any visit to a physician that results in the nondiagnosis of a subsequent condition could trigger the no-fault liability. The failure to detect a single cancer cell would be culpable under the statute, although not in ordinary discourse. So even the most thoroughgoing defenders of the no-fault principle recognize that "it is not possible to design a system for pure no-fault-compensation," lest all missed diagnosis cases are compensable.[39]

Once these exceptions are recognized, what virtue attaches to a hybrid system in which some compensable losses require proof of negligence whereas others do not? The mixed signals will, if anything, reduce the capacity of the liability system to inform other physicians and the public at large about the significance of adverse judgments. The rational patient should not be troubled if a courageous surgeon is hit by a heavy no-fault judgment in the course of a difficult treatment. But that same patient should react very differently to a botched procedure that results in early death. Because one system awards equal judgments in both cases, no one can draw easy inferences from liability to performance, thus undercutting the available information on physician performance. In the end, the demands of the subject show that the broad no-fault formula that works with industrial accidents does not carry over here. That result should come as no surprise. Workers' compensation for industrial accidents started in voluntary programs—the precise path down which no medical institution or insurance company is prepared to travel.

The inability to frame broad definitions of compensable events blocks off only one possible no-fault approach. It does not, however, prevent the implementation of a system that supplies no-fault coverage by preparing a long and comprehensive list of the types of adverse events that will trigger payment for each individual operation and procedure. Unfortunately, with the change in focus a different set of difficulties intervene. Medicine moves too rapidly for a single list to last one year, let alone a decade; and the truly big cases often have no obvious precedent and thus could be left off the lists entirely. The tasks of keeping the list up to date and finding agreement as to the class of compensable events impose heavy costs of decision for disputes that might never come to a head. So to the spotty nature of the coverage, we have to add a new set of heavy front-end administrative costs just to get the program up and running, long before any assessment can be made of its practical efficacy.

These tight definitions of compensable events under a no-fault system face a second set of practical difficulties familiar to workers' compensation cases, but which assume a far greater role here. The proof of injury does not end a causal inquiry—someone still has to determine whether this injury arose from physician care. A heart attack that occurs on the job could easily be attributed to the stress of a recent divorce or a death in the family. Conversely a heart attack at home could easily be attributed to exhaustion after a major business negotiation. It is just these difficulties of causation that prompted the designers of the early voluntary plans to limit coverage to "personal injury by accidents," thereby excluding broad disease classes with multicausal origins. The same difficulty arises with adverse medical outcomes as well, which is why the New Zealand plan kept the "personal injury by accident" language and excluded from coverage diseases and medical accidents not attributable to misadventure. Bad outcomes do not have distinct pedigrees. All sorts of conditions and diseases have genetic, traumatic, or environmental causes, so that it is speculation to assume that a heart attack or case of cerebral palsy was induced by the flawless (or even flawed) performance of a surgeon or anesthesiologist, let alone which.

It is in this context that the crude logic of the negligence system takes on added weight. Although causation might not separate medical from nonmedical injuries, the line between customary and substandard care might. Thus, in the stranger cases, physical causation (hitting, setting traps, and the like) weeds out most frivolous suits; but in medical settings, causation cannot do that job. Only a negligence standard can keep the number of litigated cases down to acceptable and measurable levels. Because this negligence standard also has some deterrent and hence efficiency justification, it is not open to the objection that all its costly functions can be discharged by a system of first-party compensation. The bottom line, therefore, is that analogies across no-fault systems do not survive a closer examination of their institutional detail. But this is not to offer a defense of the status quo. It is to make the more limited, but important claim, that the workers' compensation variation of strict liability fails for medical injuries. Doctors fear it; lawyers don't quite understand it; and patients are puzzled by it. Not a winning combination.

Every general proposition gives birth to at least one exception. In this instance, it is the Virginia Injured Infant Act, a no-fault statute whose coverage formula reads as follows:

> Birth-related neurological injury means injury to the brain or the spinal cord of an infant caused by the deprivation of oxygen or mechanical injury occurring in the course of labor, delivery or resuscitation in the immediate post-delivery period in a hospital which renders the infant permanently motorically disabled and (i) developmentally disabled or (ii) for infants sufficiently developed to be cognitively evaluated, cognitively disabled.[40]

The law allows physicians and hospitals unilaterally to opt into the statutory plan without, it appears, disclosing their decision to their patients. The statute also bars the traditional medical malpractice action for accidents that fall under this definition of "birth-related neurological injuries." In its stead comes a compensation program administered by the state Industrial Commission, which is normally charged with handling workers' compensation claims. In any damages action before that body, recovery is limited to medical expense plus lost earnings on reaching maturity, calculated at 50 percent of the state's average weekly wage. The program allows no recovery for pain and suffering, and payments from collateral sources reduce the compensation award, dollar for dollar.[41] Funding for the plan comes from a $5,000 annual charge against participating physicians; a $50 charge per delivery to all hospitals, with provision for supplemental funding from other physicians; and from general insurance carriers, even those that write no medical malpractice insurance.[42]

The plan was implemented in response to the crushing verdicts that were sometimes handed down in medical malpractice cases for this sort of birth-related neurological injury. The plan has been in operation for about six years, and the most apparent feature is a paradox: the number of paid claims under the statute appears to be very small—around three or four—yet the state actuaries have required additional funds to be placed into the plan today to offset the risk of insolvency tomorrow. As best we can figure out,[43] the key to this paradox lies in the word "permanently." As drafted, the statutory award is not set once and for all by the infant's status at birth. Instead the word "permanently" has been read to suggest that if an injured infant outgrows the bad conditions at birth, he will then be allowed bring an ordinary medical malpractice law action for the injuries suffered, including those that would have been covered by statute if the plaintiff's condition had never improved. Claims under the Injured Infants Act and ordinary malpractice claims may be brought until age 18, so many lawyers adopt a wait and see attitude, and for good reason. An immediate claim under the Injured Infants Act yields low damages, nothing for pain and suffering, and the big setoff for collateral damages. If the condition remains unchanged, tort damages are available in larger numbers; and if not, claims for compensation are still timely.

Under this view, the potential liabilities for both medical malpractice and statutory damages seem considerable. Yet at the same time, because claims cannot be either deferred or revived, the statute blocks suits for infants who have died at or shortly after birth. For the claims that remain, however, compensation under either tort or no-fault is far from guaranteed because the causation hurdle must be overcome, albeit years after the initial incident took place. In both systems, the physician or hospital can defend on the ground that the injury was *not* "caused by the deprivation of oxygen or mechanical injury occurring in the course of labor, delivery or resuscitation" but rather that it originated in either some neurological or drug-induced condition. In the medical malpractice arena, all the negligence defenses are available as well.

The entire system could only be justified because it cleanses the system of unmeritorious claims against physicians or hospitals. Erroneous recoveries serve neither the end of deterrence nor that of corrective justice. The situation could be corrected, at least in part, by a shorter statute of limitations to control the waiting game, but even that reform leaves untouched the refusal to award compensation for deaths attributable to physician negligence. The Virginia statute has had more than its fair share of unintended consequences. It is hardly a model for a more comprehensive statutory reform.

CONTRACT

The rejection of the no-fault alternative thus sets the stage for a return to the contract solution so unceremoniously banished from public discussion more than 30 years ago. The key benefits of that system should be more apparent in light of the failed alternatives. As a theoretical matter, the strongest defense of voluntary contracts is that they work to the mutual benefit of both sides. Any informational deficits can be handled with disclosure, which could be made routinely by written materials and oral discussions, and supervised (perhaps) by a tort liability for informed consent. The rights of infants and incompetents could be protected not by state decree, but by allowing guardians to represent their wards on all aspects of the doctor-patient relationship, including compensation for adverse events, subject only to the standard duties of loyalty and fair play. These cases do not present difficult external harms questions found, say, when two individuals wish to take the property of a third; nor do they involve any difficult collective action problems in the funding of public goods, such as national defense or civil peace. Ordinary liability cases are issues where the basic logic of contracting works well.

Some intensely practical reasons also support the use of contract to handle liability. Virtually every reform—from low-level tinkering to the creation of alternative compensation systems—raises tricky issues of cost and effectiveness. Yet no academic and no government agency can acquire the information necessary to make these judgments at the wholesale level. Nor can they update the previously acquired information to respond to changes in the composition of their target population, in medical technology, in moral sensibility, or in legal practice. Every reform inspires debates over what will happen and whether that happening is desirable. In the end, these matters turn on playing the "edges," on making marginal adjustments.

When all is said and done, the true strengths of markets are not found in the formal models that show how perfect competitive markets yield the optimal outcomes in the best of all possible worlds. Rather, they are found in the arena in which markets are so frequently attacked: what should be done when information is imperfect and asymmetrical. Now someone has the incentive to collect the needed information and to turn it to his own advantage. If one system of liability rules outperforms another, others can imitate the successful system and disregard the other. In contrast to state regulation, if one system works well for low-income clinics and another works well for high-tech research institutions, the two groups can go their separate ways. Neither will be forced into a procrustean bed ill suited to its needs. If one clinic has needs that differ from those of a second, it can tailor its rules to take into account those differences. So, too, with research institutions. Variations in response are thus possible both within and across classes. And if none of these variations is adopted, we can be confident that the single solution that does emerge has prevailed because it works better than its rivals, and not for any extraneous or parochial reason. Over and over again, regulation, whether of judicial or legislative origin, always rests on the implicit assumption that one size fits all, and that some bureaucrat knows which size that is. The far better result is one that is agnostic to both issues. There should be no preconceptions on the uniformity of needed terms nor on what those terms should be. The information generated by uncoordinated institutions will fill that gap more quickly and more authoritatively than any academic study.

In reply, it could be said, no commentator should be allowed to stand above the fray. Rather, some hint might be made as to what arrangements will be adopted when people are allowed to take the law into their own hands and to fashion voluntary agreements under which care will be supplied. Paul Weiler takes the view that these contracts will inevitably lead to a complete release from all liability for accidental harms, including harms caused by all forms of negligence. That pattern has been observed in the past, and perhaps the past is a prologue to the future.[44] In his view, once a patient is offered a lower price for reduced legal protection, the outcome is sealed, no matter how much regret comes after the fact.

A more optimistic and more accurate view of the situation suggests otherwise. Any change in the terms of medical liability will not be a casual affair, but will (so long as contracts are secure) be decided at the highest levels within the firm. The standard contract will not be sprung on a patient at the last moment, but it will evolve from genuine deliberation between suppliers of health care and their major customers. Individual consumers are not ideal candidates to take the lead position in negotiating these arrangements. That role will in all likelihood fall on intermediates: employers groups, unions, and health care plans of all sorts. The chances that these parties will move reflexively to a simple solution of no liability is remote if both sides have something to gain from preserving some limited form of liability. In an age of competitive health care, it is not sufficient for a firm to limit liability after injury, at the back end. It is also necessary to induce groups and individual patients to enter the system at the front end. A simple reform could be to substitute enforceable arbitration arrangements for litigation. That one reform could reduce the delays in claim resolution by taking cases out of the judicial queues. It could stabilize outcomes by removing some of the unwanted variation that comes from jury selection. It could simplify the rules of evidence, thereby reducing the cost of litigation. Even without any stated substantive change, the entire range of outcomes could shift, and shift for the better.

It hardly follows that the only possible changes are procedural. A standard contract could adhere to the standard of customary care and then give some content to the term by specifying the decision rule when technology is rapidly shifting or when a genuine dispute arises as to the proper mode of attack. Likewise, damage awards could be subject to formula limitations including those that are less crude than the simple caps now introduced in some states. After all, if the level of trust in decision makers increases, more complicated formulas become viable.[45]

Now suppose that *none* of these reforms is adopted by any key institutional players. That, too, supplies us with information. It suggests that the deterrence does not work in the context of case-by-case judgments, even with arbitration. But the message also has a positive side. A broad consensus has formed around the proposition that tort litigation does not yield reliable measures of medical malpractice. If so, we should expect interested parties to redouble their efforts to measure quality of care in other ways. One reason why malpractice actions could be left quiescent is that these methods yield better information, not only about the occasional bad cases, but about the routine levels in cases that do not come close to malpractice territory. So long as institutions are involved in providing medical services, they can and will develop brand-name reputations to secure their position in the market. Various employer and consumer groups can rank institutions on everything from user friendliness to surgical outcomes, and they can do so without legal intervention.

Action is also possible at the individual level. When people move into a new town, they can ask their neighbors and coworkers who is a good physician. When people are ill, they talk to others who have had experience with doctors and institutions, and they learn from what they hear. In more recent years, they can consult special bulletins on the Internet to share information with other persons in similar situations. They can also resort to the services of internists or general practitioners who can run interference inside large organizations. If subject to chronic illnesses, they often obtain a general mastery of the field and become in some cases involved in charitable activities that give further clues as to what has happened. Less energetic, intelligent, or well-situated people can free-ride on the decisions of others.

This assemblage of information is somewhat haphazard, and surely it is not completely reliable. But it would be a mistake for any armchair thinker to assume that people who face serious health problems choose to remain ignorant when knowledge is at hand. It is the knowledge of repeat players in the system that stamps its character, not the knowledge of those who rarely avail themselves of its services. In light of these features, perhaps we might be better off in a world with reduced costs and enhanced access, even if liability is sharply curtailed or totally eliminated. Recall the high costs of running the malpractice system and the low level of payouts and reliability it yields. I don't know for certain whether this is the case; nor does anyone else. Although that ignorance is fatal to any program of direct regulation, it best explains why we need open markets, with fully enforceable contracts, no ifs, ands, or buts, to find the best levels of legal protection against adverse medical outcomes.

Weaving Access and Choice Together

The health care business constitutes now nearly one-seventh of the national economy. The issues canvassed throughout this book run the length of that vast enterprise, but in the end they do converge on a common theme. The grand task for all legal and social institutions is to try to find some way to arrange for human affairs to secure the largest net benefit to the public at large. It is not to serve the provincial or parochial ends of any one group, however discrete and powerful. Rights in this regard are instruments of human well-being, not ends in themselves. The rights and duties that are created in any part of the legal system should mesh with those created elsewhere. Health care is not special, so that proposition holds true with the questions of access and choice that have dominated this book.

So the two themes come together. Speak about matters of self-determination, and they all depend in part of the resource base that is available to persons within the health care system. The issue of organ transplantation deals with the question of scarcity every bit as much as the question of comprehensive care. Any person who worries about the proper rules for death and dying must ask whether physicians and families might be induced to cut short the lives of the sick and defenseless in order to save on costs that the system must otherwise spend. The prolonged debate over liability for medical accidents may appear directed to problems of risk allocation for accidents, but it also impinges on critical issues of access. Institutions—public or private, profit-making or charitable—that cannot find ways to fund their potential liabilities will have to shut their doors, excluding those who benefit from the services.

What then is the ideal mix of access and choice? On this the dominant wisdom is to impose all sorts of misguided limitations in the domain of choice, and then to look for external sources of funding to pay for the added costs. If it turns out that a rural health clinic cannot pay its medical malpractice premiums, we should increase its budget allocation from the state to make good the shortfall. No one thinks that it should be allowed to condition access to its services on a waiver of the right to sue. But today's dominant approach will not do in the long run. The increased tax revenues have to come from somewhere, and the unobserved contraction in economic activities counts as a real cost, even if it is hidden from public view. How large it is may be difficult to compute or demonstrate, but we should not lull ourselves into the happy conclusion that costs are small because they are indirect. No one can identify the new drugs that have not been developed because of the high cost of complying with FDA regulations. But no one should assume that the problem does not exist because the smoking gun cannot be found. Health care raises similar issues. The desirable transactions that do not take place are not easily recorded, but their loss should be entered on the overall social ledger.

Today's dominant approach seeks first to limit choice and then to subsidize access. A second path links choice and access in a different way. We should strive to lower the costs of running a health care system. Once costs are down, access will increase not by state decree, but in accordance with the usual economic principle that the lower the cost for a given service, the higher the demand. Folks will come back into the marketplace because they know that the bargains that they reach will not be blown out of the water by legislative decree or judicial fiat. The change here is a radical one in orientation. It allows people, for example, to contract out of medical malpractice liability. And it speaks against mandated items of coverage for given procedures, or against legislative initiatives that require certain stays in hospital for certain procedures, such as the recent statutes to require minimum two-day hospital stays in obstetric cases. Both parts of this program contemplate less government control, not more.

It is easy—perhaps, too easy—for academics to make proposals for major structural reforms that link choice and access in this way. But before dismissing this new approach, we should remember that in the world of public affairs, academics occupy a very different niche from business managers. Our job is to describe and prescribe, and to show how the descriptions we give support the prescriptions that we propose. The tools of legal and economic analysis are designed to outline the structure of the rules of the game. They are not a manual of how to play the game or a prediction of the particular outcomes that will follow once the rules of the game have been redefined. But to anyone who is impatient with the general direction of health care delivery in the United States and elsewhere, the obvious challenge is this: If you're so smart, why don't you try your hand at running the system yourself?

A fair invitation, but one that should be declined, and for good reason. Part one of that answer stems from a respect for the division of labor. The comparative advantage of the academic perch is its ability to describe the global consequences that will follow from the choice of the rules of the game. Those conclusions depend largely on abstract considerations of how incentives shape the conduct of individuals who are primarily, but not exclusively, interested in advancing their own self-interest. From that lofty perch, it is possible to indicate how certain private behavior will have adverse social consequences for the group, and to indicate what realignment of incentives is likely to reduce (but never eliminate) the tendencies to undertake asocial behavior.

The set of skills involved in management are vastly different, and, if anything, more difficult to master. The successful manager starts from the assumption that the dike contains three holes, for which only two plugs, which don't quite fit, are available. The name of that game is to decide which plug should be placed in which hole at what time. Victory in the game never depends on keeping water from flowing through the dike. It depends on keeping the rate of flow low enough so that productive activity does not sink below the waves. The constant theme is working the tradeoffs that are implicit in all decisions. Given that the currency of the realm is not cold cash, but a set of intangibles (good will, morale, and wear and tear) which are difficult to estimate but crucial to estimate correctly; how much of this activity do we want to exchange for how much of that? Making the wrong choices could result in an aggregation of small errors that allow the flow to swamp the ship. Making the right choices keeps the freight dry above the waterline. But the size of the holes are not constant, the plugs wear out, and new plugs are manufactured and found.

The solutions that work today may not work tomorrow. The task is to have the wisdom and courage to know when and how to change doing business. Getting it right depends on the kind of local knowledge that Hayek praised, and which is acquired only through experience, hunch, and analogy. The academic who wants to leave it to the market to decide makes that recommendation on impersonal grounds. He is sometimes the last person anyone would choose to be that market actor.

That level of dynamic is surely at work in the health care scene in the United States. Side by side with the balky and erratic legal and regulatory developments is a visible and massive revolution in the trenches. The day-to-day delivery of medical services has been greatly transformed in the last ten—make that five—years. The sole-practitioner who provides medical care from a suite of offices on a fee-for-service basis has not become extinct and will always occupy some select segment of the market. But the signal development in medicine has been the coming of age of managed care or group practice. Managed care has been defined roughly as a system that "integrates the financing and delivery of medical care through contracts with selected physicians and hospitals that provide comprehensive health care services to enrolled members for a predetermined monthly premium."[1] Managed care plans covered about 10 million people in 1976; that number reached close to 35 million in 1990, crossed 50 million enrollees in 1995, and may double yet again in the next five or so years.[2] Even these numbers understate the rate of transformation of medical care because, in addition to hard core managed care organizations, a veritable array of physician networks and preferred provider groups have mushroomed over the past years, each competing for a niche of the ever more competitive market—which is just as it should be.

The movement to managed care has not been regret-free. The traditional doctor-patient relationship was predicated in theory on the sense of individualized commitment to patient welfare. In its most ideal vision, the physician was more than a dispenser of medicine and a master of procedure. The physician understood how to take a case history of the person, not the ailment; to empathize with a patient; and to attend to psychological needs that interconnected with specific treatment choices. The dominant paradigm in today's medical schools still celebrates this form of individualized patient care, but the ever larger units into which physicians old and young are drawn march to different imperatives that depend less on empathy and more on economics.

Some brutal truths dominate medical practice in the modern marketplace. First, medicine can actually do some good in crisis situations. Let a patient subject to an acute illness or injury make it through the next 48 hours in the ICU and he can make it through the next 40 years. But for most healthy individuals, medical interventions are both mercifully infrequent and regrettably costly. Only a tiny sliver of the population has at its command the liquid assets needed to pay for major hospitalization and physician services. Most certainly, they do not have Medicare to back them up. Trying to save for a rainy day helps, but it does not cure the problem. For the "lucky," disease and accident may strike after funds put aside for 30 years have grown into a sizable nest egg. Yet for some, accident and disease hit far earlier in the cycle. Insurance, not savings, is the only mechanism to cope with the risk.

True to form, insurance brings new complications of its own. It is easy for insureds to spend other people's money. It is easy for physicians to assist them achieve that lofty end by lavishing endless care on patients who are willing to endure the inconvenience and pain of treatment. Some system of deductibles and copayments could dampen the enthusiasm for additional treatment, but the verdict is now in. Standing alone, these financial devices do not do the job. A system that leaves most of the financial risk on the insurer and places most of the business discretion in the hands of the physician and patient is a system headed for a fiscal crash.

Enter cost control devices of one sort of another. The price today of insurance is that the provider dictates the patterns of coverage and supervises the provision of services in exchange for lower premiums. It need not be that way for people who want to pay $1,000, $2,000 or $5,000 extra for medical services per year. But that kind of money is just not in the budget of the typical American family with an income of under $40,000. So, when faced with the choice between cash savings and individualized services, the typical patient picks cash savings.

The choice has real consequences, many of which are beneficial. Managed care companies are quite quick to note all the advantages that come out of a system of managed care.[3] Unnecessary care is not just something that takes time. It is something that poses an inevitable risk to every patient placed under anesthesia for surgery. Yet there is lots of it, and the problem may well be exacerbated by the traditional doctor-patient relationship. If payment depends on doing risky procedures, more of these will be done than seem necessary. To the extent that managed care companies can track the success and failure of different protocols, their interests are well aligned with those of their patients. Who can object to saving money while reducing risks of harm?

Managed care operations have another real advantage. In many cases they bond themselves automatically to solid performance. The risk allocation system accounts for the result. The managed care operation that does not detect incipient illness cannot wash its hands of the sick patient. It must treat that patient down the road, using technologies that are not only more risky for the patient but also more expensive for the managed care operation. The organization, therefore, has a powerful incentive to structure its well-patient care to pick up the early signs of future illnesses. Routine pap smears and mammograms will be in its interest in large portions of its patient base. Immunizations against common diseases are encouraged. Yet even here it is important to be careful. The greater the turnover within the network—and turnover rates are around 15 percent—the weaker the incentives for the HMO to provide preventive and diagnostic services for long-term health disabilities. So paradoxically, the less secure the regulatory framework in which they operate, the less satisfactory their performance is likely to be. Yet even with these qualifications, the assumption of risk by the HMO provider will, relative to fee-for-service medicine, increase the likelihood of solid forward-looking care. And the planning element is likely to be stronger with respect to the treatment of HMO physicians. The managed care group that charts its physician competence does not have to rely on the vagaries of the malpractice system to determine the effectiveness of various treatment options. It can track the pattern of illness over time, within a controlled population, and evaluate both physicians and protocol accordingly. Information is power; so the power lies in the system.

Yet it would be a mistake to argue that the use of managed care eliminates all conflicts between patient and physician. No contract could ever achieve that result. It is easy to identify the pressure points in the system. A patient would like an extra day to recover in the hospital, but the plan sends her home. A sick patient wants an experimental treatment that is not offered within the group. Should the group pay an outside specialist to try the procedure even if the chances of its success are minute? Should the group be under an obligation to disclose all the alternatives that are available, even if it will not fund them?[4] Desperate patients will not make dispassionate reckoning of the odds; they will grab at every last opportunity. It is not easy to say no in the moment of crisis even after flagging the potential conflict in the literature that is delivered to patient subscribers. The point has not been lost on HMOs that have inserted the notorious "gag clauses" in their contracts, which, in one form or another, limit the amount of information a doctor may disclose to patients about treatment options that are not covered under the plan. The resistance to these clauses has been widespread—they undermine the traditional fiduciary duty between doctor and patient and they make it harder for patients find out about options for which they might be prepared to pay out of pocket. The torrent of abuse hurled at these gag clauses will not go unheard. The problem of high-cost, low-return, last-ditch treatment will not disappear under any form of health care delivery, and it seems clear that fierce consumer resistance in the marketplace will force modification of crude gag clauses. It is not as though HMOs can open up their checkbooks at the demand of desperate patients, but some system of mediation or arbitration, with or without additional copayments, may be able to meet the challenge. Increased reliance on process to respond to sharp disagreements is common in other business settings, so we should not be surprised to see HMOs evolve in that direction. Here again, it is critical to see these embedded conflicts as costs—heavy costs—but not as fatal blows to the new system of patient care. All contractual arrangements have conflicts of interest. The key question is to choose that system that works best on average.

That mission is thoroughgoing. Once the risk of further treatment is shifted to a managed care operation, it is no longer possible for the patient and physician to conduct their relationship in a void. The physician becomes an employee or part owner of the practice. The accountants search for ways to squeeze out costs while still providing essential services. Old practices and conventions fall by the wayside. With some exaggeration, perhaps, it has been reported that standard office visits in California now take four minutes—hardly time to generate empathy and trust, but enough time to look into a pair of ears or check for a sore throat. Why should we expect otherwise? The soft stuff may work, but its effectiveness is hard to verify. Physicians are paid for the time they spend; their technical training is the expensive input. Their psychological insights can be duplicated by others whose hourly rate is far less. In other businesses, services are unbundled so that high-priced labor does not tarry over tasks that less talented labor can provide. The chief loan officer at a bank does not have to sit behind a teller's window or make $1,000 loans. With time, more and more routine tasks are done by machines. ATMs are one manifestation, but only one. Today, complex computer programs can pass on loan applications in hours instead of days. The real skill is in setting up the mechanism, not in delivering the services in the individual case.

Medicine is not immune from those technological pressures. The advances in technology allow the design at the center of new diagnostic tests that can be applied across the board. The better the test, the less interpretation and evaluation is required. The physician becomes ancillary to the dominant sources of knowledge, and empathetic intuitions are pushed aside by hard data. To have a physician chat with each patient for five minutes out of an hour may not seem like much, but over a year it amounts to a month of time. To allow physicians to order additional tests is to increase the need for space, laboratory technicians, record keeping services, and the like. Indeed, to allow a physician to give *free* care after hours is also expensive, if heat, electricity, insurance, and record keeping are accurately reckoned in the bill. Once again, the managers remind everyone that these collateral costs can never be ignored. In the end, the essential services are both transformed and preserved, but the nature of the doctor-patient relationship will be changed, unless and until it can be shown that the traditional doctor-patient relationship controls costs, detects disease, or both. The process becomes more impersonal, but patients do not leave the system because they value the savings more than they fear the costs. Physicians do not leave the system because the patients will not follow them.

In examining the inexorable cost pressures that drive the system today, we might casually assume that all patients are herded into the same kind of medical arrangements. But that cannot be the case. Different providers seek to occupy different niches to best exploit variations in demand. If an HMO insists that all its enrollees see only its own panel physicians, it runs the risk of defection by patients who want to retain some control over the selection of their primary care physician. The plan whose designers think that fixed-physician panels supply it with market invincibility is a prime candidate for extinction. Open panel practices and looser affiliations might win out with some groups of patients who think that the better service is worth the higher price. But then again it might not. Some groups might obtain reputations for their ability to

weed out physicians that do respond to patient needs. If the levels of satisfaction are high in certain closed plans, they could prosper by offering
a quality guarantee that more open plans cannot in practice match.

Competition is not limited to one dimension. The same process
takes place day after day with each element of the standard contract: the
schedule of benefits, the location and hours of offices, the policies on
specialization and hospitalization, the mailing of news bulletins and
pointers, and the provision of support services, billing practices, and
advertisements. It may be an unyielding constant of modern group practices that residual risks are assumed by providers, not by customers, and
not by their employers. But within that single constraint, it's anyone's
guess as to what plans will succeed, and why. No one should try to pre-
judge the outcome before the race has run its course because they are
likely to be wrong. Just as American government cannot pick out "good"
industries for an "industrial policy" to subsidize, so it cannot pick out the
winning mix of coverage and restraint in health care.

The success of HMOs has been in the marketplace. The vulnerabil-
ity of HMOs has been in both the press and in politics. One strategy is
attack on the operation of HMOs by anecdote. HMOs care for millions
of patients each year. The law of large numbers guarantees some mix-
ups, no matter how sound their overall procedures may be. So find the
anecdote and use it to condemn the system as a whole, without the
slightest concern for the soundness of the sampling procedures. Thus
Bob Herbert, writing in the *New York Times*, titles a recent outburst
against HMOs "Mugged in Hospital."[5] It recounts the conflict between
the treating physician who ordered the patient to stay in hospital after
serious complications from a hysterectomy and the HMO functionary
who refused to pick up the tab after a "concurrent utilization review."

The confrontation is typical of what can happen under capitation.
Yet Herbert's story would have had more punch if the early dismissal
from the hospital had resulted in avoidable harm to the patient, but the
patient did just fine. But even if the story had a bad ending, single coun-
terexamples do not undermine general practices. The ultimate issue must
concern the distribution of outcomes *in aggregate*, a framework in which
the harrowing anecdote becomes but one case among many. From the
position of the patient or firm choosing a health plan, the odds ex ante,
not the isolated horror story, is what drives a sound purchasing decision.
The issue is the alignment of long-term incentives. Yet the persistent

shifts in fundamentals do not stop the flood of recent publications, such as George Anders, *Health Against Wealth: HMOs and the Breakdown of Medical Trust,* whose very title trumpets the conflicts of interest between HMOs and their patients, while overlooking the major ways in which plan and patient interests are in alignment. It is only when that side of the picture is given equal billing that it becomes possible to explain why, for all their flaws, HMOs have grown in size and influence notwithstanding their bad press.

The second line of attack has been through legislation. The launching of this initiative is virtually inevitable in the American setting. There are no constitutional barriers against regulation that limit the imaginations of those who resort to politics to limit or reverse market outcomes. As with every major institutional change, this one has produced a fair share of losers who will try to recapture some of their gains through politics. Physicians, for example, often lose when HMOs insist that they retain complete control over the physicians who join their staffs. The excluded physicians have countered in a number of states by securing the passage of "any willing provider laws" which, when the complexities are stripped away, provide generally that "no hospital, physician or health care provider willing to meet the terms and conditions offered to it or him shall be excluded from the preferred provider arrangement."[6] It is not that the plan has to agree to hire anyone; it just has to agree to work with physicians who are willing to abide by its rules.

The effect of the "any willing provider laws" is to make the health plan work like a common carrier for its physicians. As such, these statutes in effect make it impossible for new health care organizations to determine the shape and scope of their staff. The only protection that they receive is from the requirement that all new physicians meet the standards of those already employed, whether desired or not. The crimp on managerial discretion, however, makes it more difficult to administer the program overall, to manage the way in which cases are handled, to monitor the behavior of all the participating physicians, and to ensure that each physician has a sufficient volume of cases to justify his or her position on the payroll. Such statutes will throw into the courts difficult disputes over whether certain physicians do meet the standards, or are capable of meeting them if given the same kind of training and instruction that are provided to group members. Formal equality in state terms is not the same as equal effectiveness in practice. The law of diminishing returns can take its toll long before the pool of potential physicians is employed, but the statute proceeds as though each additional physician is worth as much to the firm, and its customers, as the one before. Once again we see the violation of the autonomy principle in terms of a mandate for forced professional association. No other business is forced to expand its roster of employees in quite this fashion, and we can be confident that the market process will be sharply slowed down if these statutes continue to proliferate in larger markets.

The attack on managed care also comes from the patient side. Once again anecdotes can drive the case. Many plans have sent mothers home from the hospital shortly after delivery.[7] In some cases, that decision could have been a mistake, but is it one that justifies the "drive-through delivery" laws that have become the recent rage: 26 states have enacted them since 1995, and in 1996 the United States followed suit.[8] These statutes typically require that managed care plans keep newborns and their mothers in the hospital for at least 48 hours after delivery, with 96-hour minimums for cesarean births. The proponents of the bill stressed the sharp reduction in hospital time after births, which decreased for vaginal deliveries from 3.9 to 2.1 days, and from 7.8 to 4 days for cesarean deliveries. It set its norms at the lower edge of normal current practice. However, this exercise pressupposes that the reduction in hospital time should be regarded as further evidence for the deterioration of medical care; it could just as easily be read as a sign of improvement in patient management. To be sure, any overall assessment is likely to be mixed. But lest we harp on the hard cases with poor outcomes, it turns out to be much more difficult to identify some optimum hospital stay after birth[9] or to explain why the state should decide to spend plan resources on this form of care when other kinds of care might yield more payoff for the dollar. The management decisions are systematically placed in the wrong hands, where they are largely immune from correction and modification except by painful legislative deliberation.

Other more comprehensive measures are afoot. In California, about 13 of 32 million people are enrolled in HMOs and similar type plans. The political resistance to these plans has long been intense and on its November 1996 ballot, California residents voted on two union-led propositions, 214 and 216, that promised to alter the relationships between HMOs and their members[9]. Both propositions attacked the heart of the current managed care revolution—the capitation system.

Thus both propositions sought to prohibit HMOs from paying their physicians on a capitation system (so much for each patient treated), on the ground that it is improper to give physicians a financial incentive to skimp on the treatment of their patients. But imperfections come from all directions. Once physicians must be paid, in effect, on a fee-for-service system, all the old conflicts of interest are reintroduced. This makes it problematic for the firm—how can it continue to offer its contract on a capitation system when it is unable to control its own costs? Thus it is perhaps not wholly surprising that both propositions were defeated at the polls, along with a similar measure in Oregon.[10]

Popular referenda are not the only source of potential interference with market behavior. Courtesy of Medicare and Medicaid, the United States is still the largest payor for medical services in the United States, and it has recently flexed its power to limit the fee structures that HMOs can employ in dealing with Medicare and Medicaid patients. Under rules first issued in March of 1996, and effective as of January 1, 1997, the Department of Health and Human Services decreed that no more than 25 percent of a physician's total compensation may be linked to financial incentives for reducing the overall level of services provided.[11] Its public statements in support of that rule illustrate the unwarranted confidence that government officials have in the own ability to fine-tune the delivery of medical services. One the one hand, they could not deny the enormous cost-containment problems that pervade both programs. But that acknowledged, a government spokesman insisted that "We want to ensure that managed care does not limit necessary care, and that patients are not hurt in the process of curtailing costs."[12]

Once again the argument misses its mark. The division between necessary and unnecessary care is not a line, let alone a line etched in stone. It is a continuum, such that there is no way to control costs across the board without denying care in some cases where, all things considered after the fact, one wished it had been supplied. In a world of inevitable error, however, the only relevant question is what institution has the better knowledge to make the relevant tradeoffs and the stronger incentives to adjust the margins correctly in a world where more care comes at higher cost. As best one can tell, HHS plucked its 25 percent figure from the air, without examining the percentage figures found in different plans, many of which are far in excess of that amount. The net effect of the government intervention is to split off Medicare and Medicaid patients from the rest of the consuming public and to induce switches in behavior that might on aggregate cause more mischief than they cure.

Legislative programs of this sort are most conspicuous for their effort to transfer control over HMOs from management to government. That result might be defensible in markets with single suppliers, but it hardly makes sense where alternative providers can and do offer different plans for different segments of the market. There is no need to prescribe terms for firms that operate in competitive markets. All sorts of individuals and groups enter into these HMO contracts having made the decision that the cut in price is worth the reduction in service. Their overt decisions speak more about the soundness of the program, warts and all, than any stated dissatisfaction with the programs in political initiatives launched at them from without. The point is doubly true when much of the opposition to the plans comes not from its customers, but from unions, physicians, nurses, and consumer advocate groups that seek, for their own reasons, to dictate the kinds of care provided to other workers. Job preservation may be a motivation to regulate managed care operations, but hardly a justification. Once again the breach of the autonomy principle in the absence of monopoly has its price.

This last point is critical because the transformation of medicine from an honorable profession to a mass production business invites the obvious retort. If the private provision of medical care has been taken over by corporate America, why fight so hard to limit the role of government service? The similarities are there. As Max Weber pointed out long ago, certain bureaucratic imperatives constrain the options of both governments and businesses. Both are large and impersonal. Both are the work of abstract directives and general principles. Both feature an internal hierarchy that stresses chain of command and stable reporting relationships pegged more to the role than to the person.

Fair enough, but organizations not only have structures, they also have actors and these actors respond to incentives. A government department has a harder time identifying its own bottom line. If it fails to make a profit, it can appeal to the legislature to make the appropriations so desperately needed to carry on work so vital to the community. If its workers mess up, they are protected by a set of civil service procedures that immunize them from responsibility for their own decisions. If they succeed, their promotions chances are limited and their raises are kept within narrow bureaucratic bands.

Most of all, government bureaucrats have a captive audience. The managed care firm that does not perform can be held accountable. Its officers have to explain the firm's losses to a Board of Directors or to a group of disgruntled shareholders. Raiders lurk in the distance to take over ill-managed firms. Individual group members can quit, but more important, large employers' groups can play one plan against another and do so armed with knowledge of price and quality of service that rises above the anecdotal and impressionistic. The similarities in *structure* between private and government operations cannot conceal such palpable differences in *incentives.* The firm that does not give its customers more than it charges them will not have customers for long. Government officials offering tax-subsidized services rarely want for business. The impact on behavior should be clear. We can expect firms to institute cumulative changes, large and small, at an ever more feverish pace. Prices can drop sharply, and service packages can be continually redefined. It is quite amazing what can be done when price changes do not require, as with Medicare, the approval of both houses of Congress.

Yet what of charitable care? In one sense, this juxtaposition is welcome because it completes the circle of analysis. But in a second sense, it is odd, being much out of favor with the temper of the times. Charitable care was a dominant feature of American medicine all the way through the 1950s. It took place in the home office and in the hospital ward. It was rewarded by a set of informal practices that have long since decayed. It seems odd, therefore, to think that it could ever play any significant role in the medical universe of the future. The spring has been stretched so far that it has been bent out of shape, its resilience lost. If it is, some government system of assistance seems to be required to fill the gap where markets, even efficient markets, leave off.

Perhaps the turnaround can take place if given the chance. Hospitals still give out large amounts of charitable care, notwithstanding their obsession with the bottom line. The rise of new technology has not dimmed the ardor of private donors whose attention could perhaps be turned back to patient service and care. Individual physicians may work full time at the managed care facility and still fill in at a storefront operation run by a local church or neighborhood group. No set of private support can hope to match the lavish level of funding that the federal government now delivers. But the hope is that it becomes possible to do more with less. The charitable incentives to economize on care and to pick the right cases to help are insistent and powerful. The medical services could be combined with counseling to reduce the need for utilization. A few well-chosen refusals to help could plant a needed recognition that charities know how to exercise the discretion that they (should) enjoy under law. The sharp contraction of government would be as profound a shift as the rise of managed care, and perhaps more so. We need not assume that all other aspects of the situation will remain unaltered when so big a piece of the puzzle is removed. With time and with conviction, it might just be possible to restore some of the older wisdom that allowed commercial and charitable operations to work side by side.

Our system of state regulation has brought with it a host of unintended consequences, mainly bad. It has brought about a level of dependence that places the welfare of the general population in mortal peril. The evidence of failure and frustration is around us. Perhaps we can understand that the path we need to take reverses the path already taken. How ironic it is that the advances in medicine at the end of the twentieth century have far surpassed any futuristic vision at the end of the nineteenth century. Yet on matters of law and political economy, the reverse has been true. It is ironic that the legal arrangements prized by the reflective nineteenth-century theory of laissez-faire—strong autonomy rights, strong property rights, widespread contractual freedom, and powerful charitable institutions—have proved superior to the more complex legal and administrative edifice that have displaced them. How ironic indeed!

❖   ❖   ❖

ENDNOTES

TABLE OF CASES

INDEX

ENDNOTES

❖　❖　❖

INTRODUCTION

1. See, e.g., Allen Buchanan, "The Right to a Decent Minimum of Health Care," *Phil. & Pub. Affairs* 13 (1984): 54. Norman Daniels, *Just Health Care* (1985).

2. See Einer Elhauge, "Allocating Health Care Morally" *Calif. L. Rev.* 82 (1994): 1452, 1465–66, duly noting but not solving the difficulty.

3. Kenneth J. Arrow, "Uncertainty and the Welfare Economics of Medical Care," *Am. Econ. Rev.* 53 (1963): 941.

4. For the numbers on social security, see Matthew Miller, "Uh-Oh," *The New Republic* (April 15, 1996): 20–26.

5. See, e.g., Robert Nozick, *Anarchy, State and Utopia* (1974): Ch. 7, with its extensive attack on so-called "patterned" theories of justice, that is, theories that postulate some preferred ultimate distribution of goods and services.

6. On the tradeoffs between them, see Chapter 1.

7. For a more expanded treatment of these welfare rights, see Carl Wellman, *Welfare Rights* (1982). For my criticism, see Richard A. Epstein, "The Uncertain Quest for Welfare Rights," *Brig. Young U. Law Rev.* 201 (1985), reprinted with changes in G. Bryner and N. Reynolds, eds., *Constitutionalism and Rights* (1987). For an application of this distinction in connection with euthanasia, see Leon Kass, "Is There a right to Die?" *Hastings Center Report* 34 (Jan.-Feb. 1993): 35; also discussed in Chapter 13.

8. This position is rejected in much of the philosophical literature that embraces a more extensive view of the right to life. See, e.g., H. J. McCloskey, "Rights," *Phil. Quart.* 15 (1965): 115.

> My right to life is not a right against anyone. It is my right and by virtue of it, it is normally permissible for me to sustain my life in the face of obstacles. It does give rise to rights against others *in the sense* that others have or may come to have duties to refrain from killing me, but is essentially a right of mine, not an infinite list of claims, hypothetical and actual, against an indefinite number of actual, potential, and as yet non-existent human beings.

McCloskey does not give any account of the "obstacles" our rights might permit us to overcome, nor does he quite say that his views would impose affirmative obligations of support on others.

9. See, e.g., Tarleton v. McGawley, 170 Eng. Rep. 153 (K.B. 1793).

10. For elaboration, see Richard A. Epstein, *Simple Rules for a Complex World* (1995).

11. Ibid., 54-59.

12. Thomas Hobbes, *Leviathan*, (Oakeshott ed. 1962): Ch. 13, p. 101.

13. John Rawls, *A Theory of Justice* (1971).

14. See Chapter 15 for a discussion of this question in connection with assisted suicide.

15. For discussion, see Melvin Eisenberg, "Donative Promises," *U. Chi. L. Rev.* 47 (1979): 1 and Andrew Kull, "Reconsidering Gratuitous Promises," *J. Legal Stud.* 21 (1992): 39.

16. For the common law position, see Buch v. Amory Manufacturing Co., 44 A. 809 (N.H. 1897).

17. See, e.g., Ploof v. Putnam, 71 A. 188 (Vt. 1908). See also Soldano v. O'Daniels, 100 Cal. Rptr. 310 (Cal. App. 1983): (owner of a bar must allow person to enter premises to use a pay telephone to call police to stop killing nearby).

18. See, e.g., Vincent v. Lake Erie Transportation Co., 124 N.W. 221 (Minn. 1910): (ship may tie up to dock to avert disaster, but must pay just compensation for losses).

19. See Munn v. Illinois, 94 U.S. 113 (1876).

20. Allnut v. Inglis, 104 Eng. Rep. 206 (K.B. 1810).

21. Ibid.

22. For a good account of the economic costs associated with price discrimination, see David Friedman, *Price Theory* (2d ed. 1990): 255–263.

23. The Robinson-Patman Act, 15 U.S.C. §13 (1973–1989 Supp.) that governs price discrimination recognizes the need to take into account cost differentials: "[n]othing herein contained shall prevent differentials which make only due allowance for differences in the cost of manufacturer, sale, or delivery result from the differing methods or quantities in which such commodities are to such purchasers sold or delivered." The reference to "due allowance" is designed to prevent a $1 of cost difference from justifying $100 of monopoly profits.

24. See, e.g., Harold Demsetz, "Why Regulate Utilities?", *J. Law & Econ.* 11 (1968): 55.

25. See Smyth v. Ames, 169 U.S. 466 (1898); Federal Power Commission v. Hope Natural Gas, 320 U.S. 591 (1944); and Duquesne Light Co. v. Barasch, 488 U.S. 299 (1989).

26. The application of the antitrust rules to hospitals, physician, and other health care providers is a well-developed and active field. See James H. Sneed and David Marx, *Antitrust: Challenge of the Health Care Field* (1990).

27. Boston Ice Co. v. Potter, 123 Mass. 28, 30 (1877).

28. McDonald v. Massachusetts, 120 Mass. 432 (1876). "All cannot participate in its [the hospital's benefits]; the trustees are those to whom is confided the duty of selecting those who shall enjoy them, and prescribing the terms on which they shall do so."

CHAPTER I

1. Bernard Williams, "The Idea of Equality," in P. Laslett and W. Runciman, eds., *Philosophy, Politics and Society,* (1962): 110, 121; Williams offers no demonstration for this broad proposition, save an appeal to Aristotle's principles of "distributive justice."

2. See Gene Outka, "Social Justice and Equal Access to Health Care," *J. Religious Ethics* 2 (1974): 11, 12.

3. Alain Enthoven, *Theory and Practice of Managed Competition in Health Care Finance* (1988): pp. 2–4.

4. Henry Simons's standard definition of income is "Personal income may be defined as the algebraic sum of (1) the market value of rights exercised in consumption and (2) the change in the value of the store of property rights between the beginning and the end of the period in question." *Personal Income Taxation* 50 (1938). His analysis showed that tying the definition of income to receipts is incorrect. Appreciation in share value counts as income even before sale. Nonetheless Simons was concerned only with changes in net worth—a pure wealth concept. In particular, consumption was measured by the market value of the goods and services consumed, *not* the subjective value (usually greater than cost) obtained from their consumption. No system of taxation could work off of subjective value, even if it could register changes in market value when sale or other disposition is not present.

5. Richard A. Epstein, "Taxation in a Lockean World," *Soc. Pol. & Philo.* 4 (1986): 49.

6. Thomas Hobbes, *Leviathan* (Oakeshott ed. 1962): Ch. 15, p. 117.

7. Richard A. Posner, *Economic Analysis of Law* (4th ed. 1992): 13.

8. Ibid., 12–13.

9. I discuss the externality problem in greater detail in connection with restraints on alienation in Chapter 9.

10. Posner, *Economic Analysis of Law*, 459.

11. See Rosemary Stevens, *In Sickness and in Wealth* (1990): 20, which details the outpouring of charitable activities in the early part of the century. For the level of activities more generally, see Marvin Olasky, *The Tragedy of American Compassion* (1992).

12. See, e.g., Restatement (Second) Contracts, §§ 1, 71; Dougherty v. Salt, 125 N.E. 94 (N.Y. 1919).

13. Allen E. Buchanan, "The Right to a Decent Minimum of Health Care," *Phil. & Pub. Affairs* 13 (1984): 54, 69-72.

14. See *Encyclopedia Americana*, 1836, under the entry "Joseph Story, Natural Law," reprinted in James McClellan, *Joseph Story and the American Constitution* (1971): 313.

15. This was common in early charitable activities with hospitals. See Stevens, *In Sickness and in Wealth* (1990).

CHAPTER 2

1. Perhaps the first demonstration of the many problems of running health care markets is in Kenneth Arrow, "Uncertainty and the Welfare Economics of Medical Care," *Am. Econ. Rev.* 53 (1963): 941

2. For a discussion of the various claims in issue, see Mark Kelman, "Health Care Rights: Distinct Claims, Distinct Justifications," *Stanford Working Paper* No. 77, March 1991.

3. See Chapter 3 for a discussion of demanded care.

4. See John Locke, *The First Treatise of Government* (1689), ¶141-142 (P. Laslett, ed. 1960).

5. See, e.g., the liver transplant case, discussed in Clark Havighurst and Nancy M. P. King, "Liver Transplantation in Massachusetts: Public Policy as Morality Play," in J. Blumstein and F. Sloan, eds., *Organ Transplantation Policy: Issues and Prospects* (1989): 229.

6. See, e.g., the rent supplement program of San Jose, discussed in Pennell v. City of San Jose, 485 U.S. 1 (1988).

7. The classic account is still Charles Murray, *Losing Ground* (1984). His basic conclusion as of that date was "Overall, civilian social welfare costs increased by twenty times from 1950 to 1980, in constant dollars. During the same period, the United States population increased by half." Health and medical costs increased sixfold during that period. The basic patterns were slowed down somewhat in the Reagan years, but growth renewed in both the Bush and the Clinton Administrations.

8. Ibid., 8. His objections to complete equality rest on the efficiency costs that it imposes (which are great with minimum standards), and on the opposition that such equality will raise from those denied the opportunity to increase their expenditures (who can also be expected to oppose a tax on their resources).

9. See Chapter 16.

10. *"The element of cross-subsidy is essential."* Enthoven, *Theory and Practice of Managed Competition in Health Care Finance*, 5 (italics in original).

11. See the account of community rating, Chapter 6.

12. HSA § 1101(a) sets all the items for inclusion and exclusion. § 1141, under the heading of "Medical Necessity" states, "The Comprehensive benefit package does not include—(1) an item or service (other than services referred to in paragraph (2)) that is not medically necessary or appropriate." This provision seems to refer to classes of procedures, and not to individual decisions on whether a given recipient should receive a given treatment.

13. For a discussion, see, Richard A. Epstein, "A Clash of Two Cultures: Will Tort Law Survive Automobile Insurance Reform?" *Valparaiso University Law Review* 25 (1991): 173, and Benjamin Zychar, "Automobile Insurance Regulation, Direct Democracy, and the Interests of Consumers," *Regulation* 67 (Summer 1990).

14. Stressed in Stevens, *In Sickness and in Wealth*, and in Olasky, *The Tragedy of American Compassion*.

15. Robert C. Ellickson, "The Homelessness Muddle," *The Public Interest* 99 (Spring 1990): 45.

16. The statistics is this paragraph are collected from *Statistical Abstract of the United States*, No. 115, (1995): 88 and *Historical Statistics, Colonial Times to 1970*, (Bicentennial Edition, series B): 116–125.

17. For a recent account of the numbers, see Michael Tanner, *The End of Welfare: Fighting Poverty in Civil Society*, 1–31 (1996).

CHAPTER 3

1. See H. Tristram Engelhardt, Jr. and Michael A. Rie, "Intensive Care Units, Scarce Resources, and Conflicting Principles of Justice," *JAMA* 255(1986): 1159, 1161. Their data suggests that for the 1978–1979 budget year, the Massachusetts General Hospital had 7.3 percent of its beds in the ICU, but devoted some 18.4 percent of its total cost to these beds.

2. See, e.g., E. Haavi Morreim, "Profoundly Diminished Life: The Casualties of Coercion," *Hastings Center Report* 24 (1994): 33–42 and Robert D. Truog, Allan S. Brett, and Joel Frader, "The Problem with Futility," *NEJM* 326 (1992): 1560.

3. In Re Conservatorship of Wanglie, No PX-91-283 (Minn. Dist. Ct., June 28, 1991), discussed at length in Cathaleen A. Roach, "Paradox and Pandora's Box: The Tragedy of Current Right-To-Die Jurisprudence," *U. Mich. L. Ref.* 25 (1991): 133, 145–150.

4. Alex M. Capron, "In Re Helga Wanglie" *Hastings Center Report* 21(No. 5): 26–28. See, e.g., Marcia Angell, "A New Kind of 'Right to Die Case,'" *NEJM* 325 (1991): 511–512 and Steven H. Miles, "Informed Demand for 'Non-Beneficial' Medical Treatment, *NEJM* 325 (1991): 512–515.

5. Steven H. Miles, "Interpersonal Issues in the Wanglie Case," *Kennedy Institute of Ethics Journal,* 2 (1992): 61, 63. The hospital did not bring the case because it, as an institution, formed no medical judgment on its merits.

6. See, e.g., Harris v. McRae, 448 U.S. 297 (1980).

7. For support of funding, see Owen M. Fiss, "State Activism and State Censorship," *Yale L. J.* 199 (1991): 2087. For my skeptical views, see Richard A. Epstein, *Bargaining with the State* (1993): 306–311.

8. See, e.g., "Guidelines on the Termination of Life-Sustaining Treatment and the Care of the Dying," *Hastings Center Report,* (1987): 4 and "Society for Critical Care Medicine, Consensus Report on the Ethics of Foregoing Life-Sustaining Treatments in the Critically Ill," *Crit. Care. Med.* 18 (1990): 1435–39, both concluding that it is an excessive use of resources to supply intensive care treatment to persons in a permanent vegetative state.

9. See Robert D. Truog, "Triage in the ICU," *Hastings Center Report,* 22 (No. 3) (1992): 13.

10. Norman G. Levinsky, "The Doctor's Master," *NEJM* 311 (1984): 1573–1575.

11. James Lubitz and Ronald Prihoda, "The Use and Costs of Medicare Services in the Last 2 years of Life," *Health Care Financing Review* 5 (1984): 117.

12. Ibid., 119.

13. The data is summarized in Ezekiel Emanual and Linda Emanual, "The Economics of Dying—The Illusion of Cost Savings at the End of Life," *NEJM* 330 (1994): 540–544. See also, James Lubitz and G. Riley, "Trends in Medicare Payments in the Last Year of Life," *NEJM* 328 (1993): 1092–1096.

14. D. R. Waldo, S. T. Sonnefeld, D. R. McKusick, and R. H. Arnett III, "Health Expenditures By Age Group, 1977 and 1987," *Health Care Finance Rev.* 10(4) (1989): 111.

15. Emanual and Emanual, "The Economics of Dying," note that the figures do not differ much for patients who do or do not have DNR orders.

16. The treatment is called "extracorporeal membrane oxygenation," or ECMO. See Truog, "Triage in the ICU," 13.

17. Truog, "Triage in the ICU."

18. See, e.g., Mohr v. Williams, 104 N.W. 12 (Minn. 1905).

19. For this observation in the context of tort damages, see David Friedman, "What is 'Fair Compensation' For Death or Injury?" *Int'l Rev. of Law & Econ.* 2 (1982): 81.

20. Sullivan v. Old Colony Street Ry. 83 N.E. 1091, 1902 (Mass. 1908): "The rule of damages is a practical instrumentality for the administration of justice. The principle on which it is founded is compensation. Its object is to afford the equivalent in money for the actual loss caused by the wrong of another."

21. Zibbell v. Southern Pacific Co., 116 P. 513, 520 (1911).

22. Patricia M. Danzon, "Tort Reform and the Role of Government in Private Insurance Markets," *J. Legal Stud.* 13 (1984): 517, 522–524, noting the restrictions in pay-outs in various first-party plans.

23. Tom Tomlinson and Howard Brody, "Futility and the Ethics of Resuscitation," *JAMA* 264 (1990): 1276, 1277.

24. Truog, Brett, and Frader, 1563.

25. William A. Knaus, "A Controlled Trial to Improve Care for Seriously Ill Hospitalized Patients," *JAMA* 274 (1995): 1591.

26. J. Teno, J. Lynn, R. Phillips, et al., "Do Advance Directives Save Resources?" *Clin. Res.* 41 (1993): 551A (abstract).

27. See Emanual and Emanual.

28. For a detailed exposition, see William A. Knaus, et al., "The APACHE III, Prognostic System: Risk Prediction of Hospital Mortality for Critically Ill Hospitalized Adults," *Chest* 100 (1991): 1619. The earlier forms of APACHE contained somewhat different variables and offered a somewhat lower level of predictive ability when tested in a variety of clinical settings. See William A. Knaus, Elizabeth A. Draper, Douglas P. Wagner, and Jack E. Zimmerman, "APACHE II: A Severity of Disease Classification System," *Crit. Care* 13 (1985): 818, and R. W. S. Chang, S. Jacobs, and Bernie Lee, "Use of APACHE II Severity of Disease Classification to Identify Intensive-Care-Unit Patients Who Would Not Benefit From Total Parenteral Nutrition," *The Lancet* (June 28, 1986): 1483.

29. It is worth noting that the name itself changed. The earlier versions of the test called it the Acute Physiology and Chronic Health Evaluation. The newer versions strip out the "and" and add "age," so that APACHE now stands for "Acute Physiology, Age, Chronic Health Evaluation."

30. Knaus et al, "APACHE II," 1630, referring to the study of Schneiderman et al.

31. Ibid., 1619.

32. See Lawrence J. Schneiderman, Nancy S. Jecker, and Albert Jonson, "Medical Futility: Its Meaning and Ethical Implications," *Annals of Internal Medicine* 112 (1990): 949, 951.

33. Truog, Brett, and Frader, 1561.

34. Bryan Jennett, "Inappropriate Use of Intensive Care," *British Medical Journal* 289 (No. 6460) (1984): 1709–1711.

35. See, e.g., Michael J. Strauss, et al., "Rationing of Intensive Care Unit Services: An Everyday Occurrence," *JAMA* 255 (1986): 1143, noting that when beds are in short supply, access to them is curtailed and reserved for more serious cases.

36. See Daniel E. Singer, Phyllis L. Carr, Albert G. Mulley, and George E. Thibault, "Rationing Intensive Care—Physician Responses To a Resource Shortage," *NEJM* 308 (1983): 155.

CHAPTER 4

1. Hurley v. Eddingfield, 59 N.E. 1058 (Ind. 1901).

2. Ibid.

3. State ex rel. Wood v. Consumers's Gas Trust Co., 61 N.E. 674, 678 (Ind. 1901).

4. Boston Ice Co. v. Potter, 123 Mass. 28 (1877), already quoted in the Introduction.

5. 120 Mass. 432, 435 (1876). See also Birmingham Baptist Hospital v. Crews, 157 So. 224, 225 (Ala. 1934). ("Defendant is a private corporation, and [is] not a public institution, and owes the public no duty to accept any patient not desired by it.")

6. Indeed in the earlier days, the rule was so strong that the charitable immunity prevented suits for medical malpractice by patients admitted to the hospital who received care free of charge. See *McDonald*, 120 Mass. at 436.

7. 174 A.2d 135 (Del. 1961).

8. Ibid., 139. See Restatement (Second) Torts, § 323.

9. 174 A.2d at 140. For similar analysis involving flag men at railroad crossings, see Erie Ry. v. Stewart 40 F.2d 855 (6th Cir. 1930). The railroad was under no duty to place a

flagman at the intersection in the first place, but once it chose to do so, liability could follow. Note that judges divided on the question as to whether generalized public reliance was enough, or whether the injured person had individually to rely on the custom in order to recover—the precise ambiguity found here.

10. 537 P.2d 1329 (Ariz. 1975).

11. Ibid., 1331.

12. Ibid., 1332.

13. For a fuller discussion of these issues, see Epstein, *Bargaining with the State*, (1993): 196–202.

14. See Truax v. Raich, 239 U.S. 33, 41 (1915) ("It requires no argument to show that the right to work for a living in the common occupations of the community is of the very essence of the personal freedom and opportunity that it was the purpose of the [fourteenth] Amendment to secure.") Alas, it does.

15. Lovell v. Griffin, 303 U.S. 444 (1938) (striking down license on distribution of handbills); Freedman v. Maryland, 380 U.S. 51 (1965) (invalidating licensing requirement for motion pictures). See generally, Thomas Emerson, "The Doctrine of Prior Restraint," *Law & Contemp. Probs.* 20 (1955): 648.

16. 637 F. Supp. 684, 706 (D. Mass. 1986), aff'd 815 F.2d 790 (1st Cir. 1987) (Breyer, J.). The statute provided: "The [Board of Registration in Medicine] shall require as a condition of granting or renewing a physician's certificate of registration, that the physician, who if he agrees to treat a beneficiary of health insurance under Title XVIII of the Social Security Act [Medicare], shall also agree not to charge or collect from such beneficiary any amount in excess of the reasonable charge for that service as determined by the United States Secretary of Health and Human Services." Mass. Ann. Laws, ch. 112 §2 (1995).

17. For a further discussion, see Chapter 7.

18. See, e.g., Duquesne Light Co. v. Barasch, 488 U.S. 299 (1989). For the constitutional bridge between public utility regulation and physician rate regulation, see Thomas Merrill, "Constitutional Limits on Physician Price Controls," *Hastings Const. L. Quart.* 21 (1994): 635. Merrill rejects, as do I, the proposition that price controls are permissible as a matter of course so long as individuals have no legal obligation to serve the market, and notes that this theory does not protect the specific investments that individuals make in human capital. See generally, Oliver Williamson, "The Logic of Economic Organization," *J. L. Econ. & Org.* 4 (1988): 5.

19. Whitney v. Heckler, 780 F.2d 963, 972 (11th Cir. 1986). See also Minnesota Ass'n. of Health Care v. Minnesota Department of Public Works, 742 F.2d 442, 446 (8th Cir. 1984) (upholding a state rule prohibiting nursing homes that received Medicaid payments from charging non-Medicaid patients 10 percent more than Medicaid recipients).

20. See, 42 U.S.C. § 1395j. For a general discussion of Medicare, see Chapter 7.

21. 42 U.S.C. § 1395t. The appropriations are regulated in accordance with the complex formulas of § 1395w.

22. See, e.g., United States v. Bethlehem Steel Corp., 315 U.S. 289 (1942) (government defense of economic duress rejected it was sued on cost-plus contracts for the construction of submarines shortly after the American entry into World War I). The dissent of J. Frankfurter spells out the exaction possibilities, which could lead to inefficient outcomes.

23. 42 U.S.C. § 1395dd. COBRA is another acronym commonly used for the statute. It stands for Consolidated Omnibus Budget Reconciliation Act of 1986, Pub. L. No. 99-272, 100 Stat. 82 (1986), of which EMTALA is a part. Both acronyms are in use. COBRA is more venomous, but EMTALA is more precise and is more commonly used.

24. 42 U.S.C. § 1395cc.

25. 42 U.S.C. § 1395dd (a).

26. Ibid.

27. 32 U.S.C. § 1395dd(b)(1).

28. 42 U.S.C. § 1395dd (c)(1)(A) (ii).

29. 42 U.S.C. § 1395dd (a) (2) & (3).

30. 42 U.S.C. § 1395dd (b) (2) & (3).

31. 42 U.S.C. § 1395dd (d)(1)(B).

32. 42 U.S.C. § 1395dd (d)(1)(B).

33. 42 U.S.C. § 1395dd (d)(2).

34. 42 U.S.C. § 1395dd (d)(C)(2)(A).

35. Gatewood v. Washington Healthcare Corp. 933 F.2d 1037 (D.C. 1991).

36. 42 U.S.C. § 1395dd (d)(C)(2)(B).

37. 42 U.S.C. § 1395dd (e).

38. Equal Access to Health Care: Patient Dumping: Hearing Before the Subcommittee on Human Resources and Intergovernment Relations of the House Committee on Government Operations, 100th Cong. 1st Sess. 14–20 (1987). [Hereafter House Hearing on Patient Dumping]

39. See Robert L. Schiff, David A. Answell, James E. Schlosser, et al., "Transfers to Public Hospital: A Prospective Study of 467 Patients," *NEJM* 314 (1986): 552.

40. Karen H. Rothenberg, "Who Cares? The Evolution of the Legal Duty to Provide Emergency Care," *Hous. L. Rev.* 26 (1989): 21. The quoted passage is a summary of the testimony offered by Zettie Mae Hill, House Hearing on Patient Dumping, 14–21.

41. See Rothenberg, "Who Cares?" See also Andrew J. McClurg, "Your Money or Your Life: Interpreting the Federal Act Against Patient Dumping," *Wake Forest L. Rev.* 24 (1989): 173. Erik J. Olson, "No Room at the Inn: A Snapshot of an American Emergency Room," *Stan. L. Rev.* 46 (1994): 449.

42. House Hearing on Patient Dumping, 23.

43. See Mark A. Hall, "The Unlikely Case for Patient Dumping," *Jurimetrics J.* (Summer 1988): 389.

44. GAO, HRD 91–57 (May, 1991), 31–35.

45. Ibid., title page.

46. Ibid., 2.

47. Ibid., 4.

48. Ibid., 36.

49. See Olson "No Room at the Inn," 449, 451, quoting Irene Wielawski, "County Proposal Targets 16 Health Care Clinics for Closing," *L.A. Times,* (September 1, 1992): B1, B4.

50. Olson, "No Room at the Inn," 449, 458, citing Emily Friedman, "The Sagging Safety Net: Emergency Departments on the Brink of Crisis," *Hospital,* (Feb. 20, 1992): 26, 28.

51. Olson, "No Room at the Inn," 465.

52. Gary P. Young, Michele B. Wagner, Arthur L. Kellerman, et al., "Ambulatory Visits to Hospital Emergency Departments: Patterns and Reasons for Use," *JAMA* 276 (1996): 460. For an earlier study pointing in the same direction, see Kevin F. O'Grady, Willard G. Manning, Joseph P. Newhouse, and Robert H. Brook, "The Impact of Cost Sharing on Emergency Department Use," *NEJM* 313 (1985): 484.

53. Robert M. Williams, "The Costs of Visits to Emergency Departments," *NEJM* 334 (1996): 642.

54. Laurence C. Baker and Linda S. Baker, "Excess Cost of Emergency Department

Visits for Non-Urgent Care," *Health Affairs* 15 (1994): 162 ($5.4 billion); Health Care Advisory Board, "Redefining the Emergency Department: Five Strategies for Reducing Unnecessary Visits" (1993) (14.1 billion).

55. Robert S. Stern, Joel S. Weissman, and Arnold M. Epstein, *JAMA* 266 (1991): 2238.

56. Joe V. Selby, Bruce H. Fireman, and Bix E. Swain, "Effect of a Copayment on Use of the Emergency Department in a Health Maintenance Organization," *NEJM* 334 (1996): 635.

57. Ibid., 640.

58. Olson, "No Room at the Inn," 468–470.

59. Claire Spiegel and Irene Wielawski, "Care Rationed at Overcrowded County-USC," *L.A. Times* (Dec. 16, 1991): A1, A39.

60. See, e.g., David W. Baker, Carl D. Stevens, and Robert H. Brook, "Patients Who Leave a Public Hospital Emergency Department Without Being Seen by a Physician: Causes and Consequences," *JAMA* 266 (1991): 1085. Their study reports that some 8.2 percent left the emergency room without being seen, some 46 percent of whom were thought to need prompt medical attention. The average wait in the emergency room was over six hours, both for those who were seen and those who were not. Excepted from the sample were persons in unstable conditions who were taken as promptly as possible.

See also, Andrew B. Bindman, Kevin Grumbach, Dennis Keane, et al. "Consequences of Queuing for Care at a Public Hospital Emergency Department," *JAMA* 266 (1991): 1091. This study reports that 15 percent of their enrolled patients left without being seen by a physician, but most of these had less acute problems than those who chose to stay.

61. Or more precisely, "an anemic response to the problem of the medically uninsured." See Hall, "The Unlikely Case for Patient Dumping," 393.

62. Claire Ansberry, "Dumping the Poor: Despite Federal Law, Hospitals Still Reject Sick Who Can't Pay," *Wall Street Journal*, (Nov. 29. 1988): A1.

63. 16 F.3d 590 (4th Cir. 1994).

64. Ibid., 598.

65. GAO Study, 27–28.

67. Sally L. Satel, "Examining Entitlements for the Mentally Ill," *Wall Street J.* (January 28, 1992): A14.

68. Ibid.

CHAPTER 5

1. See, e.g., *Webster's Collegiate Dictionary*, 384.

2. See, e.g., Nippert v. Richmond, 327 U.S. 416, 425 (1946) "[N]ot all burdens on commerce, but only undue or discriminatory ones are forbidden."

3. See Introduction.

4. 42 U.S.C. §2003 et seq.

5. The literature is vast. For my account of these developments, see Richard A. Epstein, *Forbidden Grounds: The Case Against Employment Discrimination Laws* (1992).

6. Age Discrimination in Employment Act of 1967, 29 U.S.C. 621 § (b).

7. McDonnell Douglas Corp., v. Green, 411 U.S. 792 (1973)(protected classes); Steelworkers v. Weber, 443 U.S. 193 (1979).

8. See, e.g., Rebecca Dresser, "Wanted: Single, White Male for Medical Research," *Hastings Center Report* (January/February 1992): 24. Dresser's study is highly critical of

the practices that often exclude women and members of racial minorities from human subjects health research. The incidence, patterns, and treatment of disease often vary by sex and by racial groups, and studies on white men give an insufficient database, which may not be justified by the lower cost necessary to run these trials. One reason to privatize medical research is to avoid having to make these protocols uniform across all studies and all projects. Those groups that want broader inclusion can take the risk of weaker conclusions, and vice versa.

9. See Chapter 12.

10. See Chapters 1 and 2.

11. Richard J. Zeckhauser and W. Kip Viscusi, "Risk Within Reason," *Science* 248, (1990): 559.

12. Jack Hadley and Anthony Osei, "Does Income Affect Mortality? An Analysis of the Effects of Different Types of Income on Age/Sex/Race-Specific Mortality Rates in the United States," *Medicare Care* 20 (1982): 901.

13. John C. Shanahan and Adam D. Thierer, "How to Talk About Risk: How Well-Intentional Regulations Can Kill," *Heritage Talking Points* 13, (April 23, 1996): 6.

14. See, e.g., Ronald Dworkin, "Is the Clinton Plan Fair," *New York Review of Books,* (Jan. 13, 1994).

15. For a sympathetic account of these ambiguities, see Mark Kelman, "Concepts of discrimination in 'general ability' job testing," *Harv. L. Rev.* 104 (1991): 1157.

16. See Clinton Administration Description of President's Health Care Reform Plan, American Health Security Act of 1993, dated Sept. 7, 1993, obtained by BNA (Sept. 10. 1993): 10–11. For a more detailed description see Chapter 8.

17. John Rawls, "A Theory of Justice," 285.

18. For a further discussion of the point, see Richard A. Epstein, "Justice Across Generations," *Texas L. Rev.* 67 (1989): 1465.

19. For a discussion of the background of the plan, see Robert Pear, "Plan to Ration Health Care is Rejected by Government," *New York Times,* (August 4, 1992).

20. See, e.g., "A Bold Medical Plan, Derailed," New York Times, (August 6, 1992): 10 (Editorial).

21. See letter from Louis W. Sullivan, Secretary of Health and Human Services, to Governor Barbara Roberts, State of Oregon, dated August 3, 1992, with accompanying memo. The memo also attacked the reliance on telephone surveys that were thought to be "stereotypic assumptions about persons with disabilities," page 1, a point that will not be examined further here.

22. Ibid., Memo page 1.

23. Ibid., Memo page 2.

CHAPTER 6

1. Lindenau v. Desborough, 108 Eng. Rep. 1160, 1162 (1828). For other sentiments of the same view, see Lord Mansfield's earlier opinion in Carter v. Boehm, 97 Eng. Rep. 1162 (K.B. 1766); London Assurance v. Mansel 11 Ch.D. 363, 367 (1879), holding that an insured must disclose all that is known to him, even if he does not understand what the information is material to the evaluation of the risk. "Whether it is life, or fire, or marine assurance, I take it good faith is required in all cases."

2. Marine Insurance Act, 1906, s. 18(1).

3. See, e.g., HSA § 1384. (A) Application of Community-Rated Premiums.—The premiums charged by a corporate alliance for enrollment in a corporate alliance health

plan shall . . . vary only by class of family enrollment . . . and by premium area."

4. Ch. 501 McKinney's (N.Y.) §3231(a) (1992). "For the purposes of this section, 'community rated' means a rating methodology in which the premium for all persons covered by a policy or contract form is the same based on the experience of the entire pool of risks covered by that policy or contract form without regard to age, sex, health status or occupation."

The phrase "policy or contract form" does not refer to the policy or contract issued to a given insured, but to all insureds who receive insurance under the same basic type of policy or contract.

5. Ibid.

6. See, e.g., 24-A Maine R.S. § 5011.1.1.A, "Rates for policies subject to this subsection may not vary based on age, gender, health status, claims experience, policy duration, industry or occupation." This provision applies to Medicare Supplement Policies. A more general statute allows age, sex, and geographical location to be taken into account, 24-A Maine R.S. § 6059(2), but limits the variation in organizational rates to 150 percent of a standard rate. § 6059(3).

See also Mass. Ann. Laws Ch. 495. Same restrictions as New York, with additional provision, excluding "any other factor which the commissioner may specify by regulation."

7. N.J. Stat. Ann. § 17B :27A-2, A-4 (1993).

8. Fla. Stat. § 627.6699(m).

9. American Academy of Actuaries, quoted in Pear, "Plan to Ration Health Care," 22.

10. See Robert Pear, "Pooling Risks and Sharing Costs in Effort to Gain Stable Insurance Rates," *New York Times* (May 22, 1994): 14, col. 1.

11. Ibid., 22, col. 5. Cecil D. Bykerk, Mutual of Omaha, Chief Actuary.

12. Ibid., 22, col. 1.

13. Ibid., 22. "If their health insurance is community rated, businesses say, they will not get the benefit of savings they achieve through efficient management of their health plans and through programs promoting healthy behavior by employees." To make the statement fully accurate, the word "full" should be inserted before "benefit."

14. Ibid., 22, col. 5.

15. Ibid., 22, at cols. 3 and 4. Statement of Alice Rosenblatt, actuary at Coopers & Lybrand.

16. Ch. 501 McKinney's (N.Y.) §3233.

17. See Mark V. Pauly, Patricia Danzon, Paul J. Feldstein, and John Hoff, *Responsible National Health Insurance* (1992): 11.

18. HSA § 1402 (B). No Limits on Coverage; No pre-Existing-Conditions Limits.— A health plan may not—(3) exclude coverage of an alliance eligible individual because of existing medical conditions; (4) impose waiting periods before coverage begins.

19. P.L. 104–191 (104 Cong. 2nd Sess).

19a. Ibid., § 301. Internal Revenue Code, U.S.C. § 220.

20. "Kassebaum Recommends Limited MSA Program for Health Insurance Bill," *BNA Health Care Daily*, June 6, 1996.

21. A representative clause from New England Mutual Life Insurance Co., as reproduced in Bullwinkel v. New England Mut. Life Ins. Co., 18 F.3d 42, 430 (7th Cir. 1993) reads:

> No benefits are payable for a condition, sickness, or injury for which you or your dependent were seen, treated, diagnosed, or incurred medical expenses in the six-month period just before insurance starts until the earlier of: . . . for you or your dependent, the end of a period of twelve consecutive months after insurance starts.

22. Kirk v. Provident Life and Acc. Ins. Co., 942 F.2d 504 (8th Cir. 1991)(symptoms of bacterial endocarditis before period, diagnosis made afterward).

23. Hughes v. Boston Mutual Life Insurance Co., 26 F.3d 267 (1st Cir. 1994).

24. Brewer v. Protexall, Inc., 50 F.3d 453 (7th Cir. 1995) (no requirement to disclose health risks if comparable insurance in force during transition period, which could be read to include temporary coverage supplied by former employer).

25. See, e.g., Paul Starr, "The Framework of Health Care Reform," *NEJM* 329 (1991): 1666. "Without [regional health alliances, or if they are only voluntary, insurers will continue to be able to cherry-pick the healthy and shun the sick."

26. HSA, § 1115, which makes benefits available to any person who has in the previous year "a diagnosable mental or substance abuse disorder," and who is "experiencing, or is at significant risk of experiencing, functional impairment in family, work, school, or community activities." Which just about covers the waterfront.

27. Paul R. Billings, Mel A. Kohn, Margaret de Cuevas, and Jonathan Beckwith, "Discrimination as a Consequence of Genetic Testing," *American J. of Hum. Genetics* 50 (1992): 476.

28. For my general views on these issues, see Richard A. Epstein, "The Legal Regulation of Genetic Discrimination: Old Responses to New Technology," *Boston U. L. Rev.* 74 (1994): 1. The issue is also of great importance in the law of marriage and adoption.

29. In addition to Billings et al., "Discrimination as a Consequence," see Joseph S. Alper and Marvin R. Natowicz, "Discrimination as a Consequence of Genetic Testing," *Am. J. Hum. Genet.* 50 (1992): 465; and Larry Gostin, "Genetic Discrimination: The Use of Genetically Based Diagnostic and Prognostic Tests by Employers and Insurers," *Am. J. of Law & Med.* (1991): 109.

30. Huntington's disease, a fatal condition that sets in after reproductive years, is carried by a single dominant gene, which can now be identified by genetic testing. For discussions of the various legal and ethical issues about the gene, see Gwen Terrenoire, "Huntington's Disease, and the Ethics of Genetic Prediction," *J. Med. Ethics* 18 (1992): 79; and Natalie Angier, "Researchers Locate Gene That Triggers Huntington's Illness," *New York Times,* (March 24, 1993): T1, reporting on the discovery of the gene.

31. For one impassioned statement, see Susan Weiner, "Genetic Testing: The Perils of Cracking the Code," *Chicago Tribune,* (December 5, 1995): § 1, p. 25, col. 1.

32. For the basic constitutional blessing, see Block v. Hirsh, 256 U.S. 135 (1921). For the protest murmur, see Pennell v. City of San Jose, 485 U.S. 1, (1988) (Scalia, J. concurring).

33. Paul Starr, "The Framework of Health Care Reform."

34. See John H. Cochrane, "Time-Consistent Health Insurance," *J. Pol. Econ.* 103 (1995): 445.

35. Ch. 501 McKinney's § 3231 (1993).

36. Ibid.

37. Ibid., § 3232(a). The statute does not allow the credit in all cases, but provides: "Such credit shall apply to the extent that the previous coverage was substantially similar to the new coverage." It does not address what should be done when the earlier limits have been exhausted.

38. Ibid., § 3232(b). The section also gives a somewhat narrower definition of a preexisting condition, which covers only those conditions that would lead "an ordinary prudent person to seek medical advice, diagnosis, care or treatment," or one for which any of these in fact had been received in the previous six months.

39. Ibid., § 3232. "In determining whether a pre-existing condition provision

applies to an eligible person, the small group policy or individual health insurance policy shall credit the time the person was previously covered under a previous health insurance plan or policy or employer-provided health benefit arrangement, if the previous coverage was continuous to a date not more than sixty days prior to the effective date of the new coverage."

40. Ibid., § 3234.

41. Ibid., § 3233.

42. Pub. L Law No. 101-336, 104 Stat. 327, 42 U.S.C. §§ 12101-12213, 47 U.S. C. § 225 and § 611.

43. Ibid., § 12112(d)(2)(A).

44. Ibid., § 12112(d)(2)(B).

45. Ibid., § 12112(d)(3)(A).

46. Ibid., § 12112(d)(3)(B).

47. For further elaboration, see Richard A. Epstein, *Forbidden Grounds: The Case Against Employment Discrimination Laws* (1992): 493–494.

48. HIPAA, Pub. L. 104–191, codified as part 7 of The Employee Retirement Security Act of 1974, 29 U.S.C. § 702(a).

49. Ibid., § 703.

50. Ibid., § 2711.

51. Ibid., § 2712.(c).

52. Ibid., § 702.

53. HIPPA, § 110(a).

54. Ibid., § 103(b)(10).

CHAPTER 7

1. See Steven Hayward and Erik Peterson, "The Medicare Monster: A Cautionary Tale," *Reason* 19 (January 1993) for an excellent account of the early history.

2. Legislative History, Social Security Amendments of 1965, S.R. Rep. 404, 89th Cong., 1st Sess. (1965), reprinted in 1965 U.S.C.C.A.N. 1943, 1997. [Hereafter Medicare LH]

3. Ibid., 1979 and 2002.

4. See Hayward and Peterson, "The Medicare Monster."

5. See John C. Liu and Robert E. Moffit, "A Taxpayer's Guide to the Medicare Crisis," *The Heritage Foundation*, (September 27, 1995). Somewhat different numbers are found in Medicare LH, 2008, Table D, but the differences are unimportant. The Senate Report also included estimates of the trust fund balance, which was to rise to around $10 billion in 1990. The actual figure was $100 billion. The sums do not represent invested dollars but charges on future generations of taxpayers.

6. Medicare LH, 2011.

7. Ferrara.

8. Ibid., 1964–1965.

9. For my views, see Epstein, *Forbidden Grounds*.

10. For a contemporary account of the prevailing ethos from a supporter of the bill, see Michael Sovern, *Legal Restraints on Racial Discrimination in Employment* (1966).

11. On these lobbying efforts, see Robert Pear, "Health Industry Leads Budget Lobbying," *New York Times* (Oct. 24, 1995): A 24.

12. For a clear exposition of the basic rules, see Barry R. Furrow, Thomas Greaney et al., *Health Law*, (1995): 560–602.

13. 42 U.S.C.A. § 1395t: "Such [trust fund] investments may be made only in inter-

est bearing obligations of the United States or in obligations guaranteed as to both principal and interest by the United States." For discussion, see John Goodman and Gerald L. Musgrove, *Patient Power: Solving America's Health Care Crisis* (1992): 405.

14. See 1995 Annual Report of the Board of Trustees of the Federal Hospital Fund, 17. [Hereafter 1995 Report]

15. 42 U.S.C. § 1395(x)(u).

16. 42 U.S.C. § 1395(x)(m).

17. Ibid., § 1395x(a).

18. Ibid., § 1395d(a).

19. Ibid.

20. Ibid., § 1395cc(a)(1)(I).

21. Ibid., § 1395cc(b)(2).

22. Medicare LH, 2002.

23. Ibid., 2002. See also Table A, p. 1998, noting that for the 1955–1963 period hospitalization costs were increasing at 6.7 percent relative to a general inflation rate of 4.0 percent.

24. Ibid., 1947, 2005, Table B.

25. Ibid., 2000.

26. Ibid., 2001.

27. Hayward and Peterson, "The Medicare Monster," 21–22.

28. My thanks to David M. Cutler for supplying me with a learned overview of the evidence.

29. Willard Manning, Joseph Newhouse, Naihua Duan, et al., "Health Insurance and the Demand for Medical Care: Evidence from a Randomized Experiment," *Am. Econ. Rev.* 77 (1987): 251.

30. Alan Garber, Victor Fuchs, and James Silverman, "Case Mix, Costs and Outcomes," *NEJM* (May 10, 1984): 1231.

31. Jack Wennberg, J. J. Freeman, and W. J. Cyulp, "Are Hospital Services Rationed in New Haven or Over-Utilized in Boston?" *Lancet* 1 (May 23, 1987): 1185–1188.

32. For an exhaustive discussion of the details of this history other payment systems, see David M. Frankford, "The Complexity of Medicare's Hospital Reimbursement System: The Paradoxes of Averaging," *Iowa L. Rev.* 78 (1993): 517.

33. Donald F. Beck, *Principles of Reimbursement in Health Care* (1984), which contains advice on how proceed.

34. For an earlier discussion, see Charles E. Phelps and Lenhard Resinger, "Unresolved Risk Under Medicare," in M. Pauly and W. Kissick, eds., *Lessons From the First Twenty Years of Medicare* (1988): 117, 120–123.

35. See 42 U.S.C. § 1395(v)(1)(A). Parallel provisions for hospital services are found in ibid., 42 U.S.C. § 1395(v)(5)(A).

36. See, e.g., Frankford, "The Complexity of Medicare," 540–541.

37. See 42 U.S.C. § 1395ww(b).

38. Ibid. § 1395ww(d)(5)(A)(1).

39. William B. Schwartz, "The Inevitable Failure of Current Cost-Containment Strategies," *JAMA* 257 (1987): 220.

40. Doug Bandow and Michael Tanner, "The Wrong and Right Ways to Reform Medicare," Cato Policy Analysis Number 230, June 8, 1995. *New York Times* (May 12, 1996): Business section.

41. See, generally, 42 U.S.C. § 1395x(b); 42 C.F.R. § 410.26. See Furrow et al., *Health Law,* 566–568, for the full list.

42. Bandow and Tanner, "The Wrong and Right Ways to Reform Medicare," 11.

43. See John C. Goodman and Gerald L. Musgrave, *Patient Power: Solving America's Health Care Crisis* (1992) for account.

44. See John C. Goodman, "A Healthy Choice for Sick Patients," *Wall Street Journal,* (October 17, 1995): A18.

45. Goodman and Musgrave, *Patient Power,* 406–405, citing Karen Davis and Diane Rowland, *Medicare Policy: New Directions for Health and Long-Term Care* (1986).

46. See the so-called Baucus amendment, Pub. L. 96-265, § 507, 94 Stat. 476 (1980). See, generally, Richard M. Scheffler, "An Analysis of 'Medigap' Enrollment: Assessment of Current Status and Policy Initiatives," in *Lessons,* 1818. Goodman and Musgrove, *Patient Power,* 455.

47. See, e.g., Goodman and Musgrave, *Patient Power,* Table 8.4, 237. The table shows that it becomes ever more expensive to provide an additional dollar of insurance protection as deductibles are reduced. Thus, to reduce the deductible from $2,000 to $1,000 adds costs of about $150 for a single person aged 30 and about $500 for a single person between 60 and 64.

48. "A broad range of studies show that physicians with high practice costs or in markets with strong private demand see fewer Medicaid Patients, assign fewer Medicare claims, and are less likely to choose formal Medicare participant status." Stephen Zuckerman and John Holahan, "The Role of Balance Billing in Medicare Physician Payment Reform," in H.E. Frech III, ed., *Regulating Doctors' Fees: Competition, Benefits, and Controls under Medicare* (1991): 143, 165.

49. Ibid., 167, Table 6-3.

50. Mass. Gen. L. Ann. ch. 112 § 2 (Lawyer's Coop. 1991). The statute was upheld against various challenges in Massachusetts Medical Soc. v. Dukakis, 815 F.2d 790 (1st Cir. 1987)(Breyer, J.). For criticism of the program as an abuse of the licensing power, see Chapter 5.

51. Health Care Practitioners Medicare Fee Control Act, Pa. Stat. Ann. tit. 35, § 449.31 et seq. (Purdon Supp. 1993), sustained in Pennsylvania Medical Association v. Marconis, 942 F.2d. 842 (3rd Cir. 1991).

52. See 42 U.S.C. § 1395u(b)(3)(B).

53. 42 U.S.C. § 1395u(j)(1)(A).

54. Zuckerman and Holahan, "The Role of Balance Billing," Table 6-1. The variation was quite broad: Thus, in Rhode Island, participation moved from 0.90 in 1983, to 0.92 in 1985, to 0.95 in 1997. The corresponding figures for Illinois were 0.36, 0.55, and 0.63.

55. Omnibus Budget Reconciliation Act of 1986, Pub. L. No. 99-509, 100 Stat. 1874 42 U.S.C. § 1395u(j)(1)(B)(i).

56. U.S.C. § 1395w-4(g)(1-2).

57. See Garelick v. Sullivan, 987 F.2d 913 (2d Cir. 1993). The voluntariness argument had been previously accepted in *Massachusetts Medical Society,* and in Whitney v. Heckler, 780 F.2d 963 (11th Cir. 1986).

58. 42 U.S.C.A. § 1395w-4(g)(3).

59. 42 U.S.C.A. §§ 1395w-4(a)-(j).

60. William C. Hsiao, "Objective Research and Physician Payment: A Response from Harvard." *Health Aff.* 8 (4) (1989): 72–75, quoted in Iglehart, "The New Law on Medicare's Payments to Physicians," *NEJM* 322 (1990): 1247, 1248.

61. For a description of the plan, see Furrow et al., *H* 583–588.

62. John K. Iglehart, "The New Law on Medicare's Payments to Physicians," *NEJM* 322 (1990): 1247.

63. John Locke, *A Second Treatise of Government,* ¶ 27.

64. Presidential Veto of H. R. 2491, *Cong. Quarterly* 3762, December 9, 1995.

65. See, e.g., Martin Feldstein, "What the '93 Tax Increases Really Did," *Wall Street Journal,* October 26, 1995, "Because taxpayers responded to the sharply higher marginal tax rates by reducing their taxable incomes, the Treasury lost two-thirds of the extra revenue that would have been collected if taxpayers had not changed their behavior."

66. H.R. 2491, Title VIII, *Cong. Rec.* (House), 12582–12598.

67. H.R. 2491 § 8001, proposing new section 1851(a).

68. For a defense of the program, see Einer Elhauge, "Medi-Choice," *The New Republic* (Nov. 13, 1995): 24 .

69. Presidential Veto of H. R. 2491, *Cong. Quarterly* 3762, December 9, 1995.

70. Codified in 47 U.S.C. 151 et seq. For an initial overview of the statute, see Peter W. Huber, Michael K. Kellogg, and John Thorne, *The Telecommunications Act of 1996* (1996).

71. Telecommunications Act of 1996, 47 U.S.C. § 254.

72. H.R. 2491 § 8001, proposing new section 1854(a)(1)(A).

73. Lui and Moffit, *A Taxpayer's Guide to the Medicare Crisis,* (1995): 32–35.

74. Cal. Ins. Code § 1861.

75. See, Chapter 3.

76. Goodman and Musgrave, *Patient Power,* 439–460.

77. See Adam Clymer, "Health Care Bill Fails Over Dispute Between Parties," *New York Times* (June 8, 1996): A1.

CHAPTER 8

1. Theda Skocpol, *Boomerang: Clinton's Health Security Effort and the Turn against Government in U.S. Politics* (1996).

2. James Fallows, "A Triumph of Misinformation," *Atlantic Monthly* (January 1995): 26.

3. Alan Brinkley, "Reagan's Revenge: As Invented by Howard Jarvis," *New York Times Magazine* (June 19, 1996): 36–37. Jarvis was the lead author of California's Proposition 13, a tax limitation initiative.

4. Skocpol, *Boomerang,* 176.

5. See Paul Starr, *The Logic of Health Care Reform 4* (1994).

6. For a profile, see Erik Eckholm, "The Uninsured: 37 Million and Growing," *New York Times,* (July 11, 1993): § 4, p. 5.

7. Ronald Dworkin, "Will Clinton's Health Plan be Fair." *New York Review of Books,* (Jan. 13, 1994): 20, 22. The key passages read as follows:

> Conservative economists . . . say we should create a free market in health care by removing all tax benefits and subsidies so that people can have only the care that they can afford. While that is, of course, an unacceptable solution, it is important to see why. It is unacceptable for three reasons. First, wealth is so unfairly distributed in America that many people would be unable to buy substantial health insurance at market rates. Secondly, most people have very inadequate information about health risks and medical technology; they do not know what the risk of breast cancer is before the

age of fifty, for example, or how much, if any, routine mammography before that age would add to their life expectancy. Third, in an unregulated market, insurance companies would charge some people higher premium rates because they were greater health risks (as, indeed, many insurance companies now do) so that people with a poor health history, or who were members of ethnic groups particularly susceptible with certain disease, or who lived in areas where the risk of violent injury was greater, would be charged prohibitive rates.

But if reform succeeds—if we finally end the national disgrace of being alone among prosperous nations in cheating citizens of life and health—we may be able to build on this success. We may rediscover a national sense that justice is worth its price in tax and government. We might then win greater justice in education, housing, jobs, all the other goods and chances we now distribute so unfairly; we might begin to end the ever greater disgrace that dooms on some of us, at birth, to a bleaker life than the rest of us with think unendurable.

8. See, e.g., Dan W. Brock and Norman Daniels, "Ethical Foundations of the Clinton Administration's Proposed Health Care System," *JAMA* 271 (1994): 1189.

9. For these numbers, see John Cassidy, "Who Killed the Middle Class," *New Yorker* (October 16, 1994): 113, which never considers either regulation or redistribution as a potential source of the current malaise.

10. For an insider's account, see Starr, *The Logic of Health Care Reform,* xiii–xxii. See also Skocpol, *Boomerang,* 1–17.

11. See "Navigating the Health Swamp: A Primer," *New York Times,* (June 12, 1994): Section 4A, p. 3.

12. Skocpol, *Boomerang,* at 168–171, on public ambivalence to managed care.

13. For a contemporary account, see Steven Waldman and Bob Cohn, "The Lost Chance," *Newsweek,* (September 19, 1994): 73. For a retrospective, see Lance K. Stell, "A Postmortem for ClintonCare," *Managed Care Medicine* 2 (April, 1995): 19.

14. For a discussion of the administrative structure, see Ass'n of American Physicians & Surgeons v. Clinton, 997 F.2d 898 (D.C. Cir. 1993). For a defense of the role of Mrs. Clinton and Magaziner, see Skocpol, *Boomerang,* 9–10, 54–55, and indeed everywhere else in her book.

15. Alain Enthoven, a "Good Health Idea Gone Bad," *Wall Street J.* (October 17, 1993): A18.

16. Ass'n of American Physicians & Surgeons v. Clinton, 997 F.2d 898 (D.C. Cir. 1993), holding among other points that the Federal Advisory Committee Act did not require opening the meetings of the Task Force the public. The meetings could be kept closed because Mrs. Clinton fell within the class of "full-time officers or employees" of the United States, by virtue of her White House duties, even though she was not a civil service employee of the United States.

17. CCH, President Clinton's Health Care Proposal (1993).

18. Recounted in Skocpol, *Boomerang,* 1–5.

19. Gallup/CNN/ *USA Today* poll. (Storrs, Conn.: Roper Center for Public Opinion Research, 9/24/93).

20. Laurence Gostin, "Health Care Reform in the United States," *J. Law & Medical Ethics* 21 (1992): 6.

21. "Your Future Health Plan" (letter), *Wall Street Journal* (October 13, 1993): A22.

22. Martin Feldstein, "What's Wrong With the Clinton Health Plan," *Wall Street Journal* (July 14, 1993): A12.

23. American Academy of Actuaries, *A Review of Premium Estimates in the Health Security Act (#7)* (July, 1994).

24. Skocpol, *Boomerang*, 156–157.

25. For the grudging recognition of the effectiveness of these programs, see Skocpol, *Boomerang*, 134–139.

26. Quoted in Skocpol, *Boomerang*, 146.

27. Ibid., 153–157.

28. "Clinton Health Plan Loses Support in Poll," *Chi. Trib.* (March 2, 1994): A4.

29. Skocpol, *Boomerang*, 102–106.

30. See, Chapter 6.

31. Letter of October 27, 1993, set out in CCH, xxix, xxx.

32. Kenneth E. Thorpe, "The Best of Both Worlds: Merging Competition and Regulation," *J. Am. Health Policy* (July/August 1992): 20–24.

33. Working Group Draft, A-4, echoed again in Brock and Daniels, "Ethical Foundations."

34. HSA §§ 1151-1154.

35. Working Report, A-18.

36. Ibid.

37. HSA § 1403.

38. HSA, A-5.

39. A-4, A-5. HSA, § 1001(c).

40. Nadine Strossen, "National Health Care: Will Big Brother's Doctor be Watching Us?" *Cornell J. of Law & Pub. Pol.* 4 (1995): 438. Strossen's views have extra weight because her remarks, short and to the point, were delivered in her capacity as President of the American Civil Liberties Union.

41. See Plyler v. Doe, 457 U.S. 202 (1982).

42. Quoted in Stell, "A Postmortem," 21.

43. Ibid., 21.

44. Skocpol, *Boomerang*, 145.

45. Elizabeth McCaughey, "No Exit: What the Clinton Plan Will Do for You; Health Care Reform," *The New Republic* 6, (February 7, 1994): 21.

46. Skocpol, *Boomerang*, 153.

47. Elizabeth McCaughey, "She's BAAACK! Clinton's Plan on the Ropes," *The New Republic* 9, (February 28, 1994): 17.

48. See HSA § 1321 (b) (1). A regional alliance is not required under this section to offer a contract with a health plan—(1) the alliance finds that the proposed premium exceeds 120 percent of the weighted-average premium within the alliance." Note that the imposition of overall budget caps under the program makes it difficult for these more expensive plans to gain approval. See Elizabeth McCaughey, "She's BAAACK," 20–21.

49. Skocpol, *Boomerang*, 153.

50. Robert Pear, "Clinton Fails to Get Endorsement of Elderly Group of Health Plan," *New York Times* (February, 25, 1994): A1, A15. Skocpol, *Boomerang*, 92–95.

51. AP, "The Health Care Debate: The Constituencies: Directors' Vote of Support Angers Members of Retiree Group," *New York Times* (August 12, 1994): 18A, Col. 1.

52. HSA §§ 4104-4106 (Hospitalization); §§ 4111-4116 (professional fees); §§ 4131-4135 (both).

53. A-7. HSA §§ 1111-1128.

54. HSA §§ 2001-2009.

55. Strossen, "National Health Care," 439.

56. Harris v. McRae, 448 U.S. 297 (1980).

57. Rust v. Sullivan, 500 U.S. 173 (1991), upholding the regulation that imposed the restriction.

58. HSA § 1116. Query: does "voluntary family planning services" cover abortions?

59. For a statement of its position, see Strossen, "National Health Care," 440.

60. HSA § 1162.

61. Strossen, "National Health Care," 444.

62. See, e.g., Corporation of Presiding Bishop of the Church of Jesus Christ of Latter-Day Saint v. Amos, 483 U.S. 327 (1987) (upholding the exemption of religious organizations from the employment discrimination laws).

63. Skocpol, *Boomerang*, 116–117.

64. Memo from consultant Stan Greenberg to Ira Magaziner, September 14, 1993, about the September 22, 1993 speech. Quoted in Skocpol, *Boomerang*, 117.

65. HSA §§ 6202.

66. HSA §§ 1322(b)(2)(B).

67. HSA § 1322(c)(2).

68. For the inconclusive debate, see Skocpol, *Boomerang*, 30–35.

69. HSA §§ 1221-1224.

70. HSA § 1323.

71. HSA §§1321-1323.

72. HSA § 1381.

73. HSA § § 1384(a).

74. HSA § 1384 (b)(3).

75. HSA § 1385.

76. HSA § 1384(d).

77. HSA § 7111.

78. Martin Feldstein, "What the '93 Tax Increases Really Did," *Wall Street Journal* (October 26, 1995).

79. HSA §§ 3001-2051.

80. HSA § 3013(c)(2).

CHAPTER 9

1. Under current law, the Uniform Anatomical Gift Act allows the donor to specify the recipient, UAGA § 2a.

2. For a discussion of the conflict, see Blumstein, "Government's Role in Organ Transplantation Policy," in J. Blumstein and F. Sloan eds., *Organ Transplantation Policy: Issues and Prospects* (1989): 5, 30.

3. For discussion, see Chapter 12.

4. Andrew Kull, "Reconsidering Gratuitous Promises," *J. Legal Stud.* 21 (1992): 39, 49–50. The expression "sterile transaction" derives from the work of a Frenchman, Claude Bufnoir, Propriété et Contrat 487 (2d ed., 1924). The want of a productive element has led to some legal uneasiness about the enforceability of a promise to make a gift. See, generally, Melvin Aron Eisenberg, "Donative Promises," *U. Chi. L. Rev.* 47 (1979): 21 and Richard A. Posner, "Gratuitous Promises in Economics and Law," *J. Legal Stud.* 6 (1977): 411.

5. See Ronald H. Coase, "The Problem of Social Cost," *J.L. & Econ.* 3 (1960): 1.

6. For discussion, see Richard A. Epstein, "Unconscionability: A Critical Reappraisal," *J.L. & Econ.* 18 (1975): 293.

7. See E. Allan Farnsworth, *Contracts,* 2d ed. (1990): 679–700.

8. Ibid., 283–287.

9. For a discussion of these holdout problems, see Richard A. Epstein, *Bargaining with the State* (1993): Ch. 3 .

10. David D. Friedman, *Price Theory* 2d ed. (1990): 465–469.

11. For further discussion, see Richard A. Epstein, "Surrogacy: The Case for Full Contractual Enforcement," *Va. L. Rev.* 81 (1995): 2305, 2323–2325.

12. See Margaret Radin, "Market Inalienability," *Harv. L. Rev.* 100 (1987): 1849.

13. See, e.g., Catharine MacKinnon, "Pornography, Civil Rights, and Speech," *Harv. Civ. Rights- Civ. Liberties L. Rev.* (1985): 1.

14. See American Booksellers Association v. Hudnut, 7720 1 F.2d 323 (7th Cir. 1985) (invalidating the MacKinnon-inspired Indianapolis antipornography ordinance).

15. See, Harry Kalven, Jr., *A Worthy Tradition* (1988).

16. I have taken just this line with respect to various forms of hurt that flow from individual actions of discrimination. See Richard A. Epstein, *Forbidden Grounds: The Case Against Employment Discrimination Laws,* (1992): 498–499. "Given the limits of our own knowledge, I believe that the best way to take into account the full range of symbols, good and bad, noble and vain, is for the legal system to *ignore* them all—mine and yours alike." Indeed if the only justification for the antidiscrimination laws were to curtail their symbolic effects, they should be declared unconstitutional under the first amendment.

17. See, e.g., Muller v. Oregon, 208 U.S. 412 (1908) (upholding statute preventing women from working in factories more than 10 hours per day).

18. Reed v. Reed, 404 U.S. 71 (1971) (invalidating preferences for males in the administration of estates).

19. See Lori B. Andrews, "Beyond Doctrinal Boundaries: A Legal Framework for Surrogate Motherhood," *Va. I Rev.* 81 (1995): 2343, 2349 2350.

20. Field, *Surrogate Motherhood,* 75–83.

21. Ibid., 184. The figure is 495 out of 500 contracts.

22. Elizabeth Anderson, *Valuation in Economics and Philosophy* (1993): 172.

23. Ibid., Chapter 8. For an effective critique on her position, from which I have learned much, see Richard J. Arneson, "Commodification and Commercial Surrogacy," *Phil. and Pub. Aff.* 21 (1992): 132.

24. Farnsworth, *Contracts,* 809–817.

25. As could happen in cases of surrogate parents. See the account of a surrogate baby with a brain defect who was rejected when the adopting couple had divorced in the interim. Recounted in Field, *Surrogate Motherhood,* 1–2.

26. For a poignant illustration, see K.H. through Murphy v. Morgan, 914 F.2d 846 (7th Cir. 1990).

27. Anderson, *Valuation,* 175, asking "Is Women's Labor a Commodity?"

28. See Lori B. Andrews, "Surrogate Motherhood: The Challenge for Feminists," *Law, Med. & Health Care* 16 (1988): 72.

29. Matter of Baby M, 537 A.2d 1227, 1241–42 (N.J. 1988). Its key passage reads as follows:

> The prohibition of our statute is strong. Violation constitutes a high misdemeanor, a third-degree crime, carrying a penalty of three to five years

imprisonment. The evils inherent in baby-bartering are loathsome for a myriad of reasons. The child is sold without regard to whether the purchasers will be suitable parents. The natural mother does not receive the benefit of counseling and guidance to assist her in making a decision that may affect her for a lifetime. In fact, the monetary incentive to sell her child may, depending on her financial circumstances, make her decision less voluntary. Furthermore, the adoptive parents may not be fully informed of the natural parent's medical history.

Baby-selling potentially results in the exploitation of all parties involved. Conversely, adoption statutes seek to further humanitarian goals, foremost among them the best interests of the child.

30. See e.g., Steven Pressman, "The Baby Brokers," *California Lawyer* 30 (July 1991).

CHAPTER 10

1. One of these was the theft of corpses for use in medical instruction, a common offense during the nineteenth century. See, e.g., Charles Dickens, *A Tale of Two Cities* (1859), and his portrayal of Jerry Cruncher, a specialist in the business.

2. Leon Kass, "Organs for Sale? Propriety, Property and the Price of Progress," *The Public Interest* 107 (Spring 1992): 67.

3. For its most vivid documentation, see Lloyd R. Cohen, "Increasing the Supply of Transplant Organs: The Virtues of a Future Market," *Geo. Wash. L. Rev.* 58 (1989): 1, 3–6 (advocating a limited market for organ transplants). Cohen has since expanded and updated his article in book form: *Increasing the Supply of Transplant Organs: The Virtues of an Option Market* (1995). I shall refer on occasion to both. See, also, Judith Areen, "A Scarcity of Organs," *J. Legal Educ.* 38 (1988): 555.

4. Cohen, "Increasing the Supply," 4–5; updated in his book, Cohen, *Increasing the Supply,* 5–7. There has been no major relief to the shortage between 1989 and 1995. For similar estimates, see James F. Blumstein, "Government's Role in Organ Transplant Policy," in James F. Blumstein and Frank A. Sloan, eds., *Organ Transplantation Policy, Issues and Prospects* (1989): 5, 12–13, from whose critical review of present organ transplantation policy I have greatly profited.

5. For these figures, see Elisabeth Rosenthal, "Parents Find Solace in Donating Organ," *New York Times* (May 14, 1993): B5, B8. The article describes how the decision to donate the organs of a child can help the healing process for the parents. The story gave no hint of the increased shortages over time as it extolled the virtues of voluntary donations.

6. The major source of organs for transplantation do come from accidental death to young persons, usually male. K. Bart et al., "Cadaveric Kidneys for Transplantation," *Transplantation* 31 (5) (1981): 379. K. Bart et. al., "Increasing the Supply of Cadaveric Kidneys for Transplantation," *Transplantation* 31 (5) (1981): 383.

7. "In September 1991 UNOS estimated that approximately 8.7% of patients needing a liver transplant died while waiting for a transplant. In the 3 months ending September 30, 1991, the number of patients who died while with heart transplants was 211; kidney transplants, 264; heart-lung transplants, 13; and pancreas transplants, 9. These are probably minimum estimates of deaths. Some patients are withdrawn from the transplant waiting list because they have become too ill, but are not routinely reported to UNOS if they die at some later time." J. G. Turcotte, "Supply, Demand and Ethics of Organ Procurement: The Medical Perspective," *Transplantation Proceedings* 24 (1992): 2140–2142.

8. Pub. L. No. 98-507, 98 Stat. 2339 (1984), codified at 42 U.S.C.A. § 274e (West 1991).

9. Ibid.

10. Ibid.

11. Ibid.

12. Organ Transplant Act, Pub. L. No. 98-507. 1984 U.S. Code Cong. & Admin. News 3982, confirmed in the report of the joint committee that noted the decision to make these sales lawful.

13. B. A. Virnig and A. L. Caplan, "Required Request: What Difference Has it Made?" *Transplantation Proceedings,* 24 (1992): 2155, 2158.

14. For further evidence, see Cohen, *Increasing the Supply,* 12.

15. Turcotte, "Supply, Demand and Ethics," 2140. "The 1-year graft survivals for cadaveric kidney transplants increased from approximately 50% to 85%. The actuarial patient survivals following heart and liver transplantation increased from 25% to 85 and 75, respectively."

16. See Omnibus Budget Reconciliation Act of 1986, Pub. L. No. 99-50-9, § 9318.

17. Arthur Caplan, "Organ Procurement: It's Not in the Cards," *Hastings Center Rep.* 14 (1984): 9.

18. See 1986 Budget Reconciliation Act, Pub. L. No. 99-509, Soc. Security Act, § 1138(a)(1)(A): All protocols for organ donations must "assure that families of potential organ donors are made aware of the option of organ or tissue donation and their option to decline."

19. See, e.g., Cal. Health and Safety Code, § 7184)West 1988 Supp. (duty to notify family of the option); Ind. Code Ann., § 29-2-16-10 (West 1988 Supp) (duty to notify legal representation of the option to donate organ). The California Statute provides that "each general acute care hospital shall develop a protocol for identifying potential organ and issue donors. The protocol shall require that any deceased individual's next of kin . . . at or near the time of notification of death be asked whether the deceased was an organ donor. . . . If not, the family shall be informed of the option to donate organs and tissues.

20. See Jeffrey M. Prottas, "The Organization of Organ Procurement," in James F. Blumstein and Frank A. Sloan, eds., *Organ Transplantation Policy, Issues and Prospects* (1989): 41 and Oh U Uniewski, "Enhancing Organ Recovery by Initiation of a Required Request Within a Major Medical Center," *Transplantation Proc.* 18 (1986): 426 (reporting a 300 percent increase).

21. See Cohen, *Increasing the Supply,* 21.

22. See Virnig and Caplan, "Required Request," 2158.

23. See Rosenthal, "Parents Find Solace," B8, comments of Dr. Norman Shumway.

24. Peter H. Schuck, "Government Funding," *Organ Transplantation Policy,* 171, n.7. For a well-known case of a refusal to turn off life-support systems after brain death, see Strachan v. John F. Kennedy Memorial Hospital, 538 A.2d 346 (N.J. 1988) (allowing a claim for intentional infliction of emotion distress).

25. Proposed in Arthur L. Caplan, "Sounding Board: Ethical and Policy Issues in the Procurement of Cadaver Organs for Transplantation," *Human Organ Transplantation* (1987): 272, 275.

26. Judith Areen, "A Scarcity of Organs," *J. Legal Educ.* 38 (1988): 555, 565.

27. See Rosenthal, "Parents Find Solace," B8.

28. Ibid. The size of that increase has been disputed. Cohen, *Increasing the Supply,* 39 (denying that the increase is "significant").

29. 497 So. 2d 1188 (Fla. 1986).

30. Fla. Stat. 932.9185.

Corneal removal by medical examiners.—(1) In any case in which a patient is in need of corneal tissue for a transplant, a district medical examiner or an appropriately qualified designee with training in ophthalmologic techniques may, upon request of any eye bank authorized under s. 732.918, provide the cornea of a decedent whenever all of the following conditions are met:

(a) A decedent who may provide a suitable cornea for the transplant is under the jurisdiction of the medical examiner and an autopsy is required in accordance with s. 406.11.

(b) No objection by the next of kin of the decedent is known by the medical examiner.

(c) The removal of the cornea will not interfere with the subsequent course of an investigation or autopsy.

(2) Neither the district medical examiner nor his appropriately qualified designee nor any eye bank authorized under s. 732.918 may be held liable in any civil or criminal action for failure to obtain consent of the next of kin.

31. See William Prosser, *The Law of Torts*, (1st ed. 1955): 43–44.

32. Dougherty v. Mercantile-Safe Deposit & Trust Co., 387 A.2d 244 (Md. Ct. App. 1978).

33. *Powell*, 497 So. 2d, 1191.

34. Ibid., 1192.

35. Ibid., 1189–1992.

CHAPTER II

1. See, e.g., Lori Andrews, "My Body, My Property," *Hastings Center Rep.*, (Oct. 1986): 28, James Blumstein, "The Case for Commerce in Organ Transplantation," *Transplantation Proceeding* 24 (1992): 2190; M. Brams, "Transplantable Human Organs: Should Their Sale Be Authorized by State Statutes?" *Am J. L. & Med.* 3 (1977) 183; Lloyd R. Cohen, "Increasing the Supply of Transplant Organs: The Virtues of a Future Market," *Geo. Wash. L. Rev.* 58 (1989): 1, 3–6, reissued and updated as *Increasing the Supply of Transplant Organs: The Virtues of an Option Market* (1995); Henry Hansmann, "The Economics and Ethics of Markets for Human Organs," in James F. Blumstein and Frank A. Sloan, eds., *Organ Transplantation Policy, Issues and Prospects* (1989); Jack Kevorkian, "A Controlled Auction Market is a Practical Solution to the Shortage of Transplantable Organs," *Med. and L.* 47 (1992).

2. Richard Schwindt and Aidan R. Vining, "Proposal for a Future Delivery Market for Transplant Organs," *J. Health Politics, Policy & Law* 11 (1986): 483, 489.

3. Henry Hansmann, "Markets for Human Organs" 57, 61–66.

4. Cohen, *Increasing the Supply*, 33–34 (arguing that his proposal has lower transaction costs than the Hansmann rival).

5. Jesse Dukeminier, "Supplying Organs for Transplantation," *Mich. L. Rev.* 68

(1970): 811, 863.

6. Cohen, *Increasing the Supply,* 92.

7. Hastings Center, Ethical Legal and Policy Issues Pertaining to Solid Organ Procurement: A Report of the Project on Organ Transplantation (1985): 11–12.

8. The 1987 amendments to the UAGA specifically state that a gift of an organ "does not require the consent or concurrence of any other person after the death of the donor."

9. James Blumstein, "The Case for Commerce in Organ Transplantation," *Transplantation Proceedings* 24 (1992): 2190.

10. Tentatively endorsed in Hansmann, "Markets for Human Organs," 71–77.

11. For a discussion of these issues, see Peter A. Singer, Mark Siegler, John D. Lantos, Jean C. Emond, Peter F. Whitington, J. Richard Thistlewaite, and Christoph E. Broelsch, "The Ethical Assessment of Innovative Therapies: Liver Transplantation Using Living Donors," *Theoretical Medicine* 11 (Stockholm) (1990): 87. The live liver transplantation program began at the University of Chicago with transplants from relatives to infant donees, on average 15 years of age. Early reports indicate a 90 percent survival rate from the program. Mark Siegler, "Liver Transplantation Using Living Donors," *Transplantation Proceedings* 24 (1992): 2223. Siegler notes: "We refused to implement the study unless there were some benefits to the recipient that could not be obtained utilizing the traditional cadaveric source of donor livers." Ibid., 2224, which there were. The condition, however, seems to be too restrictive. So long as disclosure is given to the donor, that consideration should be mentioned, but not be regarded as dispositive. And often the critical point is the expansion of the supply of organs and the reduction in waiting time for others.

12. For a brief summary of the relevant medical information, see Chapter 12.

13. See, Cohen, *Increasing the Supply,* 60, n109.

14. For a good refutation of most of the antimarket arguments, see Hansmann, "Markets for Human Organs," 71–78.

15. Lloyd Cohen takes this line for ordinary cadaveric transfers (Cohen, *Increasing the Supply,* 61) but deviates from it in dealing with live sales on the ground that "it raises the depressing prospect of the poor selling their organs in desperation. Ibid., 59, n109.

16. W. A. Cramond, J. H. Court, B. A. Higgins, P. R. Knight and J. R. Lawrence, "Psychological Screening of Potential Donors in a Renal Homotransplantation Programme," *Brit. J Psychiatry,* 113 (1967): 1213, 1219, quoted in Dukeminier, "Supplying Organs," 812, n3.

17. See Task Force, 36 (Table II-1).

18. 226 N.W. 2d 180 (Wis. 1975).

19. Ibid., 181.

20. Richard Titmuss, *The Gift Relationship: From Human Blood to Social Policy* (1971).

21. For a call for heavier reliance on the tort mechanism, see Ross D. Eckert, "The AIDS Blood-Transfusion Cases: A Legal And Economic Analysis of Liability," *San Diego L. Rev.* 29 (1992): 203.

22. Thomas H. Murray, "Gifts of the Body and the Needs of Strangers," *Hastings Center Rep.* 17 (1987): 30, 35.

23. On which see, Marvin Olasky, *The Tragedy of American Compassion* (1992).

CHAPTER 12

1. Here I rely heavily on James Blumstein's excellent article, "Government's Role in Organ Transplant Policy in Organ Transplantation Policy: Issues and Prospects," in James F. Blumstein and Frank A. Sloan, eds., *Organ Transplantation Policy, Issues and Prospects* (1989): 5.

2. 42 U.S.C. § 274(b)(2)(D).

3. Blumstein, "Government's Role," 19 (footnotes omitted) (emphasis in original).

4. Before 1990, the decisions of UNOS were routinely backed up by HHS even though they did not follow the procedures set out, for example in the administrative procedure act. Blumstein, "Government's Role," 20. Since that time, HHS has modified its position so UNOS policies are subject to review and approval by HHS, and its proceedings must now meet the rule-making requirements of the Administrative Procedure Act on notice, comment, and publication. See 54 Fed. Reg. 51802 (1989). In addition, noncompliance with UNOS regulations no longer means automatic exclusion from Medicare or Medicaid. But HHS has yet to formulate its own guidelines as to what sanctions are appropriate for noncompliance.

5. Blumstein, "Government's Role," 26.

6. Ibid., 24–26.

7. Task Force on Organ Transplantation, xxi.

8. Ibid., xxi.

9. Ibid., 87.

10. Ibid., 89.

11. Ibid., 89.

12. Martin Benjamin et al., "What Transplantation Can Teach Us about Health Care Reform," *NEJM* 330 (1994): 858.

13. For a detailed description of the point system on which this account is based, see Ian Ayres, Laura G. Dooley and Robert S. Gaston, "Unequal Racial Access to Kidney Transplantation," *Vand. L. Rev.* 46 (1993): 805. A shorter statement of their views can be found in Robert S. Gaston, Ian Ayres, Laura Dooley, and Arnold Diethelm, "Racial Equity in Renal Transplantation: The Disparate Impact of HLA-Based Allocation," *JAMA* 270 (1993): 1352. See also Lloyd Cohen and Melissa Michelsen, "The Efficiency/Equity Puzzle in Kidney Allocation: A Reply to Ayres, et al and UNOS" (forthcoming *Annual Review of Law and Ethics* 1996).

14. Blumstein, "Government's Role," 29.

15. UNOS Policy 3.4. For discussion, see Ayres, Dooley and Gaston, "Unequal Racial Access," 821–822, 841–842. Cohen and Michelsen, The Efficiency/Equity Puzzle, 25–27.

16. Cohen and Michelsen, "The Efficiency/Equity Puzzle," 50–55.

17. For discussion, see Richard A. Posner, *Aging and Old Age* (1995): 51–65, noting both explanations.

18. For a defense on grounds of desert in conditions of scarcity, see Alvin H. Moss and Mark Siegler, "Should Alcoholics Compete Equally for Liver Transplantation," *JAMA* 265 (1991): 1295. The authors argued, inter alia, that the even if there were a genetic predisposition to the condition, the ability to check it before it became chronic should count. The Moss/Siegler proposal brought forth strong objections. See, e.g., Carl Cohen and Martin Benjamin, "Alcoholics and Liver Transplantations," *JAMA* 265 (1991): 1299, one of a half dozen critical articles.

19. "UNOS will review the activities of any transplant center that exceeds the 10 per-

cent ceiling guideline recommended by the National Task Force on Organ Transplantation for the number of organ transplants performed on foreign nationals." Wayne B. Arnason, "Directed Donation—The Relevance of Race," *Hastings Center Report* (Nov.-Dec. 1991): 13, 17. In addition, the UNOS guidelines bans exports outside of Canada "unless a well-documented and verifiable effort, coordinated through UNOS, has failed to find a suitable recipient for that organ in the United States or Canada." UNOS Policy 6.5.1. See also Task Force, 10. See also the original 1986 Task Force recommendation, page 10, which urges this position, in part because of the suspicion that hospitals have given priority to nonresident aliens because of their willingness to pay. "If money is the real reason for assigning priority to non-immigrant aliens, then some transplant institutions are selling organs that have been donated to them without charge." Task Force, 93.

20. For an elaboration, see Richard A. Epstein, "Altruism—Universal and Selective," *Soc. Serv. Rev.* 67 (1993): 388.

21. Gerhard Opelz et al., "Influence of Race on Kidney Transplant Survival," *Transplantation Proc.* 9 (1977): 1237; Paul Terasaki, et al., "Long Term Survival of Kidney Grafts," *Transplantation Proc.* 21 (1989): 615; Arnason, "Directed Donation," 14.

22. See, e.g., Arnason, "Directed Donation."

23. United States Renal Data System, 1988 Annual Data Report.

24. Office of the Inspector General, The Distribution of Organs for Transplantation: Expectations and Practices (1991): 8.

25. See Ayres, Dooley, and Gaston, "Unequal Racial Access," 825–836.

26. See Ayres, Dooley, and Gaston, "Unequal Racial Access," 833–836.

27. L. G. Hunsicker and Philip J. Held, "The Role of HLA Matching for Cadaveric Renal Transplants in the Cyclosporine Era," *Seminars in Nephrology* 12 (1992): 293 (small gains); Donald E. Butkus et al., "Racial Differences in the Survival of Cadaveric Renal Allografts," *NEJM* 327 (1992): 840 (significant differences); Cohen and Michelsen, "The Efficiency/Equity Puzzle," 28–37.

28. David Gjertson et al., "National Allocation of Cadaveric Kidneys by HLA Matching," *NEJM* 324 (1991): 1032, where the authors propose the national pool because it increases the likelihood of good matches.

29. Ayres, Dooley, and Gaston, "Unequal Racial Access," 849–850. Arnason, "Directed Donations."

30. Ayres, Dooley, and Gaston, "Unequal Racial Access," 845.

31. Ibid., 846. A draft version of their paper did urge the explicit racial classification. "To counterbalance the disparate impact of mandatory six 6 antigen sharing and partial antigen points, all potential black recipients would receive a fixed number of points, calculated to provide cadaveric kidneys for blacks in proportion to black representation in the ESRD population." Mss., 57.

32. Ibid., 842–843.

33. UNOS Policies 3.5.6.1 & 3.5.6.2 (1995).

34. Ayres, Dooley, and Gaston, "Unequal Racial Access," 820–822.

35. See Cohen and Michelsen, "The Efficiency/Equity Puzzle," 53–56.

36. Cohen and Michelsen, "The Efficiency/Equity Puzzle," 51–56.

37. Adam Smith, *A Theory of Moral Sentiments* (1759).

CHAPTER 13

1. For an exhaustive history of the ebbs and flow, see Ezekiel J. Emanuel, "The History of Euthanasia Debates in the United States and Britain," *Ann. Internal Med.* 121

(1994): 793.

2. William Knaus et al., "A Controlled Trial to Improve Care for Seriously Ill Hospitalized Patients," *JAMA* 274 (1995): 1591.

3. Gina Kolata, "Organ Shortage Leads to Nontraditional Transplants, and Ethical Concerns," *New York Times* (June 2, 1993): A6.

4. The two most quoted judicial passages read: "No right is held more sacred, or is more carefully guarded, by the common law, than the right of every individual to the possession and control of his own person, free from all restraint or interference of others, unless by clear and unquestionable authority of law." Union Pacific Ry Co. v. Botsford, 141 U.S. 250, 251 (1891); "Every human being of adult years and sound mind has a right to determine what shall be done with his own body; and a surgeon who performs an operation without his patient's consent commits an assault, for which he is liable in damages." Schloendorff v. Society of New York Hospital, 105 N.E. 92, 93 (N.Y. 1914). Only *Schloendorff* was directly concerned with unauthorized treatment. *Botsford* upheld the right of a plaintiff to resist a physical examination to determine the extent of her injuries, which is now routinely allowed. See Fed. Rules of Civ. Proc. rule 35.

5. These may be withdrawn under current AMA guidelines, Opinion 2.18 of the Current opinions of the Council on Ethical and Judicial Affairs (1986), cited in Cruzan by Cruzan v. Harmon 760 S.W.2d 408, 423 n.18 (Mo. 1988).

6. 801 P.2d 617 (Nev. 1990).

7. For similar decisions, see State v. McAfee, 385 S.E.2d 651 (Ga. 1989) (same); In Matter of Farrell, 529 A.2d 404 (N.J. 1987); Bouvia v. Superior Court, 225 Cal. Rptr. 297 (1986) (termination of life support allowed in case of severe cerebral palsy, quadriplegia, and degenerative and crippling arthritis).

8. Cited in McKay v. Bergstedt, 801 P.2d 617, 621 (Nev. 1990) and universally followed.

9. Consider the oft-quoted language from Bouvia v. Superior Court of Los Angeles County, 225 Cal. Rptr. 297 (Cal. App. 1986):

> Here Elizabeth Bouvia's decision to forego medical treatment or life-support through a mechanical means belongs to her. It is not a medical decision for her physicians to make. Neither is it a legal question whose soundness is to be resolved by lawyers or judges. It is not a conditional right subject to approval by ethics committees or courts of law. It is a philosophical decision that, being a competent adult, is hers alone. 225 Cal. Rptr. at 305.

10. See, e.g., Matter of Quinlan, 355 A.2d 647 (N.J. 1976); Superintendent of Belchertown State School v. Saikewicz, 370 N.E.2d 417 (Mass. 1977); Brophy v. New England Sinai Hospital Inc., 497 N.E.2d 626 (1986). See, generally, Nancy K. Rhoden, "Litigating Life and Death," *Harv. L. Rev.* 102 (1988): 375 (dealing with incompetents, but noting the dominance of the autonomy standard with competent patients).

11. Every state in the union and the District of Columbia has a general durable power of attorney statute. For a list, see Cruzan v. Director, Missouri Department of Health, 497 U.S 261, 292 n.3. And 13 states and the District of Columbia have statutes that authorize a durable power of attorney to deal with matters of health care. *Cruzan*, n.2.

12. Sanford Kadish, "Letting Patients Die: Legal and Moral Reflections," *Cal. L. Rev.* 80 (1992): 857.

13. Franklin G. Miller, Timothy E. Quill, Howard Brody, et al., "Regulating Physician-Assisted Death," *NEJM* 331 (1994): 119.

14. See David Margolick, "Jurors Acquit Dr. Kevorkian in Suicide Case," *New York*

Times (May 3, 1994): A1. Two years later, the story is much the same. Jack Lessenberry, "Jury Acquits Kevorkian in Common-Law Case," *New York Times* (May 15, 1996): A14, noting his acquittal in the last three cases and suggesting that no further charges are likely to be brought.

15. For a similar view, see Dan Brock, "Voluntary Active Euthanasia," *Hastings Center Report*, 22 (1992): 10 n.2. See also, T. E. Quill, C. K. Cassel, and D. E. Meier, "Care of the Hopelessly Ill: Proposed Clinical Criteria for Physician-Assisted Suicide," *NEJM* 327 (1992): 1383.

16. William A. Prosser and W. Page Keeton, *Law of Torts* (5th ed., 1984): § 56.

17. See, e.g., for an early attack, James Barr Ames, "Law and Morals," *Harv. L. Rev.* 22 (1908): 97, 110–113, urging repudiation of the distinction.

18. Pridgen v. Boston Housing Authority, 308 N.E.2d 467 (Mass. 1974) (duty of care owed to known trespasser in position of peril).

19. For discussion, see Richard A. Epstein, "A Theory of Strict Liability," *J. Legal Stud.* 2 (1973): 151, 198–200, attacking Ames, "Law and Morals," and stating my earlier arguments against the duty to rescue strangers.

20. See also discussion in Introduction.

21. Glanville Williams, "Euthanasia," *Medical-Legal J.* 41 (1973): 14, 21; George Fletcher, "Prolonging Life," *Wash. L. Rev.* 42 (1967): 999. See also James Rachels, "Active and Passive Euthanasia," *NEJM* 192 (1975): 78.

22. See Barber v. Superior Court, 195 Cal. Rptr. 484 (1983).

23. See Cruzan by Cruzan v. Harmon, 760 S.W.2d, 408, 421 (Mo. Bank. 1988). "Since *Quinlan,* the medical profession moved to abandon any distinction between extraordinary and ordinary treatment in considering the propriety of withdrawing life sustaining treatment." For a recent confirmation of this view, see Yale Komisar, "Active v. Passive Euthanasia: Why Keep the Distinction?" *Trial* (March 1993): 32, 34.

24. Daniel Callahan, *What Kind of Life?* (1990): 233.

25. Restatement (Second) of Torts, § 431 (1965): "The actor's negligent conduct is a legal cause of harm to another if (a) his conduct is a substantial factor in bringing about the harm." For application, see, e.g., Mitchell v. Gonzales, 819 P.2d 872 (Cal. 1991) (death by drowning is not sole cause of harm to excuse negligent supervision by adult).

26. E. Haavi Morreim, "Whodunit? Causal Responsibility of Utilization Review for Physicians' Decisions, Patients' Outcomes," *Law, Medicine and Health Care* 20 (1992): 40, 46, stressing causal liability for omission where care is undertaken, but not otherwise. For a more general discussion, see H. L. A. Hart and Tony Honoré, *Causation in the Law* 2d ed. (1985): 11–12 (the distinction between cause and condition) and 138–140 (medical omissions as acts).

27. For an explicit approval of this position, see the statement of the American Thoracic Society, where section 1 provides: "Respect for patient autonomy is the primary basis for withholding and withdrawing life-'sustaining therapy.'" *Am. Rev. Respir. Dis.* 144 (1991): 726, 726 and notes, with suitable references that "[w]ithholding and withdrawing life-sustaining therapy, with or without palliative sedation or analgesia, are generally, but not universally, considered to be ethically and legally distinct from assisted suicide and active euthanasia. The latter is the administration of a lethal agent for the purpose of causing death. Physician involvement in assisted suicide and active euthanasia, even if requested by the patient, is not endorsed by the ATS." Ibid., 727.

28. Leon Kass, "Is There a Right to Die," *Hastings Center Report* (Jan.-Feb. 1993): 34.

29. John Locke, *Second Treatise on Government,* ¶ 27.

30. For my criticisms, see Richard A. Epstein, "Possession as the Root of Title," *Ga. L. Rev.* 13 (1979): 1221 and Richard A. Epstein, "On the Optimal Mix of Common and Private Property," *Soc. Phil. and Pol.* 11 (No. 2) (1994): 17.

31. *Second Treatise on Government,* (1689): Chapter 5, ¶ 23. Yet even here, Locke appears to bend a little, by allowing in the same paragraph the slave the option to commit suicide "whenever he finds the hardship of his slavery out-weigh the value of his Life." But he returns to this theme in explaining the limitations on the power of the legislature to take property or life arbitrarily in Ch. 11, paragraph 135.

32. Ibid., Ch. 4, paragraph 23.

33. Immanuel Kant, *The Metaphysical Principles of Virtue* (trans. by James Ellington, 1964): 83–84.

34. Discussed in Callahan, *What Kind of Life?*, 228–229.

35. For discussion, see Richard A. Epstein, *Simple Rules for a Complex World* (1995): Chapters 3 and 8.

36. See Canterbury v. Spence, 464 F.2d 772 (D.C. 1972), which builds on *Schloendorff.*

CHAPTER 14

1. Daniel Callahan, *What Kind of Life?* (1990): 230.

2. Thomas Hobbes, *Leviathan,* (Oakeshott ed. 1962): Ch. 14, p. 105. "As first a man cannot lay down the right of resisting them, that assault him by force, to take away his life; because he cannot be understood to aim thereby, at any good to himself."

3. John Locke, *Second Treatise on Government,* (1689): Ch. 10, paragraph 138. "The *supreme power cannot take* from any man any part of his *property* without his own consent; for the preservation of property being the end of government, and that for which men enter into society, it necessarily supposes and requires, that the people should *have property,* without which they must be supposed to lose that by entering to society, which was the end for which they entered it; too gross an absurdity for any man to own." In the absence of any real transaction, there are no counterweights to the rational calculations captured by such terms as "necessarily" and "absurdity."

4. See, generally, Farnsworth, *Contracts* § 4.27.

5. For the literature on Bayes's rule, see Amos Tversky and Daniel Kahneman, "Causal Schemas in Judgments under Uncertainty," in Martin Fishbein, ed., *Progress in Social Psychology* (1980): 117. For legal implications, see David Kaye, "The Law of Probability and the Law of the Land," *U Chi. L. Rev.* 47 (1979): 34.

6. For a case that displays all these ambiguities, see Knight v. Jewett, 834 P.2d 696 (Cal. 1992). The case involved a coed touch football game in which the female plaintiff asked the male defendant to stop playing so rough, only for him to injure her on the next play. His conduct was probably consistent with the background norm, but inconsistent with her request (to which his assent was, at best, evasive). The majority of the court upheld the assumption of risk defense (consent for accidents, as it were), while a dissent wanted the jury to pass on the evidence of the specific case.

7. For discussion, see Jonathan J. Koehler and Daniel Shaviro, Veridical Verdicts: Increasing Verdict Accuracy Through the Use of Overtly Probabilistic Evidence and Methods," *Cornell L. Rev.* 75 (1990) 247.

8. For a graphic illustration of this problem, see Hubert Smith, "Relation of Emotions to Injury and Disease: Legal Liability for Psychic Stimuli," *Va. L. Rev.* 30 (1944): 193, who examined all the decided cases where the plaintiff sought to recover for physical injuries attributable to emotional distress and concluded that the overcompensation for

plaintiffs was so great that the legal system would have been both cheaper and more accurate "had all courts denied damages for injury imputed to psychic stimuli alone." Ibid., 285.

9. For the troubled history of prize-fighting, see Hudson v. Craft. 204 P.2d 1 (Cal. 1949).

10. For evidence, see Richard A. Posner, *Aging and Old Age* (1995): 239, as part of his defense of assisted suicide.

11. "Neither for Love Nor Money: Why Doctors Must Not Kill," *The Public Interest* 94 (Winter 1989): 25.

12. Tamar Lewin, "Doctor Cleared of Murdering Woman with Suicide Machine," *New York Times* (Dec. 14, 1990): A19.

13. Pub. Act No. 3, M.C.L. A. § 752.1027, § 7(1)(a)&(b) & 7(2)-(3).

Section 7. (1) A person who has knowledge that another person intends to commit or attempt to commit suicide, and who intentionally does either of the following is guilty of criminal assistance to suicide, a felony punishable by imprisonment for not more than 4 years or by a fine of not more than $2,000, or both.

(a) Provides the physical means by which the other person attempts or commits suicide.

(b) Participates in a physical act by which the other person attempts or commits suicide.

(2) Subsection 1 shall not apply to withholding or withdrawing medical treatment.

(3) Subsection (1) does not apply to prescribing, dispensing, or administering medications or procedures if the intent is to relieve pain or discomfort and not to cause death, even if the medication or procedure may hasten or increase the risk of death.

Note how the statute struggles to deal with cases of double effect, which arise when the administration of medicine to relieve pain is also likely or certain to cause death. Such cases cannot be called assisted suicide without throwing the entire medical profession into jail. In this regard, the Michigan statute is far narrower than the AMA's definition of assisted suicide, which covers all cases "when a physician facilitates a patient's death by providing the necessary means and/or information to enable the patient to perform the life-ending act (e.g., the physician provides sleeping pills and information about the lethal dose, while aware that the patient may commit suicide)." Council on Ethical and Judicial Affairs, American Medical Association, "Decisions Near the End of Life," *JAMA* 267 (1992): 2229–2233.

14. People v. Kevorkian, 527 N.W.2d 714 (Mich. 1994).

15. Ibid., 24.

16. Posner, *Aging and Old Age*, 243–250.

17. See the allegations of the plaintiff physicians, Timothy E. Quill, Samuel C. Klagsbrun, and Howard A. Grossman, in Quill v. Vacco, 80 F.3d 716, 719 (2d. Cir. 1996).

18. Carlos F. Gomez, *Regulating Death: Euthanasia and the Case of the Netherlands* (1991).

CHAPTER 15

1. The New York State Task Force On Life and the Law, "When Death Is Sought: Assisted Suicide and Euthanasia in the Medical Context" (executive summary) (1994): ix.

2. Uli Schmetzer, "A Catch in Australia's Suicide Law," *Chicago Tribune* (July 27, 1996): 1 (noting fierce physician and clerical resistance to the legalization of physician-assisted suicide in the Australia's Northern territories).

3. Paul Wilkes, "The Next Pro-Lifers," *New York Times Magazine* (July 21, 1996): 22.

4. Edward R. Grant and Paul Benjamin Linton, "Relief or Reproach?: Euthanasia Rights in the Wake of Measure 16," *Or. L. Rev.* 74 (1995): 449, 450.

5. Ibid., 450. George J. Annas, "Death by Prescription: The Oregon Initiative," *NEJM* 331 (1994): 1240.

6. *JAMA* 259 (Jan. 8, 1988): 272.

7. The key passages read:

It was a gallows scene, a cruel mockery of her youth and unfulfilled potential. Her only words to me were, "Let's get this over with."

I retreated with my thoughts to the nurses' station. The patient was tired and needed rest. I could not give her health, but I could give her rest. I asked the nurse to draw 20 mg of morphine sulfate into a syringe. Enough, I thought, to do the job. I was going to give Debbie something that would let her rest and to say good-bye. Debbie looked at the syringe, then laid her head on the pillow with her eyes open, watching what was left of the world. I injected the morphine intravenously and watched to see if my calculations on its effects would be correct. Within seconds her breathing slowed to a normal rate, her eyes closed, and her features softened as she seemed restful at last. The older woman stroked the hair of the now-sleeping patient. I waited for the inevitable next effect of depressing the regulatory drive. With clocklike certainty, within four minutes, the breathing rate slowed even more, then became irregular, then ceased. The dark-haired woman stood erect and seemed relieved.

It's over, Debbie.

Note that "rest" is used as a substitute for death; that "job" is used as a substitute for euthanasia.

8. Willard Gaylin, Leon R. Kass, Edmund D. Pellegrino, and Mark Siegler, "Doctors Must Not Kill" *JAMA* 259 (1988): 2139. The authors repeat their categorical opposition to euthanasia, chastise *JAMA* for publishing this anonymous piece, and urge the editors of *JAMA* to turn over all information to the proper law enforcement officials in the "pertinent jurisdictions" (which are of course unknown).

9. Kenneth L. Vaux, "Debbie's Dying: Mercy Killing and the Good Death," *JAMA* 259 (1988): 2140.

10. Ibid., 2141.

11. George D. Lundberg, "'It's Over, Debbie' and the Euthanasia Debate," *JAMA* 259 (1988): 2142, 2143. "Results of a recent Roper poll, and the responses to our publication of 'It's Over, Debbie' suggest that the general public may feel very differently from physicians about euthanasia."

12. For a convenient summary, see Gomez, *Regulating Death*, 25–48

13. For details on the case, see Gomez, *Regulating Death*, 28–32.

14. Ibid., 32–34.

15. Ibid., 36–37.

16. Necessity as a defense to a charge of murder is itself a very complex doctrine that is invoked only rarely, and usually unsuccessfully for the killing of another human being. For the classic case, see R. v. Dudley & Stevens, 14 Q.B.D. 273 (1884); and for

exhaustive commentary on the interaction between the defense and customary practices, see A. W. B. Simpson, *Cannibalism and the Common Law: The Story of the Tragic Last Voyage of the Mignonette and the Strange Legal Proceedings to which it Gave Rise* (1984).

17. For discussion, see John Keown, "On Regulating Death," *Hastings Center Report,* (March-April 1992): 39–40.

18. Gomez, *Regulating Death,* 37–44.

19. Gomez, *Regulating Death,* 44–48. See also Henk A. M. J. ten Have and Jos V. M. Welie, "Euthanasia: Normal Medical Practice?" *Hastings Center Report* (March-April 1992): 34.

20. Gomez, *Regulating Death,* 51–52.

21. These numbers are drawn from ten Have and Welie, "Euthanasia," 34–35.

22. See the comments of Herbert Hendin, an American psychiatrist and executive director of the American Suicide Foundation, deploring the Dutch practice. Paul Wilkes, "The Next Pro-Lifers," 22, 25. Hendin's position is elaborated at far greater length in Herbert Hendin, *Seduced by Death: Doctors, Patients, and the Dutch Cure* (1996). Robert Bork joined the chorus against physician-assisted suicide in Robert H. Bork, *Slouching Toward Gemorrah* (1996): 110–111.

23. Gomez, *Regulating Death,* 51–56. The results of the Remmelink Commission were reported after the completion of the Gomez book.

24. New York Task Force, 23.

25. See, e.g., Alexander Morgan Capron, "Euthanasia in the Netherlands: American Observations," *Hastings Center Reports* (March-April 1992): 31l; Keown, "On Regulating Death"; Daniel Callahan, *When Self-Determination Runs Amok,* 52; and New York State Task Force, ix and 120. ("Despite these differences about the underlying ethical questions, the Task Force members unanimously recommend that the existing law should not be changed to permit assisted suicide and euthanasia.")

26. Gomez, *Regulating Death,* 95–113.

27. Ibid., 167, n44.

28. Ibid., 57–93

29. Timothy E. Quill, "Death and Dignity: A Case of Individualized Decision Making," *NEJM* 324 (1991): 691, 694, noting his refusal to make a coroner's case where he helped his patient die. Once publicized, Dr. Quill's case was in fact brought before a grand jury which refused to indict him. The New York State Task Force, 5.

30. Gomez, *Regulating Death,* 83–84.

31. Ibid., 85–86.

32. Ibid., 181.

33. Ibid., 107–113.

34. Ibid., 185.

35. Stephen Chapman, "Dead Wrong," *Chicago Tribune* (November 12, 1995): § 1, p. 17. A. D. Ogilvie and S.G. Potts, "Assisted Suicide for Depression: The Slippery Slope in Action?" *British Medical J.* 309 (1994): 492–493.

36. Gomez, *Regulating Death,* 119.

37. Ibid., 194.

38. Wilkes, "The Next Pro-Lifers," 21, 26, reporting on the observation of Herbert Hendin.

39. Marlise Simons, "Dutch Doctors to Tighten Rules on Mercy Killings," *New York Times* (September 11, 1995): A3.

40. Cal, Referendum, § 2525.7.

41. Ibid., § 2525.5.

42. Ibid., § 2525.13.

43. Ibid., § 2525.3.

44. See, e.g., Alexander Morgan Capron, "Even in Defeat, Proposition 161 Sounds a Warning," *Hastings Center Report* (Jan.-Feb. 1993): 32. Capron was strongly against the proposal and thought that the medical profession had to make clear that (a) its was still permissible for a patient to refuse treatment, and (b) that painkillers are almost always effective in easing pain at the end of life, the latter being a hotly disputed point. These points are surely relevant to an informed choice, but go only to the issue of disclosure, not to the question of who makes the final choice.

45. Oregon Act, at § 2, codified at Or. Rev. Stat. § 127.800 et seq.

46. Ibid., § 2.

47. Ibid., § 3.06 (Safeguards).

48. Ibid., § 3.14 (Construction of Act).

49. Ibid., § 3.14.

50. Ibid., §4.01 (Immunities) and § 4.02 (Liabilities).

51. Ibid., §§ 3.12–3.13.

52. Ibid., § 3.09 (documentation) and § 3.11 (reporting requirements).

53. Gomez, *Regulating Death*, 114–116 and Table 6.

54. The New York State Task Force on Life and the Law, "When Death is Sought: Assisted Suicide and Euthanasia in the Medical Context" (1994): 203.

55. See Grant and Linton, "Relief or Reproach?" 525–534.

CHAPTER 16

1. See, e.g., Antonin Scalia, "Originalism: The Lesser Evil," *U. Cin. L. Rev.* 57 (1989): 849.

2. See, e.g. Ronald Dworkin, *Freedom's Law: The Moral Reading of the American Constitution* (1996).

3. Lee v. State of Oregon, 891 F. Supp. 1429 (D. Or. 1995).

4. Compassion in Dying v. State of Washington, 49 F.3d 586 (9th Cir. 1995).

5. Compassion in Dying v. State of Washington, 79 F.3d 790 (9th Cir. 1996).

6. Quill v. Vacco, 80 F.3d 716, 730–731 (2d. 1996).

7. Ibid., 725–730.

8. 891 F. Supp. 1429 (D. Or. 1995).

9. Ibid., 1433.

10. Ibid., 1435, n.9.

11. Ibid., 1437.

12. Stephen L. Carter, "Rush to a Lethal Judgment," *New York Times* (July 21, 1996): 28–29.

13. Grant and Linton, "Relief or Reproach?" 462. The authors give a complete compilation on pp. 462–463, nn 44–46.

14. "A person is guilty of promoting a suicide when he knowingly causes or aids another person to attempt suicide." Rev. Code Wash. 9A36.060(1). It is punishable as a felony by imprisonment of up to five years and fines of up to $10,000. Rev. Code Wash. 9A.20.020(1)(c).

15. "[A]dult persons have the fundamental right to control the decision relating to the rendering of their own health care, including the decision to have life-sustaining treatment withheld or withdrawn, in states of a terminal condition or permanent unconscious condition." The Washington Natural Death Act, Rev. Code Wash., 70.122.010 (1995).

16. *Compassion in Dying,* 49 F.3d at 594.

17. Ibid., 594.

18. *Compassion in Dying,* 49 F.3d at 591, which relied on Yale Kamisar, "Are Laws Against Assisted Suicide Unconstitutional?" *Hastings Center Report* (May 1993): 32.

19. See *Compassion in Dying,* 79 F.3d at 794–795.

20. See comments of Kathleen Foley, a neurologist quoted at length in Paul Wilkes, "The Next Pro-Lifers," *New York Times Magazine* (July 21, 1996): 45.

21. Anthony L. Back, Jeffrey I. Wallace, Helene E. Starks, and Robert A. Pearlman, "Physician-Assisted Suicide and Euthanasia in Washington State," *JAMA* 275 (1996): 919.

22. See. Uli Schmetzer, "A Catch in Australia's Suicide Law," *Chicago Tribune* (July 27, 1996): 1.

23. Northern Territories (Australia), Rights of the Terminally Ill Act, § 7.

24. Jeffrey Rosen, "What Right to Die?" *The New Republic* (June 24, 1996): 28.

25. 79 F.3d at 801–802.

26. Roe v. Wade, 410 U.S. 113 (1973).

27. 388 U.S. 1 (1967).

28. 79 F.3d. at 805–806.

29. Ibid., 825–832.

30. Ibid., 833.

31. Ibid., 806–810.

32. 79 F.3d, 845–847 (Beezer, J. dissenting).

33. See Richard A. Epstein, *Takings: Private Property and the Power of Eminent Domain* (1985).

34. See Lucas v. South Carolina Coastal Council, 505 U.S. 1003 (1992), which refused to extend the nuisance conception that far.

35. See, e.g., Lovell v. City of Griffin, 303 U.S. 444 (1938) Erzoznik v. City of Jacksonville, 422 U.S. 205 (1975).

36. See John Stuart Mill, *On Liberty* (1859)

37. 198 U.S. 45 (1905).

38. For my answer, see Richard A. Epstein, "The Harm Principle—And How it Grew," *Toronto L. J.* 45 (1995): 369.

39. Paul Wilkes, "The New Pro-Life Movement," *The New York Times Magazine* (July 21, 1996): 22, 44.

40. See, e.g., City of Akron v. Akron Center for Reproductive Health, 462 U.S. 416 (1983) (invalidating requirement of hospitalization for second trimester abortions; informed consent requirement; and 24-hour waiting period); Planned Parenthood of Central Missouri v. Danforth, 428 U.S. 52 (1976)(invalidating requirements of both spousal and parental consent); Planned Parenthood of Southeastern Pennsylvania, 505 U.S. 833 (1992)(invalidating spousal notification requirements; upholding 24-hour waiting period and informed consent requirements).

41. 80 F.3d 716 (2d Cir. 1996).

42. *Compassion in Dying,* 79 F.3d at 831. *Quill,* 80 F.3d at 718, 719.

43. Yale Kamisar, "Are Laws Against Assisted Suicide Unconstitutional," *Hastings Center Report* (May 1993): 32; Yale Kamisar, "Assisted Suicide and Euthanasia: The Cases Are in the Pipeline," *Trial,* December 1994.

44. Grant and Linton, "Relief or Reproach?" 468–474.

45. See, e.g., Franklin G. Miller, et al., "Sounding Board: Regulating Physician-Assisted Death," *NEJM* 331 (1994): 119, 120, quoted in Judge Beezer's dissent in *Compassion in Dying,* 79 F.3d at 853.

46. 80 F.3d at 831. The point was pressed in Judge Beezer's dissent.

47. 80 F.3d at 729–731.

48. Ibid., 723–725.

49. 79 F.3d at 838.

50. 80 F.3d at 731.

51. Guido Calabresi, A Common Law for the Age of Statutes (1982), cited at 80 F.3d at 735.

52. N.Y. Pub. Health Law, § 2989(3).

53. Linda Greenhouse, "High Court Hears 2 Cases Involving Assisted Suicide," *New York Times* (January 9, 1997): A1. The subheading reads: "Justices, in an Unusually Personal Session, Reveal Their Reluctance to Intervene."

CHAPTER 17

1. See Daniel Callahan, "On Feeding the Dying," *Hastings Center Report* (October, 1983): 22.

2. 497 U.S. 261 (1990).

3. Cruzan by Cruzan v. Harmon, 760 S.W.2d 408 (Mo. en banc 1988).

4. Ibid., 419.

5. Unif. Rights of the Terminally Ill Act, 9B U.L. A. 620 § 10; Mo. Stat. Ann., § 459.055 (1985).

6. Mo. Stat. Ann, § 459.055. URITA contains a similar provision that ends, however, with the word "euthanasia" and does not contain the clause "nor permit any affirmative or deliberate act or omission to shorten or end her life." URITA § 10(g).

7. On the weaknesses of these approaches, see Nancy K. Rhoden, "Litigating Life and Death," *Harv. L. Rev.* 102 (1988): 375, which points out in great detail the difficulties of both approaches.

8. *Cruzan,* 760 S.W.2d at 425.

9. See Elizabeth S. Scott and Robert E. Scott, "Parents as Fiduciaries," *Va. L. Rev.* 81 (1995): 2401.

10. 573 A.2d 1235 (D.C. App. 1990).

11. Ibid., 1244.

12. 476 U.S. 610 (1986).

13. No otherwise qualified handicapped individual . . . shall, solely by reason of her or his disability, be excluded from the participation in, be denied the benefits of, or be subjected to discrimination under any program or activity receiving Federal financial assistance. 87 Stat. 394, 29 U.S.C. § 794(a).

14. *Bowen,* 476 U.S. at 659.

15. See Weber v. Stony Brook Hospital, 456 N.E.2d 1186 (N.Y. 1983).

CHAPTER 18

1. See also Henry W. Ballantine, "Title by Adverse Possession," *Harv. L. Rev.* 32 (1918): 135, for the law of adverse possession.

2. For the question of tort remedies, see C. H. S. Fifoot, *History and Sources of the Common Law* (1949): 1–184. Medical malpractice and product liability are not listed in the torts discussed. Loss or destruction of property by bailees are included on the list, as an established form of liability both in Roman and English law. For the evolution of the actions for the recovery of land, see A. W. B. Simpson, *History of the Land Law* (2d ed. 1986): Ch. 2 and Ch. 7.

3. See Oliver Wendell Holmes, "The Common Law," Lectures III and IV (1881).

4. See, e.g., Restatement (Second) of Torts, § 282 (1965).

5. See, e.g., Losee v. Buchanan, 51 N.Y. 476, 484–485 (1873).

If I have any of these [factories, machinery, dams, canals, or railroads] upon my lands, and they are not a nuisance and are not so managed as to become such, I am not responsible for any damage they accidentally and unavoidably do my neighbor. He receives compensation for such damage by the general good, in which he shares, and the right which he has to place the same things upon his lands.

6. Hay v. Cohoes Co., 2 N.Y. 159, 160 (1848).

7. See the Thorns case, Y.B. Mich. 6 Ed. 4, f. 7, pl. 18 (1466), reprinted, in Richard A. Epstein, *Cases and Materials on Torts*, (6th ed. 1995): 88. "So, too, if a man makes assault upon me and I cannot avoid him, and in my own defence I raise my stick to strike him, and a man is behind me and in raising my stick I wound him, in this case he shall have an action against me, and yet the raising of my stick to defend myself was lawful and I wound him me invito [against my will]."

8. Brown v. Kendall, 60 Mass. (6 Cush.) 292 (1850).

9. For the evolution in perspective, see Richard A. Epstein, "A Theory of Strict Liability," *J. Legal Stud.* 2 (1973): 151; Richard A. Epstein, *Simple Rules for a Complex World*, (1995): Ch. 4.

10. See, e.g., LeRoy Fibre Co. v. Chicago, Milwaukee & St. Paul Ry., 232 U.S. 340 (1914), especially the dissent of Justice Holmes. See, generally, Mark Grady, "Common Law Control of Strategic Behavior: Railroad Sparks and the Farmer," *J. Legal Stud.* 17 (1988): 15, favoring the defense in the case put in the text.

11. See, e.g., Smith v. Baker, [1891] A.C. 325 (England); St. Louis Cordage v. Miller, 126 F. 495 (8th Cir. 1903). For the classical contemporary exposition of the doctrine, see Francis H. Bohlen, "Voluntary Assumption of Risk," *Harv. L. Rev.* 20 (1906): 14. For a modern reinterpretation, see Richard A. Epstein, "The Historical Origins and Economic Structure of Workers' Compensation Law," *Ga. L. Rev.* 16 (1982): 775.

12. Lex Aquilia, D. 9.2.29: "If you give a cup to a jeweller to be filigreed and he breaks it through a lack of skill, he is liable for wrongful damage; but if he breaks it not from lack of skill but because it was badly cracked, he may have a defense. Hence most artisans who receive things of this kind stipulate that they will not do the task at their risk, which prevents either an action on the contract or under this statute. Translated by James B. Thayer, *Lex Aquilia* (1929): 27–29. The legal position and the social practice has scarcely changed.

13. See, e.g., Mohr v. Williams, 104 N.W. 12 (Minn. 1905); Schloendorff v. Society of New York Hospital, 105 N.E. 92 (N.Y. 1914).

14. Lex Aquilia, D. 9. 2. 8: Proculus says that if a doctor unskillfully operates on a slave, either the action on the contract or that on the Lex Aquilia will lie." Thayer, 11.

15. See, e.g., the very troubled case of the "hairy hand," Hawkins v. McGee, 146 A. 641 (N.H. 1929), where the physician both solicited the business and "guaranteed" the outcome.

16. See Sullivan v. O'Connor, 296 N.E.2d 183 (Mass. 1973), warning about the dangers of transforming "optimistic" opinions into "firm promises."

17. For a discussion of the general point, see Richard A. Epstein, "The Path to the *T. J. Hooper*, The Theory and History of Custom in the Law of Tort," *J. Legal Stud.* 21 (1992): 1, 19–20.

18. Lex Aquilia, D. 9.2.8.

19. Slater v. Baker, 24 Eng. Rep. 860, 861 (K.B. 1767). The case arose under the

forms of action, where the was a "special action on the case," which could be for either contract or tort.

20. Ibid., 863. The case involved a form of experimental treatment for resetting a broken leg.

21. See Brown v. Boorman, 8 Eng. Rep. 1003 (H.L.E. 1844). The headnote describes the rule accurately as follows: "Whenever there is a contract, and something is to be done in the course of the employment which is the subject of that contract, if there is a breach of duty in the course of that employment, the party injured may recover either in tort or in contract."

22. See, e.g., Clarence Morris, "Custom and Negligence," *Colum L. Rev.* 42 (1942): 1147, 1165.

23. Allan H. McCoid, "The Care Required of Medical Practitioners," *Vand. L. Rev.* 12 (1959): 549, 608.

24. The T.J. Hooper, 60 F.2d 737 (2d Cir. 1932) which I discussed at length in Epstein, "The Path to the *T. J. Hooper*," 32–36.

25. The T. J. Hooper, 60 F.2d at 740.

26. It is a position that I have taken to greater length in other writings. See Richard A. Epstein, "Medical Malpractice: The Case for Contract," *Am. Bar Found. Res. J.* (1976): 87; Richard A. Epstein, "Contracting Out of the Medical Malpractice Crisis," *Perspective in Biology and Medicine* 20 (1977): 288; Richard A. Epstein, "Medical Malpractice: Its Cause and Cure," in S. Rottenberg, ed., *The Economics of Medical Malpractice* (American Enterprise Institute, 1977), 245.

27. Uniform Partnership Act, § 18 (1994).

28. See Richard A. Posner, "A Theory of Negligence," *J. Legal Stud.* 1 (1972): 29.

29. Ibid., 73.

30. Epstein, "The Historical Origins," 787–797.

31. Workmen's Compensation Act, 60 & 61 Vict. Ch. 37 (1897).

32. See, e.g., the Wainwright Commission Report of 1910, which led to the passage of the first New York State system in 1910, which was struck down on state constitutional grounds in Ives v. South Buffalo Ry. Co., 94 N.E. 431 (N.Y. 1911). The statute was reenacted after state constitutional amendment and was then upheld against federal constitutional challenges in New York Central R.R. v. White, 243 U.S. 188 (1916).

33. Price V. Fishback, "Liability Rules and Accident Prevention in the Workplace: Empirical Evidence from the Early Twentieth Century," *J. Legal Stud.* 16 (1987): 305, 314.

34. See, e.g., Thomas G. Shearman and Amasa A Redfield, *Treatise of the Law of Negligence* (5th ed. 1898): vi–vii.

35. See, e.g., President and Directors of Georgetown College v. Hughes, 130 F.2d 810 (D. C. Cir. 1942); Darling v. Charleston Community Memorial Hospital, 211 N.E.2d 253 (Ill. 1965). See generally, for a full-throated endorsement of the modern rules, Fowler V. Harper, Fleming James Jr., and Oscar S. Gray, 5 The Law of Torts, § § 29.16 & 29.17 (1986).

36. See Feoffees of Heriot's Hospital v. Ross, 8 Eng. Rep. 1508 (H. L. 1846), overruled in Mersey Docks Trustees v. Gibbs, [1866] L. R. 1 H.L. 93.

37. McDonald v. Massachusetts General Hospital, 120 Mass. 432 (1876).

38. For a case that disagrees, see *Georgetown College*, at 130 F.2d. at 825–826.

39. See, e.g., Powers v. Massachusetts Homoeopathic Hospital, 109 F. 294, 304 (1st Cir. 1901): "If, in their dealings with their property appropriated to charity, they [members of the hospital board] create a nuisance by themselves or by their servants, if they dig pitfalls in their grounds and the like, there are strong reasons for holding them liable to outsiders, like any other individual or corporation. The purity of their aims may not justify

their torts; but, if a suffering man avails himself of their charity, he takes the risks of malpractice, if their charitable agents have been carefully selected." The same approach was also applied to employees of the firm. Hospital of St. Vincent v. Thompson, 81 S.E. 13 (Va. 1914).

40. See, e.g., Southern Methodist Hospital and Sanitarium v. Wilson, 46 P.2d 118 (Ariz. 1935).

41. *Georgetown College*, 130 F.2d at 826.

42. Schumacher v. Evangelical Deaconess Society of Wisconsin, 260 N.W. 476 (Wis. 1935) (extending the immunity for a paying patient); Norfolk Protestant Hospital v. Plunkett, 173 S.E. 363 (Va. 1934) (no immunity, incompetent nurse); Powers v. Massachusetts Homœopathic Hospital, 109 F. 294 (1st Cir. 1901).

43. "Abolition of the immunity as to the paying patient is justified as the last short step but one to extinction. Retention for the nonpaying patient is the least defensible and most unfortunate of the distinction's refinements. He, least of all, is able to bear the burden. More than all others, he has no choice. He is the last person the donor would wish to go without indemnity." *Georgetown College*, 130 F.2d at 827. The mistake in the argument is that it assumes that the likelihood of receiving charitable care is constant, regardless of the cost of its provision. See Chapter 2.

44. See Schloendorff v. Society of New York Hospital, 105 N.E. 92 (N.Y. 1914) (Cardozo, J.), applying the general immunity to a patient whose $7 daily fee was insufficient to cover the cost of daily maintenance.

45. See, e.g., Wendt v. Servite Fathers, 76 N.E.2d 342 (Ill. App. 1947)(insurance policy that allowed insurer to plead charitable immunity only on the request of the insured).

46. See Chapter 4 for a discussion of this portion of *McDonald* supra, addressing the broader question of forced associations and the refusal to deal.

47. See Malloy v. Fong, 232 P.2d 241, 247 (Cal. 1951).

48. *Georgetown College*, 130 F.2d at 823–824.

49. Ibid., 826.

50. 383 P.2d 441 (Cal. 1963).

51. Ibid., 442. Note that a more restrictive release would excuse the hospital even for negligence in the selection of its agents.

52. The decisive passage in *Tunkl* reads:

> In placing particular contracts within or without the category of those affected with the public interest, the courts have revealed a rough outline of the type of transaction in which the exculpatory provisions will be held invalid. Thus the attempted but invalid exemption involves a transaction that exhibits some or all of the following characteristics. It concerns a business of a type generally thought suitable for public regulation. The party seeking exculpation is engaged in performing a service of great importance to the public, which is often a matter of practical necessity for some members of the public. The party holds himself out as willing to perform this service for any member of the public who seeks it, or at least for any member coming within certain established standards. As a result of the essential nature of the service, in the economic setting of the transaction, the party invoking exculpation possesses a decisive advantage of bargaining strength against any member of the public who seeks his services. In exercising a superior bargaining power the party confronts the public with a standardized adhesion contract of exculpation, and makes no provision whereby a purchaser may pay additional reasonable fees and obtain protection against

negligence. Finally, as a result of the transaction, the person or property of the purchaser is placed under the control of the seller, subject to the risk of carelessness by the seller or his agents.

Ibid., 444–446 (footnotes omitted).

53. Glen O. Robinson, "Rethinking the Allocation of Medical Malpractice Risks Between Patients and Providers," *Law and Contemp. Probs.* 49 (Spring 1986): 173, 185–188.

54. See, e.g, P. S. Atiyah, "Medical Malpractice and the Contract/Tort Boundary," *Law and Contemp. Prob.* 49 (1986): 287, 295–296.

55. Madden v. Kaiser Foundation Hospitals, 552 P.2d 1178 (Cal. 1976).

56. Manchester, Sheffield & Lincolnshire Railway Company v. H. W. Brown, 8 A.C. 703 (H.L.E. 1883) (20 percent premium to cover losses for fish and other goods lost in transit).

57. See Richard A. Epstein, "Products Liability as an Insurance Market," *J. Legal Stud.* 14 (1985): 645, for further discussion, see Chapter 6 on insurance availability.

58. See, e.g.., Olson v. Molzen, 558 S.W.2d 429 (Tenn. 1977).

59. See, e.g., Helling v. Carey, 519 P.2d 981 (Wash. 1974).

60. See, e.g., Benson v. Dean, 133 N.E. 125 (N.Y. 1921).

61. See Benjamin P. Sachs, "Is the Rising Rate of Cesarean Sections a Result of More Defensive Medicine," in Institute of Medicine, *Medical Professional Liability and the Delivery of Obstetrical Care* (1989): 27, 36–37, [Hereafter IOM, Obstetrical Care].

62. See William L. Prosser and W. Page Keeton, *The Law of Torts* (5th ed. 1984).

63. See, e.g., Anderson v. Somberg, 338 A.2d 1 (N.J. 1975).

64. See Byrne v. Boadle, 159 Eng. Rep. 299 (Ex. 1863).

65. Paul C. Weiler, *Medical Malpractice on Trial* (1991): 3 (citing Mark Peterson, Civil Juries in the 1980s (RAND Institute for Civil Justice (1987)).

66. See, e.g., Patricia M. Danzon, "The Frequency and Severity of Medical Malpractice Claims: New Evidence," Law and Contemp. Probs. 49 (Spring 1986): 57–58.

67. Weiler, *Medical Malpractice,* at page 4–5.

68. See James R. Posner, "Trends in Medical Malpractice Insurance, 1970–1985," *J. Law and Contemp. Probs.* 49 (1986): 37, 49. His data runs from 1959 to 1983, but the same trend continues afterwards. And a similar cost justification can be found for the cost of vaccines; see Richard L. Manning, "Changing Rules in Tort Law and the Market for Childhood Vaccines," *J. Law and Econ.* 37 (1994): 247. The data for the diphtheria, pertussis, and tetanus vaccine (DPT) show price increases from $0.19 per unit in 1975 to $100.62 in 1987, most of which was for insurance premiums. Since that date, contributions into the vaccine funds have reduced liability exposures, but insurance premium plus vaccine tax are still close to $10 per dosage.

CHAPTER 19

1. The conception dates from Aristotle, where it was used in opposition to distributive justice. See his *Nicomachean Ethics,* Book V, Ch. 4. For more modern commentary on the issue, see Glanville Williams, "The Aims of the Law of Tort," *Current Legal Probs.* 4 (1951): 137; Richard A. Posner, "The Concept of Corrective Justice in Recent Theories of Tort Law" *J. Legal Stud.* 10 (1981): 187, 200. The "corrective justice requires annulling a departure from the preexisting distribution of money or honors in accordance with merit, but only when the departure is the result of *an act of injustice,* causing injury."

2. See Weiler, *Medical Malpractice,* 104–105, and 218–219 at note 28.

3. See Patricia Danzon and Lee A. Lillard, "Settlement out of Court: The Disposition of Medical Malpractice Claims," *J. Legal Stud.* 12 (1983): 345.

4. Henry S. Farber and Michelle J. White, "A Comparison of Formal and Informal Dispute Resolution in Medical Malpractice," *J. Legal Stud.* 23 (1994): 777.

5. James K. Hammitt, Stephen J. Carroll, and Daniel A. Relles, "Tort Standards and Jury Decisions," *J. Legal Stud.* 14 (1985): 751.

6. Ibid., 754–755.

7. The study has been reported in many places. See, e.g., Troyen R. Brennan, L. L. Leape, M. M. Laird, et al., "Incidence of Adverse Events and Negligence in Hosptalized Patients: Results of the Harvard Medical Practice Study," *NEJM* 324 (1991): 370; A. R. Localio, A. G. Lawthers, Troyen A. Brennan et al., "Relation Between Malpractice Claims and Adverse Events Due to Negligence," *NEJM* 325 (1991): 245; Paul C. Weiler, Troyen A. Brennan, Joseph P. Newhouse, and Howard H. Hiatt, "Proposal for Medical Liability Reform," *JAMA* 267 (1992): 2355.

8. Weiler, *Medical Malpractice,* 12.

9. Richard L. Abel, "The Real Tort Crisis—Too Few Claims," *Ohio St. L. J.* 48 (1987): 443.

10. For a convenient summary of the points, see Richard E. Anderson, "'An Epidemic' of Medical Malpractice? A Commentary on the Harvard Medical Practice Study," Civil Justice Memo (Manhattan Institute, July 1996).

11. Ibid., 3.

12. Ibid., 13.

13. Ibid., 73–74.

14. Don Dewees and Michael Trebilcock, "The Efficacy of the Tort System and Its Alternatives: A Review of the Empirical Evidence,"*Osgoode Hall L. J.* 30 (1992): 57.

15. See H. Laurence Ross, *Settled Out of Court: The Social Process of Insurance Claims Adjustment* (1970): 98–100.

16. See Paul C. Weiler, "The Case for No-Fault Medical Liability," *Md. L. Rev.* 52 (1993): 908, 926 n.68. For a more detailed account from which these numbers are drawn, see Stephen D. Sugarman, "Doctor No," *U. Chi. L. Rev.* 58 (1991): 1499, which offers a sustained critique of the costliness, clumsiness and Kafkasque quality of the current system.

17. On the general point, see Epstein, *Simple Rules for a Complex World,* 30–36.

18. Paul Starr, *The Logic of Health Care Reform: Why and How the President's Plan Will Work* (1994): 20. The 1 percent of the total cost of health care translates into about 3.7 percent of physician revenue, a figure that is roughly consistent with earlier studies of the issue. See Roger A. Reynolds, John A. Rizzo, and Martin L. Gonzalez, "The Cost of Medical Professional Liability," *JAMA* 257 (1987): 2776, using a 4 percent figure, based on 1984 data.

19. See Weiler, "The Case for No-Fault Medical Liability," 911.

20. Figures supplied by Ralph Muller, President of the University of Chicago Hospitals for the 1995 year.

21. On the complications of these obligations under EMTALA, see Chapter 4.

22. Civil Justice Reform Amendments of 1995, Pub. Act 89-7735 ILCS 5/2-1115.1(a). The cap is adjusted annually by the percentage change in the consumer price index for the previous year. Ibid., 735 ILCS 5/2-1115.1(b).

23. For general discussion, see Patricia Danzon, *Medical Malpractice: Theory, Evidence and Public Policy* (1985): 146–149; Paul Weiler, *Medical Malpractice,* 85–89.

Anecdotal evidence on the pervasive nature of defensive medicine is found in the American Medical Association's Study of Professional Liability Costs (1983).

24. IOM, Obstetrical Care, 27, 36–37.

25. IOM, Obstetrical Care, 76.

26. That ratio derives from a study by Roger A. Reynolds et al., "The Cost of Medical Professional Liability," based on 1984 data.

27. IOM, Obstetrical Care, 36. He relied on the American College of Obstetricians and Gynecologists' "Professional Liability and Its Effects: Report of a 1987 Survey of ACOG's Membership" (1988).

CHAPTER 20

1. See, e.g., Civil Justice Reform Amendments of 1995, Pub. Act, 89-7, 1995 Illinois Laws 7.

2. See, e.g., Wash. Rev. Code, § 4.24.290 (1994), requiring as a response to Helling v. Carey, 519 P.2d 981 (Wash. 1974), that plaintiffs prove that physicians and other health care providers "failed to exercise that degree of skill, care and learning possessed by other persons in the same profession, and that as a proximate result of such failure the plaintiff suffered damages."

3. Nevada Rev. Stat. Ann. § 41A.100 (1993) which limits res ipsa loquitur to "foreign substances" unintentionally left inside the body, to an explosion or fire, and "unintended burn caused by heat, radiation or chemicals, or injury to a part of the body "not directly involved in treatment," and finally to surgical procedures "performed on the wrong patient or the wrong organ, limb or part of a patient's body." The most open-ended of these ground is the fourth dealing with a part of the body "not directly involved in treatment," which is in part a reference to the classic case of Ybarra v. Spangard, 154 P.2d 687 (Cal. 1944), alleging injuries to neck and shoulders from an appendectomy.

4. Fein v. Permanente Medical Group, 695 P.2d 665 (Cal. 1985) (sustaining cap on pain and suffering damages of $250,000); Kansas Malpractice Victims Coalition v. Bell, 757 P.2d 251 (Kan. 1988) (striking down statute with $1 million overall cap and $250,000 on pain and suffering).

5. For a review of the strengths and weaknesses of the alternatives, see Samuel A. Rea, Jr., "Lump-Sum versus Periodic Damage Awards," *J. Legal Stud.* 10 (1981): 131.

6. The judicial response here has been spotty. See, e.g., Powell v. Blue Cross and Blue Shield, 581 So. 2d 772 (Ala. 1990).

7. Westendorf by Westendorf v. Stasson, 330 N.W.2d 699 (Minn. 1983).

8. See. e.g., Calif. Civ. Code, § 3333.1 (allowing defendant in action for professional negligence to introduce evidence of collateral benefits, and plaintiff to introduce evidence of their cost). N.Y. Civ. Prac. L. & R. § 4545(a) (1994) (reduction by amount of collateral benefits subject to a reduction for the costs of obtaining them).

9. See Patricia Danzon, "The Frequency and Severity of Medical Malpractice Claims: New Evidence," *Law and Contemp. Probs.* 49 (Spring 1986): 57, 72.

10. Ibid., 77.

11. On the proposal, see, Kirk B. Johnson, Carter G. Phillips, David Orentlicher, and Martin S. Hatlie, "A Fault-Based Administrative Alternative for Resolving Medical Malpractice Claims," *Vand. Law Rev.* 42 (1989): 1365.

12. For a more detailed analysis, which leads to the same mild sympathy for the proposal, see Weiler, *Medical Malpractice*, 115–122.

13. See Dewees and Trebilcock, "The Efficacy of the Tort System and Its Alternatives: A Review of the Empirical Evidence," *Osgoode Hall L.J.* 30, 87–88 and 132.

14. For the frustrations of similar efforts in Medicaid, see Bonita Brodt, Maurice Possley and Tim Jones, Medicaid System in Chaos, Part 6: Policing, at § 1 (November 5, 1993).

15. See, e.g., Fla. Stat. § 766.101(3) (creating a qualified privilege "for any act or proceeding undertaken or performed within the scope of the functions" of the review committee, provided they are done "without intentional fraud") with Cal. Civil Code § 47(2) (creating an absolute privilege).

16. Pub. L. No. 99-660, 100 Stat. 3784, (codified at 42 U.S.C. §§ 11101-11152 [1986]).

17. For general discussion, see Fitzhugh Mullan, Robert Politzer, Caroline T. Lewis et al., "The National Practitioner Data Bank: Report from the First Year," *JAMA* 268 (1992): 73.

18. 42 U.S.C. §11134.

19. 42 U.S.C. § 11131.

20. 42 U.S.C. § 11132.

21. 42 U.S.C. § 11133.

22. 42 U.S.C. § 11134(c).

23. 42 U.S.C. § 11135(a).

24. 42 U.S.C. § 11135 (b).

25. Restatement (Second) of Torts, §§ 585–587 (1965).

26. See, e.g., Gregoire v. Biddle, 177 F.2d 579 (2d Cir. 1949) (charges of false arrest against Attorney General); Barr v. Matteo, 360 U.S. 564, 575 (1959) (high government officials acting "within the outer perimeter" of their duty).

27. See, e.g., Butz v. Economou, 438 U.S. 478 (1978); Harlow v. Fitzgerald, 457 U.S. 800 (1982) (only qualified privilege for high presidential aide).

28, 42 U.S.C. § § 11111(a)(1).

29. See, e.g., Patrick v. Burget, 486 U.S. 94 (1988) (peer review committees of private hospitals are not exempt from antitrust laws).

30. 42 U.S.C. at § 11111(a)(1).

31. 42 U.S.C. at § 11112(a)(3).

32. 42 U.S.C. at § 11112(a)(4).

33. For a recent balanced account, see Weiler, *Medical Malpractice* 132–158. For earlier evaluations supportive of the system, see Clark C. Havighurst, "'Medical Adversity Insurance'—Has Its Time Come?" *Duke L. J.* (1975): 1233; Laurence R. Tancredi, "Designing a No-Fault Alternative," *Law and Contemp. Prob.* 49 (Spring 1986): 277. For more critical responses, see Robert E. Keeton, "Compensation for Medical Accidents," *U. Pa. L. Rev.* 121 (1973): 590; Guido Calabresi, "The Problem of Malpractice: Trying to Round out the Circle," *U. Toronto L. J.* 27 (1977): 131; Richard A. Epstein, "Medical Malpractice: Its Cause and Cure," in Simon Rottenberg, ed., *The Economics of Medical Malpractice* (1978): 245–267.

34. See Chapter 18.

35. The results can be disastrous when the covered events are not well defined. See Gary T. Schwartz, "Waste, Fraud, and Abuse in Workers' Compensation: The Recent California Experience," *Md. L. Rev.* 52 (1993): 983.

36. An Act to Amend the Accident Compensation Act, § 2(1)(ii).(1972).

37. The quotations are from ACC v. Auckland Hospital Board, 2 NZLR 748, 751 (1980).

38. See, generally, Joseph King, "Causation, Valuation, and Chance in Personal Injury Torts Involving Preexisting Conditions and Future Consequences," *Yale L.J.* 90 (1981): 1353. For an recent summary of the use of the rule in negligence cases, see Fennell v. Southern Maryland Hosp. Center, Inc., 580 A.2d 206 (Md. 1990). All states allow recovery when the chances of recovery make it more likely than not that the death was attributable to the missed diagnosis. A majority of states now allow some limited recovery for smaller reductions in the chances of recovery.

39. See Weiler, "The Case for No-Fault Medical Liability," 930–931.

40. Va. Code Ann. § 38.2-5001 (1995). I discussed an earlier version of this statute shortly after passage in Richard A. Epstein, "Market and Regulatory Approaches to Medical Malpractice: The Virginia Obstetrical No-Fault Statute," *Va. L. Rev.* 74 (1988): 1451.

41. Va. Code Ann. § 38.2-5009 (1995).

42. Va. Code Ann. § 38.2-5020 (1995).

43. Phone conversation with Professor Jeffrey O'Connell, University of Virginia Law School, June 8, 1994. Professor O'Connell was not aware of any published material that deals with this issue.

44. Weiler, *Medical Malpractice*, 96–100, 113.

45. For the analogous proposal in products liability cases, see Paul Rubin, T*ort Reform by Contract* (1993).

POSTSCRIPT

1. John K. Iglehart, "Physicians and the Growth of Managed Care," *NEJM* 331 (1994): 1167, 1167.

2. See Paul A. Pautler and Michael G. Vita, "Hospital Market Structure, Hospital Competition, and Consumer Welfare: What Can the Evidence Tell Us?" *J. Contemp. Health L. and Policy* 10 (1994): 117.

3. See, e.g., Aetna, "Managed Care: High Quality Care at Reduced Cost" (undated, but done after 1994).

4. See, e.g., Mark A. Hall, "Informed Consent to Rationing Decisions," *The Milbank Quarterly* 71 (1993): 645 (arguing against the requirement of specific disclosures at the time of treatment); Paul S. Appelbaum, "Must We Forgo Informed Consent to Control Health Care Costs? A Response to Mark A. Hall," Ibid., 660.

5. *New York Times* (August 9, 1996): A15.

6. See, e.g., Va. Code. Ann. § 38.2-3407 (Michie 1994). For a summary of these laws and the tensions that they have with the federal ERISA statute, see Note, "ERISA Preemption of 'Any Willing Provider' Laws—An Essential Step Toward National Health Care Reform," *Wash. U. L. Quart.* 95 (1995): 227. ERISA stands for the Employee Retirement Insurance Act of 1974, 29 U.S.C. § 1001 et seq. (1988). The current legal dispute is whether ERISA's preemption of state laws that "relate to any employment benefit plan," invalidates the any willing provider laws, a conclusion that was denied in Stuart Circle Hospital Corp. v. Aetna Health Management, 995 F.2d 500 (4th Cir. 1993), which sustained the Virginia statute against this preemption challenge.

7. Newborns' and mothers' Health Protection Act of 1996, (S. 969). For discussion, see Senate Report 104-326, 104th Cong. (2d Sess.). For an illustration of the state laws, see Act of November 21, 1995, Ch. 218, §§ 1, 3-6, 8, 1995 Mass. Legisl. Serv. 726, 726–728. These bills are criticized in "Health Care Law—'Drive-Through Delivery' Regulation—Massachusetts Requires Hospital Stays of Forty-Eight Hours for New Borns and Post

Partum Mothers," *Harv. L. Rev.* 106 (1996): 2116, and defended in George J. Annas, "Women and Children First," *NEJM* 333 (1995): 1647.

8. Valerie M. Parisi and Bruce A. Meyer, "To Stay or Not to Stay? That Is the Question," *NEJM* 333 (1995): 1635 (noting that the lack of agreement covers both low and high risk cases).

9. Vincent J. Schodolski, "Alleged HMO Abuses Spur California Ballot Issues," *Chicago Tribune* (August 13, 1996): 1.

10. David R. Olmos, "Election '96: Experts Foresee More Efforts to Reform HMO Regulations," *Los Angeles Times* (November 7, 1996): D4.

11. For the proposed regulations, see Department of Health and Human Services, "Medicare and Medicaid Programs: Requirements for Physician Incentive Plans in Pre-paid Health Care Organizations," *Federal Register* (March 27, 1996) Vol. 61, No. 60, 13430.

12. See Marlene Cimons, "U.S. Acts to Ease HMOS' Cost Pressure on Doctors," *Los Angeles Times* (December 26, 1996): A1.

TABLE OF CASES*

❖ ❖ ❖

*The numbers in parenthesis refer first to the chapter, and then to the footnote within the chapter. I stands for the Introduction and P for the Postscript.

INDEX

❖ ❖ ❖

485